http://vanat.cvm.umn.edu/neurolect PDFs/
Lect Auditory sxs.

FUNDAMENTALS OF HEARING

FUNDAMENTALS OF HEARING

An Introduction

FIFTH EDITION

William A. Yost

Parmly Hearing Institute
Loyola University Chicago
Chicago, Illinois

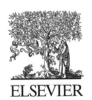

SAN DIEGO • NEW YORK • BOSTON
LONDON • SYDNEY • TOKYO • TORONTO

Academic Press is an imprint of Elsevier

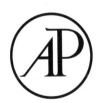

Academic Press is an imprint of Elsevier
30 Corporate Drive, Suite 400, Burlington, MA 01803, USA
525 B Street, Suite 1900, San Diego, California 92101-4495, USA
84 Theobald's Road, London WC1X 8RR, UK

This book is printed on acid-free paper.

Library of Congress Cataloging-in-Publication Data

Yost, William A.
   Fundamentals of hearing: an introduction / William A. Yost.–5th ed.
       p. ; cm.
   Includes bibliographical references and index.
   ISBN-13: 978-0-12-370473-3   ISBN-10: 0-12-370473-1 (hardcover : alk. paper)
   1. Hearing. I. Title.
   [DNLM: 1. Hearing–physiology. 2. Auditory Perception–physiology. 3. Ear–anatomy & histology.
WV 270 Y65f 2006]
   QP461.Y67 2006
   612.8′5–dc22

                                                                                    2006009427

British Library Cataloguing-in-Publication Data
A catalogue record for this book is available from the British Library.

ISBN-13: 978-0-12-370473-3
ISBN-10: 0-12-370473-1

For information on all Academic Press publications
visit our Web site at www.books.elsevier.com
Printed in the United States of America

08   09   10   9   8   7   6   5   4   3

To my friends, colleagues, and teachers:
Gilbert Johns
Don Robinson
Dave Green
Don Teas

Contents

Preface   xi

1
The World We Hear, An Introduction

Hearing   1
Normal Human Hearing and Plan
   of the Book   1
Brief History of the Study of Hearing   4
Hearing and Science   5
Summary   7
Supplement   7

I
The Auditory Stimulus: Sound

2
Sinusoids, The Basic Sound

Vibration   11
Sinusoids   13
Frequency   14
Starting Phase   15
Amplitude   17
Damped Vibrations   18
Summary   18
Supplement   19

3
Sound Transmission and Sound Propagation

Sound Propagation   21
Pressure and Sound Intensity   25
Decibels   25
Interference   27
Sound Fields   30
Summary   33
Supplement   34

4
Complex Sounds

Complex Stimuli   37
Transients   39
Beats and Amplitude Modulation   41
Square Wave   43
Frequency Modulation   45
Noise   47
Narrowband Noise, Envelope, and Fine
   Structure   49
Summary   51
Supplement   51

5
Sound Analysis

Resonators   53
Filters   55
Nonlinearities   59
Sound and Its Analysis   61
Summary   61
Supplement   61

II
Peripheral Auditory Anatomy and Physiology

6
The Outer and Middle Ears

Structure of the Outer Ear	67
Structure of the Middle Ear	68
Function of the Outer Ear	71
Function of the Middle Ear	75
Middle Ear and Inner Ear Impedances	78
Summary	80
Supplement	80

7
Structure of the Inner Ear and Its Mechanical Response

Structure of the Inner Ear	83
Mechanical Response of the Inner Ear	90
Summary	101
Supplement	101

8
Peripheral Auditory Nervous System and Hair Cells

Cochlear Potentials	103
Hair Cells, Stereocilia, Outer Hair Cell Motility, and Neural Transduction	108
Cochlear Emissions	112
Structure of the Auditory Nerve	113
Summary	118
Supplement	119

9
The Neural Response and the Auditory Code

Function of the Afferent Auditory Nerve	121
Two-Tone Suppression and Other Nonlinear Neural Responses	131
Function of the Efferent System	134
Encoding of Frequency, Intensity, and Time	134
Summary	138
Supplement	139

III
Auditory Sensation

10
Auditory Sensitivity

Thresholds of Audibility	143
Duration	147
Temporal Integration	149
Differential Sensitivity	150
Frequency Discrimination	150
Level/Intensity Discrimination	151
Temporal Discrimination	152
Temporal Modulation Transfer Functions	153
Summary	154
Supplement	154

11
Masking

Tonal Masking	159
Noise Masking	162
Critical Band and the Internal Filter	163
Relationship Between Excitation Patterns and Critical Bands	164
Temporal Masking	166

The Workbook contains suggested questions (with answers) for each chapter. Many of the PowerPoint presentations can be used to run demonstration experiments.

As in the past, this edition could not have been written without the assistance of many people, especially the faculty, staff, and students of the Parmly Hearing Institute of Loyola University of Chicago. They are: *faculty* Sheryl Coombs, Toby Dye, Dick Fay, Andy Lotto, John New, Stan Sheft, Bill Shofner, and J.D. Trout; *staff* Joe Boomer, Jim Collier, Linda Davis-Fairley, and Noah Jurcin; *students* Chris Brown, Elizabeth Chrobak, Susan Guzman, Dan Mapes-Rirodan, and Bill Whitmer. But most especially I want to thank my wife, Lee, for her love and patience, without which I could not have completed this task.

William A. Yost

1

The World We Hear, An Introduction

HEARING

Sound constantly surrounds us and informs us about many objects in our world. Our ability to determine the sources of sounds is one of our most important biological traits. Any animal's abilities to locate food, avoid predators, find a mate, navigate, and communicate often depend on being able to determine the sources of sounds. In order to determine sound sources, an animal needs to know that a sound source exists, what it is, where it is, if it is moving, and so on. Sounds from various sources are combined into one complex sound field and do not reach us as individual sounds. There are not separate "pipelines" to our senses for each potential sound source in our environment, as some ancient Greeks suggested. We receive one sound input that is made up of a sum of the sounds from all of the sources in our environment. Figure 1.1 depicts this situation for several instruments that might exist in a musical group. Whether we listen at a concert (where all of the instruments exist as sound sources) or to the radio (where the radio loudspeaker is the only source of the sound), we receive a single sound field but can determine the various instruments in the band (i.e., the sources of the music we perceive).

In order to determine sound sources, the nervous system first processes the complex sound field by translating (*transducing*) the various physical aspects of sound into a *neural code* for these physical characteristics of the complex sound field. This neural code is then further processed by the central nervous system to provide neural subsets that aid us in determining the sound sources. Finally, this auditory neural information is combined with that from other sensory systems (e.g., vision) and that provided by experience and stored in memory, to elicit appropriate behaviors and emotions in response to the presence of sound sources. The entire sequence of coding, processing, integration, and responding to sound defines *hearing*, as depicted in Figure 1.2.

NORMAL HUMAN HEARING AND PLAN OF THE BOOK

This book is primarily concerned with the neural coding of the physical attributes of sound and the direct consequences of that coding for the normal function of the auditory system. A great deal is known about neural coding of sound, but far less is known about processing, integration, and response output

1

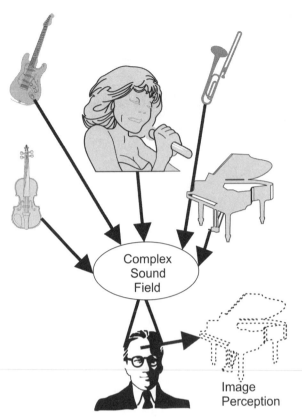

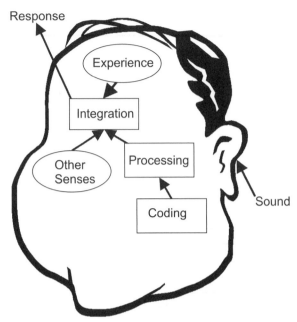

FIGURE 1.2 The stages of processing that lead to hearing. The physical attributes of sound (frequency, intensity, and time) are first coded by the peripheral auditory nervous system. This neural code is then processed by higher neural centers to help the listener determine the sources of sound. This neural information is integrated with other sensory information and that based on experience, and all of this neural processing leads to behavioral responses.

FIGURE 1.1 A schematic diagram indicating a number of objects (musical instruments) that could produce sound. The sounds from all of these sources are combined into one complex sound field that is received by the listener. The auditory nervous system of the listener first provides a neural code of the basic physical attributes of the complex sound field, and then this neural code is further processed to aid the listener in determining the various sources. The listener perceives an auditory image of each sound source (e.g., the piano).

(see Figure 1.2). To comprehend this coding, we need to understand something about the basic physical attributes of sound, which, we will learn, are *frequency, intensity,* and *time*. It will also be useful to learn a little about physical systems that process sound before we turn to a study of the biological processor, the auditory system. Thus, physical concepts of filtering and the nonlinear response to sound stimulation

will be briefly discussed. These topics, the first four chapters, constitute Part I of the book (The Auditory Stimulus: Sound). Part II (Peripheral Auditory Anatomy and Physiology) contains four chapters describing the structure (*anatomy*) and function (*physiology*) of the parts of the nervous system that provide the neural code for frequency, intensity, and time (the peripheral auditory system). The four chapters of Part III (Auditory Sensation) cover humans' sensations of the basic attributes of sound: frequency, intensity, and time. In addition, Part III covers the ability of humans to locate the source of sounds. The three chapters of Part IV (Auditory Perception of Complex Sounds, the Central Nervous System, and Auditory Disorders) provide a brief introduction to auditory *perception* of sound sources, speech, and music; the basics of the central auditory nervous system; and abnormalities of auditory processing.

As indicated previously, the book primarily describes the neural processes, sensations, and perceptions of the normal auditory system. However, Chapter 16 does provide an overview of some of the ways in which the auditory system becomes damaged. While many students and readers of this book have interests in non-normal auditory systems, the premise of this book is that an understanding of normal auditory processing is crucial to fully appreciate the abnormal system and the various ways of dealing with hearing impairment.

The general area of medicine devoted to the study of auditory problems is called *otology*, which is part of a larger area called *otorhinolaryngology* or *otolaryngology*. *Oto* refers to the ear, *rhino* to the nose, and *laryngology* to the throat; thus this area of medicine is often referred to as the ear, nose, and throat (ENT) specialty. In addition to persons with a medical degree (M.D. degree), those trained in the field of *clinical audiology* with a Masters Degree, Au.D. (Doctor of Audiology), or Ph.D. (Doctor of Philosophy) work with patients having auditory problems. The otologist undertakes special training after receiving a medical degree; the audiologist receives training as part of the work toward a Masters (M.A.) or doctoral (Au.D. or Ph.D.) degree and by meeting certification requirements. The otologist and audiologist often work together in aiding someone with an auditory problem. The audiologist provides the diagnostic testing and rehabilitation, while the otologist also provides diagnostics and any necessary medical treatment.

Hearing scientists come from just about every field of science: biology, psychology, engineering, physics, and chemistry as well as otology and audiology. However, the majority of hearing scientists are probably best labeled as *neuroscientists*, scientists who study the nervous system as the organ of behavior. Neuroscience is often divided into two main areas: *integrative and functional neuroscience*—the study of the structure and function of neurons, neural centers, and neural circuits—and *molecular neuroscience*—the study of the molecular, cellular, and genetic aspects of the nervous system. Integrative and functional neuroscience includes the study of *neural anatomy* (neural structure), *neural physiology* (neural function), and *behavioral neuroscience* (behavior of humans and other animals). Behavioral neuroscience in the study of hearing includes *psychoacoustics*—the study of the relationship between the physical attributes of sound (frequency, intensity, and time) and a subject's sensations of these physical attributes—and *perception*—the study of auditory perceptions. Most scientists who study perception are psychologists or audiologists. This book is primarily about the integrative and functional neuroscience of hearing.

Most tests for hearing impairment provided by otologists and audiologists as well as the cures and rehabilitation procedures deal with aspects of the neural coding of the basic attributes of sound. For example, a hearing aid is usually fitted based on a number of hearing tests, the most important of which is the *audiogram*, which determines an individual's sensitivity to sounds of different frequencies. The hearing aid primarily amplifies sound such that listeners are better able to detect sounds with frequencies to which they are insensitive. A firm background in the fundamentals of hearing (i.e., understanding the neural code for the basic attributes of sound) is required to understand why an audiogram measures hearing sensitivity, how and why a hearing aid might help a person hear better and to appreciate new advancements in hearing aid design.

The neural code is primarily provided by the early, or *peripheral*, stages of the auditory nervous system. Thus, the book will emphasize the anatomy and physiology of the peripheral auditory system. Again, most is known about the peripheral stages of the neural basis of hearing. You will be introduced to the *central auditory nervous system* (those neural stages that come after the peripheral ones) and complex sound processing, but we will not cover these topics in as much detail as the peripheral system and the perception of simple sounds.

The ability to communicate is perhaps the most important attribute of hearing for humans. A *communication system* is often described as consisting of a *sender*, a *message*, and a *receiver*; for humans, this is represented by *speech*, *language*, and *hearing*. This book focuses on a basic understanding of the hearing part of a communication system. With such knowledge one should be better able to understand the role hearing plays in communication, especially speech communication.

Although the book's aim is to describe the basics of normal human hearing, much of what is known about auditory processing comes from the study of hearing in other animals. A significant amount of our basic knowledge about hearing, hearing impairment, and relief for hearing impairments is a result of our ability to study a wide variety of animals. Understanding how all animals cope with their acoustic environment through the use of their auditory system provides valuable information about and insights into a wealth of crucial scientific and societal questions.

BRIEF HISTORY OF THE STUDY OF HEARING

Documentation of an interest in the senses goes back at least as far as the ancient Greeks. These scholars were fascinated with the senses, and philosopher/scientists such as Pythagoras made important contributions that are still useful today. Among other discoveries, Pythagoras worked out the relationship between the length of strings and the pitch of musical sounds. However, most of what we currently know about hearing began in the middle of the 19th century, although some of the gross anatomy of the inner ear was studied as early as the 17th century. The mid to late 1800s saw the full development of biology and the beginnings of the modern study of the behavioral sciences. During this time, refinements of the microscope provided a significant tool for biology, and the philosophical debate concerning mind/body dualism was waning, making the empirical study of behavior possible. In the early part of 20th century the developments of the oscilloscope for measuring electrical activity and vacuum tube devices that generated

sounds produced quantum increases in our knowledge of hearing.

During the late 1800s and early 1900s, physicists such as Gustav Fechner, Lord Rayleigh, and Herman von Helmholtz and biologists such as Alfonso Corti, Ramon y Cajal, and Johannes Muller performed important experiments and suggested crucial theories that form the basis of much of what we know about hearing today. A great deal of the early work on hearing, as with the other senses, began with an interest in object, or source, determination. As a part of this interest scientists and philosophers reasoned that objects were perceived because we processed the attributes of the object or attributes that the objects produced (e.g., sound). Thus, a great deal of the study of hearing hinged on the study of the attributes of sound: frequency, intensity, and time. Helmholtz crystallized this approach when he proposed a theory for auditory processing of frequency as the key ingredient of our perception of *pitch*. As we will learn, pitch perception is a crucial element of hearing. Without our ability to perceive pitch, music would be little more than drumbeats and speech would probably sound something like Morse code. The fascination with frequency coding as the key element in pitch perception permeated the field of hearing for nearly a century. Classic hearing textbooks often described "*theories of hearing*." These were really more theories of frequency processing than theories of all of hearing. But because pitch perception is such a crucial aspect of hearing, a theory of frequency processing could almost be considered a full theory of hearing. From the 1940s to the 1960s, interest in these theories focused on the *place theory* (the place in the nervous system with the most neural activity codes for the perception of pitch) of Georg von Bekesy over the *temporal theory* (*volley theory*, or a theory of the temporal properties of the neural response that determines pitch) of Glen Wever. Although Wever's volley theory was really a combination of the place and temporal theories, Wever (1949) is often cited as a proponent of the temporal theory. Von Bekesy won the Nobel Prize for Medicine and Physiology in 1961 for his work on the place theory of frequency coding,

Dependent Variable = Functional relationship ← DV and IV ✱

in particular for his work on how the biomechanics of the inner ear provides a code for frequency that can be used by the nervous system. We learn a great deal more about this work later in the book. The debate concerning theories of hearing has dwindled to arguments about details. Most hearing scientists now recognize the important role that both the place and temporal theories play in understanding hearing.

During the 1930s and '40s, a great deal of research in hearing was conducted in order to develop and improve the telephone, and thus some of the key studies were performed at Bell Laboratories. During World War II, interest in military devices such as sonar detection spurred additional knowledge of hearing, especially at the Psychoacoustics Lab and later at the Eaton Peabody Labs at Harvard University. During the 20th century, especially during the later decades, significant contributions to the hearing sciences were provided by researchers from Europe and Japan. With the development of the digital computer and its use in the biological and behavioral sciences during the 1960s, a large number of new experiments were performed and theories developed. Today the arsenal of tools available to the auditory scientist is vast, including those emerging from cell biology, molecular biology, and genetics. Our understanding of the normal and abnormal auditory system is growing rapidly. It is hoped this book provides the information you need to understand and appreciate new knowledge that is continually being added to the database of information about hearing.

HEARING AND SCIENCE

The empirical and observational methods of science are the basis for most of what we know about hearing. To fully appreciate the facts, data, and theories pertaining to hearing, it is important that you have some acquaintance with how those facts, data, and theories are acquired. There are two general ways of conducting science: the *empirical method* and the *observational method*. Empirical methods involve conducting experiments in which scientists directly manipulate the objects they want to understand. Observational methods are used when the scientist cannot directly manipulate these objects, such as in the study of astronomy (i.e., one cannot directly manipulate planets, but scientists can observe them).

Using the scientific method, a scientist determines the functional relationship between two variables: the *dependent variable* (DV) and the *independent variable* (IV). The scientist seeks the following:

$$DV = f(IV), \qquad (1.1)$$

that is, to determine the functional relationship [$f(\ )$] between the DV and the IV; or, how does the dependent variable change when the independent variable changes?

The independent variable is something the experimenter manipulates, while the dependent variable is something the experimenter measures that might vary as a consequence of changing the independent variable. Thus, a scientist who wants to know how the steepness of an incline affects the speed at which a ball rolls down the incline will vary the steepness (*slope*) of the incline (IV) and measure the speed (DV) of the rolling ball for each setting of the incline's slope. The scientist could establish the following relationship:

$$S = f(SL), \qquad (1.2)$$

where S is the ball's speed, say in meters per second, SL is the slope as a ratio of the height of the incline to the horizontal width of the incline, and $f(\ )$ is the relationship that was found (e.g., if for each unit increase in the slope, the ball rolled twice as fast, the relationship could be written as: $S = 2SL$).

In many experiments, variables in addition to the independent variable may also lead to a change in the dependent variable. These other variables are especially important if they covary with the independent variable. Suppose, for instance, that in the ball-rolling experiment, the experimenter increased the slope (IV) by keeping the width of the incline fixed and raising its height. In this case, both the slope and the height of the incline change together. Thus, the experimental outcome (equation 1.2) could be written as either $S = f(SL)$ or $S = f(H)$, where H is the incline height. If the

TABLE 1.1 Hypothetical Relationship Between the Slope of an Incline and the Speed (in meters/second) of a Ball Rolling down the Incline

Slope	Speed (m/sec)
1	2
2	4
3	6
4	8
5	10

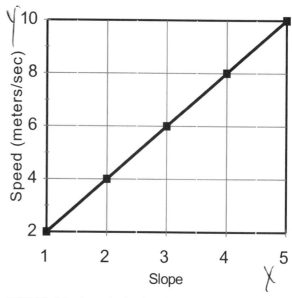

FIGURE 1.3 A graph showing the hypothetical relationship between the speed of the rolling ball (the DV) and the slope of the incline (IV). The curve is based on the relationship shown in equation (1.2) and Table 1.1.

scientist is interested in the effect of slope on the ball's speed, then the fact that height is covaried with slope means the results are confounded (one cannot be sure which variable, the intended independent variable or the confounding variable, led to the change in the DV). Thus, height becomes a *confounding variable* (CV) for this experiment.

The experimenter needs to *control* for confounding variables. In the present example this could be done in a number of ways. The experimenter could, for example, do two experiments: (1) Keep the slope the same but change the height of the incline (that is, change the width in proportion to height), and (2) keep height the same but change the slope (by changing the width). The outcome of these two experiments would indicate how the three variables affect the ball's speed. A wide variety of experimental methods exist that allow scientists to control for confounding variables in order to determine the relationship between the independent and the dependent variables without the relationship's being affected by confounding variables.

A key aspect of science is communicating the outcome of an experiment as exactly, concisely, and clearly as possible. This means displaying the functional relationship (e.g., equation 1.1) exactly, clearly, and concisely. This is usually done in one of four ways: display the raw data, tabulate the data, draw a figure of the data, or write an equation that describes the functional relationship.

Table 1.1 and Figure 1.3 show the results of the ball-rolling experiment if equation 1.2 represented

the hypothetical experimental outcome. Notice that the DV is shown as the entries in the cells of the table and along the vertical axis (the y-axis, or *ordinate*) of the graph, whereas the IVs are represented by the rows and columns of the table and along the horizontal axis (the x-axis, or *abscissa*) of the graph. If there is more than one independent variable, then one IV can be represented along the horizontal axis and the other can be represented by having different curves on the figure.

The data from experiments are used to form hypotheses, models, theories, and laws in order to account for a number of relationships between independent and dependent variables and to predict how untested relationships between independent and dependent variables might turn out. Whether a particular combination of relationships is called a hypothesis, model, theory, or law often depends on the scientist who is making the proposal. Usually the term *law* is reserved for statements that apply to a wide range of conditions and are unlikely to change very quickly. There are few laws of hearing but many hypotheses, models, and theories. All scientific hypotheses, models, theories, and laws must be testable using the scientific method. As such they are constantly changing as new experiments are performed that either confirm or reject the predictions made by the hypotheses, models, theories, and laws. Thus, our knowledge of hearing has changed, as it always will.

SUMMARY

This book concentrates on the neural coding of the physical attributes of sound, which are frequency, intensity, and time, and on the sensations and perceptual consequences of that coding. An emphasis is placed on normal human hearing so that future scientists and practitioners such as audiologists and otologists will understand the basic concepts of hearing. The study of hearing has a rich history, in which a great deal of the work over the past 100 years dealt with various "theories of hearing." Knowledge of hearing is based on the scientific method, in which scientists seek to find functional relationships between independent and dependent variables that are not confounded.

SUPPLEMENT

The book by Bregman (1990), *Auditory Scene Analysis*, the book by Yost, Fay, and Popper (2006), as well as articles by Yost (1992a, b, 1993) cover in more detail the idea that sound source determination is a crucial aspect of hearing. The Acoustical Society of America has reprinted many of the classic textbooks in acoustics, including some in hearing: Stevens and Davis (reprinted in 1983) and von Bekesy (reprinted in 1989). These are excellent books that serious students of hearing should read.

Gulick, Gescheider, and Frisina (1989) provide a brief historical review of hearing, especially of the various "theories of hearing." A detailed history of perception can be found in Boring's (1942) classic book on the history of experimental psychology. Some of Helmholtz's works have been translated by Warren and Warren (1968) and provide fascinating reading for anyone interested in the history of physics as it relates to sensory processing. The book by Shaughnessy and Zechmeister (1990) provides an excellent discussion of the scientific method used in the behavioral sciences.

The alert student would have noticed that one more control experiment is required in order to determine the exact relationship between incline slope and the speed of the rolling ball, because the two control experiments that were mentioned still leave the length of the incline as a confounding variable.

The most exact, concise, and clear method to display a functional relationship between the DV and IV is with an equation. Because it isn't always possible to write such an equation, plotting the data is the second preferred method for displaying and communicating the results of an experiment (i.e., the data).

I

The Auditory
Stimulus: Sound

2

Sinusoids, The Basic Sound

VIBRATION

In the most general sense, when we say we "hear," we usually mean we are sensitive to the sounds in our environment. Sound may be defined in either physical or perceptual terms. Let us first consider the physical definition. *Vibration* of an object makes sound possible. Any object with the properties of *inertia* and *elasticity* may vibrate and, hence, may produce sound. Thus, any vibrating object has the potential to produce sound. If we "hear" the vibration, the sound is *audible*. Vibration is the movement of an object from one point in space to another point and usually back again to or through the first point. The fact that a force must be exerted on an object to make it move defines *inertia*, whereas the ability of the object to return to a starting or initial state after it is deformed or moved by this force defines *elasticity*. In practice, almost every object has inertia and elasticity, meaning almost every object can vibrate. Few restrictions exist for the type of vibration required to produce sound. As long as an object moves, it has the potential to produce sound. The object may move regularly back and forth or randomly; it may complete a vibratory cycle in seconds or in fractions of a second, or it may move only once or millions of times. An infinite variety of vibrations are capable of producing sound.

The vibration of an object per se does not result in "hearing." Rather, the vibrating object produces a sound wave in a medium like air, and the pressure changes in this sound wave ultimately lead to auditory sensations and perceptions. This chapter deals with the properties of a vibrating object that can become a sound source. Chapter 3 covers the topic of the transmission of this vibratory information as a sound wave.

A musical cymbal or drum head can serve as an example of an object that vibrates when struck by something, such as a drumstick, and as a result produces an audible sensation. These percussive instruments vibrate when struck, and as a result a distinctive musical element is added to one's musical perception. The *mass*-and-*spring* example shown in Figure 2.1 may be used to describe, in a general way, all vibrations, including those of cymbals and drum heads. Recall that if an object has inertia and elasticity it can vibrate, leading to a possible sound. In Figure 2.1 the mass (e.g., the cymbal) would require a force (e.g., the cymbal being struck with a drumstick) to move it, which represents the property of inertia. The spring has a restoring force, which represents the property of elasticity (the opposite of elasticity is *stiffness*). If a force moves the mass out from its resting state (called *state of equilibrium*, as shown in Figure 2.1a) to the position shown in Figure 2.1b and then the

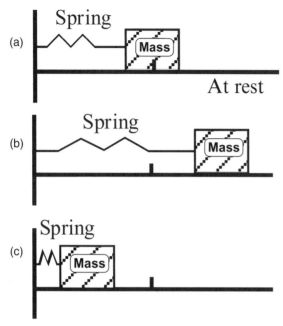

Spring

(a)

Mass

At rest

Spring

(b)

Mass

Spring

(c)

Mass

FIGURE 2.1   A diagram of the mass and inertia (spring) components necessary for sound production. When the mass is set into
motion, it will move back and forth (left and right as you view from
panels 2.1a to 2.1b to 2.1c) in a sinusoidal motion, assuming there
is no friction. This is the description of a free-vibration system.

force is removed, the spring would pull the mass back
through the point of equilibrium to a position such as
that shown in Figure 2.1c. The mass would then *oscillate* back and forth; that is, the mass would vibrate.
If there were no *resistance*, such as *friction*, to the
motion of the mass, it would continue to oscillate back
and forth forever. Thus, the example shown in Figure
2.1 is a model for vibratory systems. In this case,
because no force is applied to the system after it is set
into motion, the vibration is called a *free vibration*.

As the mass moves back and forth, its *distance*,
or *displacement*, (*d*) from the state of equilibrium is
constantly changing. Thus, $d(t)$ represents the distance
the mass has traveled from its state of equilibrium, or
resting state, as a function time (*t*). At any moment in
time *t*, $d(t)$ is an *instantaneous displacement*. Positive
values of $d(t)$ may represent displacements outward
from the resting state, while negative values of $d(t)$

would represent inward displacements. *Maximum displacement* is represented by *A* (+*A* for the maximum
outward displacement and −*A* for the maximal inward
displacement). The value of $d(t)$, therefore, varies from
zero to +*A*, back through 0 to −*A*, and this *cycle* of
oscillation is repeated. In Figure 2.2, the vibration is
depicted as starting at $d(t) = 0$, when $t = 0$ (i.e., the mass
is at its resting state when the force is first applied). The
mass may not be at its resting state [i.e., at $d(t) = 0$]
when the vibration starts (i.e., at $t = 0$). In this case,
the mass would start at this new starting position and
would move to either +*A* or −*A*, depending on the relative position of the start, and would oscillate as before
between the extremes of +*A* and −*A*. The relative starting position of the vibrating object is referred to as the
starting phase (e.g., if the starting position is such that
$d(t) = 0$ when $t = 0$, the starting phase is zero). Therefore, there are three important parameters describing
the motion of the vibrating object: the maximum
displacement, or *amplitude*, the rate, or *frequency*, at
which the object oscillates, and the *starting phase*.

The motion of the mass-and-spring model can be
described mathematically in terms of the *force* (*F*)
required to move the mass (*m*), which is opposed by
the restoring force of the spring (*s*). Force is expressed
as mass times acceleration (*a*); *F* = *ma* or, in terms of
the spring, *F* = *sa*. Because these two forces are equal
and opposite in the mass-and-spring model: *ma* = *ms*
and *ma* + *ms* = 0. One solution to this equation that
describes how the mass may vibrate is

$$d(t) = A\sin\left[2\pi\sqrt{(s/m)}t + \theta\right], \qquad (2.1)$$

where $d(t)$, *A*, *s*, *m*, and *t* are defined as previously in
this chapter. *Sin* is the trigonometric sinusoidal function (see Appendix A), and θ represents starting phase.
The term π is the Greek letter "pi," and it refers to the
fact that a sinusoidal function may be derived from a
circle (see Appendix A) and *pi radians* is the same as
180°, or half of a circle. Equation (2.1) can be written
in a more general form:

$$d(t) = A\sin(2\pi ft + \theta), \qquad (2.2)$$

where *f* is frequency. Thus, in the case of the mass-
and-spring model, $f = \sqrt{(s/m)}$. Equation (2.2) is a

[handwritten at top: 3 important parameters of vibrating objects: ① amp ③ starting phase ② freq]

general equation that has three parameters—frequency (f), amplitude (A), and starting phase (θ)—describing the instantaneous displacement [$d(t)$] of a vibrating object as a function of time (t).

The sinusoidal relationship of equation (2.2) describing a vibrating object appears in another crucial mathematical relationship that is of great value in the study of acoustics and hearing. Joseph Fourier, a Frenchman who lived during the time of Napoleon (Fourier lived from 1768 to 1830), derived important theorems for the flow of heat; his analysis can be applied to the types of vibrations described in this book. Fourier derived a theorem specifying that *any* vibration can be resolved into a sum of a particular type of vibration, the sinusoidal vibration. This sum of sinusoidal vibrations, a *Fourier series*, can describe almost any arbitrary vibratory pattern. The derivation of these sinusoids is *Fourier analysis*. Thus, sinusoidal vibrations are the basic building blocks of all vibrations and, hence, of all possible sounds.

SINUSOIDS

A sinusoid, also called a *sine wave*, describes a particular relationship between *displacement* and *time*, that is, a particular vibration (see Appendix A). Figure 2.2 is a diagram of a sinusoid as indicated by equation (2.2). Displacement simply means the distance an object moves, and a sine wave describes the continuous, regular back-and-forth displacement of a vibrating object. Notice that from the starting position [displacement $d(t) = 0$], the motion in this example goes upward to a maximum positive distance [$d(t) = +A, +A = +10$], then back to the starting position, then downward to a maximum negative distance [$d(t) = -A, -A = -10$] and finally back to the starting position over the time period of 1 sec. The sinusoidal vibration is symmetric in displacement about the resting, or equilibrium, position [*displacement* = 0], and the vibratory pattern repeats itself perfectly. Theoretically, this back-and-forth vibration can go on forever, but because it repeats itself perfectly, only one complete transition of the motion is shown. A *cycle* is one

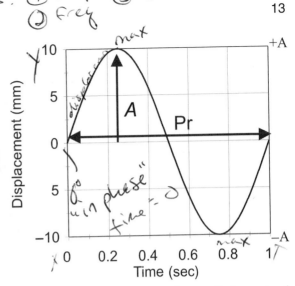

FIGURE 2.2 A sinusoidal relation between displacement and time. From the starting position at 0, the peak amplitude is +10 (A); the period (Pr) is 1 second; the frequency is 1 Hz.

complete transition of a periodic function such as a sinusoid.

Once the values of the three parameters of a sinusoid (A, f, and θ) have been specified, they have described a single sinusoid. Unless all three parameters are specified, there can be more than one sine wave. Because any vibration consists of a sum of sinusoidal vibrations, any vibration is described by the amplitude, frequency, and starting phase of each sinusoid that constitutes the vibration (see Chapter 4). Any vibration consisting of the sum of more than one sinusoid is called a *complex vibration*, whereas a single sine wave is called a *simple vibration*. Vibratory patterns are also called *waves* or *waveforms*; therefore, waves or waveforms can be simple or complex. Sinusoidal motion is also referred to as *simple harmonic motion* (see the end of this chapter and Chapter 3).

Generally, amplitude is a measure of displacement; frequency is a measure of how often per unit of time an object moves back and forth (oscillates); and starting phase indicates the relative position of the object at the instant in time it begins to vibrate. The parameters of the sine wave refer to the physical description of a vibration. A large area of the study of hearing (*psychophysics* and its subfield in hearing, *psychoacoustics*) is concerned with human perception of these parameters. On a subjective (perceptual) basis, changes in the amplitude of a sine wave are generally labeled as *loudness* and changes in frequency as *pitch*. There is not a single subjective term for starting phase because we are sensitive to changes in starting phase only under particular conditions. For instance, changes in the difference of starting phase at the two ears result in changes in the perceived location of the stimulus in space. Thus, for those conditions in which two ears are stimulated with a difference in starting phase, these changes in the starting phase may correspond to changes in the *locus*, or *location*, of the stimulus.

The relationships of the *physical* attributes to the *subjective* attributes of sound are somewhat complex. Many of these interactions are discussed in Chapter 13. Because of these complex interactions between the physical and subjective dimensions of sound, care must be exercised when describing an acoustic stimulus. In referring to the physical stimulus, the terms *frequency*, *amplitude*, and *starting phase* should be used. In referring to how a person perceives the stimulus, the subjective terms *pitch*, *loudness*, and in some cases, *perceived location* are used.

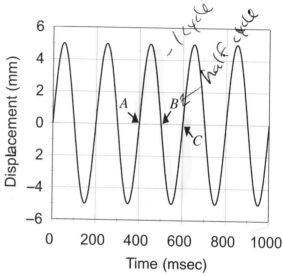

FIGURE 2.3 A sinusoid with a frequency of 5 Hz (Pr = 200 msec, f = 1000/200 msec = 5 Hz); the starting phase is 0°, the peak amplitude is +5. One period is the time between points A and C and not between points A and B or B and C.

FREQUENCY

The frequency of a sinusoid or any vibration is the *number of cycles* it completes per second. The symbol Hz, standing for *hertz* (hertz is cycles per second), is used to denote this number. If a periodic vibration, such as a sine wave, completes 100 full cycles in 1 sec, then it is said to have a frequency of 100 Hz. As mentioned previously, a complete cycle occurs when the vibratory pattern begins and ends at the same point of displacement after having taken on all possible values of $d(t)$. Thus, frequency in hertz is the same as the number of cycles per second of periodic vibration. The sinusoid in Figure 2.2 has completed one cycle in 1 sec, and so its frequency is 1 Hz.

The amount of time a vibration takes to complete one cycle is called its *period* (Pr). Thus, the period

of the sinusoid in Figure 2.2 is 1 sec. Since the periods of the vibrations that one normally experiences are short (equivalently, the frequencies are high), fractions of a second (abbreviated *sec*) are usually expressed in terms of milliseconds (thousandths of a second, abbreviated *msec*; 1 sec = 1000 msec, or 1 msec = 0.001 sec). The period of the sine wave in Figure 2.3 is 200 msec, or 0.2 sec. In Figure 2.3 the sine wave completed 5 cycles in 1000 msec (1 sec), which means that one cycle would have taken one-fifth as long or 200 msec (1000 msec/5 cycles = 200 msec). The period (Pr) of the sine wave in Figure 2.3 is 200 msec. Since the sine wave in Figure 2.3 completed 5 cycles in 1000 msec, its frequency is 5 Hz (1000/200 msec = 5 Hz).

Frequency and period are, therefore, reciprocally related:

$$f = 1/\text{Pr} \qquad (2.3)$$

when Pr is expressed in units of seconds and f in units of hertz, and

$$\text{Pr} = 1/f$$

Periodic: repeating pattern

For period measured in milliseconds the relations are

$$f = 1000/\text{Pr} \quad \text{and} \quad \text{Pr} = 1000/f \qquad (2.4)$$

Remember that period was defined in terms of one complete cycle, that is, the time between any two successive identical points on the waveform. In Figure 2.3 the period may be determined, for example, by finding the time between points A and C on the waveform since the waveform is at zero displacement and the waveform is going up after both points A and C. The time between points A and B or B and C equals only half a period. Notice that point B is not exactly like point A (the sine wave is going up at points A and C but down at point B).

Either frequency or period may be used to describe the oscillation of a periodic vibration, although it is usually easier to determine the period and compute the frequency using equation (2.3) or (2.4). These two terms (frequency and period) are also used to describe the periodic repetition occurring in many nonsinusoidal vibrations (i.e., complex vibrations). The only requirement of these nonsinusoidal vibrations is that they are periodic; whatever pattern of vibration exists, it must be repeated. The complex vibration described in Figure 2.4 is periodic, but it is not a sinusoid. Its period is 5 msec because the time between two identical successive points (such as the peaks at A and B) is 5 msec. Its frequency is 200 Hz because 200 Hz = 1/0.005 sec (or 200 Hz = 1000/5 msec) or because the vibration went through one cycle [one pattern of vibration between points A and B in 0.005 sec (5 msec)]. For complex vibrations with a periodic repetition rate, the frequency of vibration is called *repetition frequency*, and for sinusoids, *sinusoidal frequency*.

STARTING PHASE

The starting phase of a sinusoid corresponds to the point in the displacement cycle at which the object begins to vibrate. Starting phase is usually defined in terms of *degrees of angle*. A sinusoid is said to start at zero phase, or to start "in phase," when time equals zero ($t = 0$) the displacement $d(t)$ also equals zero. The

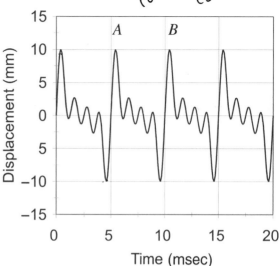

FIGURE 2.4 A complex periodic vibration that is not a sinusoid. The frequency of repetition is 200 Hz. The period is shown by the time indicated between points A and B (5 msec). Its peak amplitude is 10 mm, peak-to-peak amplitude is 20 mm.

sine wave in Figure 2.2 starts at zero phase. The sinusoid in Figure 2.5 starts one-half of a period later than the zero-starting-phase (see Figure 2.2) condition. In Figure 2.6 the starting phase is one-quarter of a period later.

The description of starting phase is the *phase angle*. This term stems from the fact that a sinusoid that has completed one cycle of vibration has completed a circle (see Appendix A). Because a circle has 360° (or 2π radians), a sine wave has gone through 360° (2π radians) when it has completed one cycle, 180° (π radians) when it has completed one-half of a cycle, 90° ($\pi/2$ radians) in one-quarter of a cycle, and so on. Thus, degrees of circular angle can define the starting phase of a sinusoid. The sinusoid in Figure 2.5 has a starting phase angle of 180°, those in Figures 2.2 and 2.4 start at a phase angle of 0°, and the one in Figure 2.6 starts at a phase angle of 90°. If the wave begins at time equal to zero when the displacement is positive, the starting phase must be between 0° and 180°, whereas if it begins at a negative displacement, the starting phase lies between 180° and 360°.

important concept!

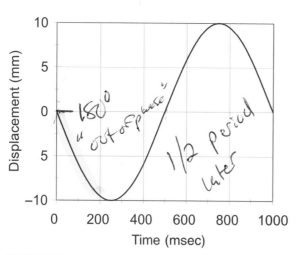

FIGURE 2.5 A sinusoid that begins at 180° starting phase. Compare this sinusoid to the one in Figure 2.2, which begins at 0° starting phase.

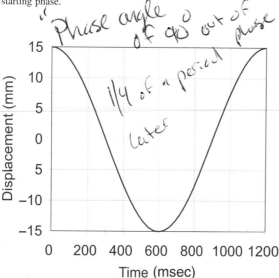

FIGURE 2.6 A sinusoid that begins at 90° starting phase. Compare this sinusoid with those in Figures 2.2 and 2.5.

The starting-phase angle is determined by noting the change in the starting displacement of a sinusoid *relative* to the 0° starting-phase condition shown in Figures 2.2 and 2.3. Starting phase is a relative term; all starting phases are stated in degrees relative to the

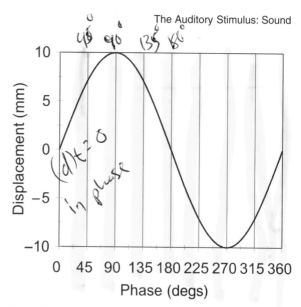

FIGURE 2.7 A sinusoid is divided into eight sections of phase, expressed relative to the zero-degree-starting-phase condition.

zero-degree-starting-phase condition. If, for instance, a sinusoid starts at maximum displacement at a time equal to zero (see Figure 2.6), then it has begun a quarter of a period later than the 0° starting-phase condition. Thus, the starting phase is one-quarter of 360°, or 90°.

Figure 2.7 shows a sinusoid divided into fractions of a period. The time, or horizontal, axis is divided into eight equal sections of phase. This type of figure can be used to determine starting phase. If the sinusoid starts at one of these eight positions when time equals zero, then the starting phase can be determined by using the appropriate value on the horizontal axis.

Sometimes two sinusoids are said to be *out of phase* with each other. If the two are out of phase and have the same frequency, then they must have different starting phases. In Figure 2.8 sinusoid *A* is 90° out of phase with sinusoid *B* because sinusoid *A* starts at 0° phase and sinusoid *B* at 90° phase. Because both sinusoids have the same frequency, however, the phase difference between them could be determined at any two points along the time axis. At both points *C* and *D*, for instance, the difference between the two waveforms is also one-quarter of a period, or 90°

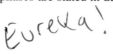

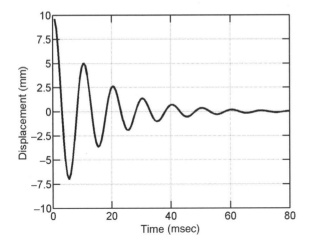

FIGURE 2.10 A plot of the amplitude of sinusoidal vibration, given there is a frictional force acting against the free vibration. Notice that the amplitude of successive peaks decreases at a constant ratio of 0.5. Friction causes the vibration to die out (damp) over time.

producing an audible sound. A mass and spring can be used to describe vibrations, and a sinusoidal relationship describes the displacement of the mass as a function of time. A sinusoid or any vibratory pattern has three physical parameters: amplitude (a measure of displacement in terms of peak, peak-to-peak, or rms amplitude), frequency (a measure in units of hertz [Hz] as the number of vibratory oscillations per second), and starting phase (usually measured in units of degrees as a relative measure of the displacement position when the vibration begins). Fourier analysis shows that all complex waves consist of a sum of sinusoids (a simple wave). The properties of mass (inertia), elasticity, and resistance all contribute to a complete description of a vibration.

SUPPLEMENT

Because sound is a well-studied area of physics, most introductory physics textbooks contain a section on sound and acoustics. Rossing (1990), Rosen and

Howell (1991, Chapters 2 and 3), and Moore (1997, Chapter 2) provide reviews of sound that go beyond the material presented in this book. For the advanced reader, the book by Hartmann (1998) provides a much more thorough discussion of sound.

A variety of topics in this chapter deserve additional discussion so that the interested student can more fully appreciate the material and be better prepared for the material in subsequent chapters. The sinusoid is not the only function or waveform that can describe sound or free vibrations. However, the sinusoidal function has a variety of properties that make it ideal for analyzing vibrations, including those that relate to Fourier's theorem (see Appendix C and Chapter 4) and harmonic motion.

In using the circular analogy (see Appendix A) to describe sinusoids, frequency can be expressed as the rate at which a point moves along a circle's circumference. Thus, ω becomes the angular velocity (angular distance divided by time) of the moving point:

$$\omega = 360°/t = 2\pi f,$$

where $360°$ is 2π, f is frequency; and t is time (recall that $f = 1/t$). For this reason the sinusoidal term is sometimes expressed as $\sin(\omega t)$. The frequency and displacement of many vibrations, simple and complex, can be described as indicated in the chapter. Starting phase is a measure that is almost always only applied to sinusoidal vibrations. However, since all vibrations can be described as the sum of sinusoidal vibrations, the measure of starting phase is implicit in the measure of all vibrations (this concept is discussed in Chapter 4).

The concepts of *velocity*, *acceleration*, and *force* have already been mentioned. Here are the definitions of these terms (see also the section at the back of this book on "Terms, Measurements, Equations, and Conversions"):

$$v = \text{velocity} = d/t,$$

where d = distance and t = time;

$$a = \text{acceleration} = v/t,$$

where v = velocity and t = time; and

$$F = \text{force} = ma,$$

where m = mass of the object and a = acceleration.

It follows that

$$a = d/t/t \quad \text{and} \quad F = mv/t.$$

These concepts helped in the derivation of a quantitative description of the free vibration shown in Figures 2.1 and 2.10. From this derivation the frequency of the mass and spring vibration was $f = \sqrt{(s/m)}$. That means that for a vibrating object the frequency of vibration is proportional to the square root of the stiffness of the restoring force and inversely proportional to the square root of the mass of the object being vibrated. Thus, increasing the mass of an object four times will reduce the frequency by a factor of one-half, and making the stiffness four times as great will increase the frequency by a factor of 2.

The magnitude of vibration as displacement [$d(t)$] was used to emphasize the point that vibration refers to a change in the displacement of an object over time. However, in most discussions of sound and acoustics, the term *amplitude* (a) is used instead of displacement and $a(t)$ refers to instantaneous amplitude. Amplitude may mean displacement, but as is seen in Chapter 3, there are also other measures of amplitude. For the purposes of this book, amplitude and displacement will be considered synonymous, but they must not be viewed as synonymous with other terms for describ-

ing the magnitude of sound, such as *level* and *intensity*, which are covered in Chapter 3.

In this chapter, the root-mean-square amplitude of a sinusoid was stated as equal to 0.707 times the peak amplitude (A). This can be seen by applying the definition of rms to a sinusoidal function and using integration:

$$A_{rms} = \sqrt{1/T \int_0^T A^2 \sin^2(\omega t)dt} = \sqrt{A^2/T \int_0^T \sin^2(\omega t)dt},$$

where A_{rms} is rms amplitude, A is peak amplitude, $\omega = 2\pi f$, and T is one period of vibration. Applying integral calculus for a sin-squared function yields

$$A_{rms} = \sqrt{(A^2/T)[t/2 - 1/4\{\sin(2\omega t)\}]}\Big|_0^T;$$

that is, the integral of $\sin^2(\omega t) = t/2 - 1/4 \sin(2\omega t)$.

The integral at $t = 0$ and $t = T$ must next be evaluated. At $t = 0$ the entire right-hand side of the equation is zero. At $t = T$,

$$A_{rms} = \sqrt{(A^2/T)[(T/2) - 1/4\sin(2\omega T)]} = \sqrt{A^2/2}.$$

That is, under these conditions, $\sin(2\omega T) = 0$, because $\sin(2\omega T) = \sin(4\pi f T)$ (recall that $\omega = 2\pi f T$ and $f = 1/T$; i.e., T is the period); thus, $\sin(4\pi f t) = \sin(4\pi T/T) = \sin(4\pi) = 0$ [see Appendix A for sinusoid tables, and note that $\sin(4\pi) = 0$].

Therefore,

$$A_{rms} = \sqrt{A^2/2} = A/\sqrt{2} = 0.707A,$$

because $1/\sqrt{2} = 0.707$.

3

Sound Transmission and Sound Propagation

SOUND PROPOGATION

In everyday life we do not hear an object vibrate directly; rather, the vibrating object causes a wave motion in air, which then causes our eardrum to vibrate, starting the process of hearing. Sound can travel through any elastic medium that has inertia. In other words, sound can travel through air, water, steel, and so on, but not through a vacuum.

Because air is the medium for sound transmission in most everyday situations, we will consider the transmission of sound through air. Air consists of molecules in constant random motion. When an object vibrates in air, the molecules tend to move in the direction the object moves rather than in random motion. The air molecules next to the object move first and then pass this movement onto adjacent molecules. The molecules themselves do not move all the way from the object to the receiver; they only pass along a wave of motion by causing molecules next them to move, these molecules in turn cause their neighbors to move, and so on. In this train-like progression (much like a falling row of dominoes) the motion of the air molecules is *propagated* (transferred) through the air toward the ear. When the air molecules next to the ear are moved by this motion, the eardrum (*tympanic membrane*) is vibrated, and this eventually results in our experiencing audible sound.

Let us examine more closely the changes that take place in air when an object is vibrated. When a vibrating object moves in one direction, air molecules are pushed in the same direction (assuming no frictional forces interfere). The molecules next to the vibrating object are compressed together as the object moves outward away from its resting state, creating an area with a greater *density* (mass per unit of volume) of air molecules. Certain laws of chemistry/physics, the *gas laws*, state that as the density of air molecules increases, the *pressure* increases. That is, pressure is proportional to density. Thus, as the object moves outward, the density of air molecules next to the vibrating object increases and creates high pressure in this area: An area of *condensation* had been generated (i.e., the air molecules are condensed). As the vibrating object moves in the opposite direction (back toward its resting state), the air molecules obey another property of the gas laws: Gases, including air, will evenly fill the space they occupy. Thus, the air molecules fill the space vacated by the vibrating object moving in the opposite direction. As the vibrating object moves back past its resting state, an even larger vacated area is generated for the air molecules to fill.

Now the density of air molecules has decreased, and, thus, the pressure is lower. An area of *rarefaction* has been generated (i.e., the density of air molecules is rarified).

The mere presence of molecules in air creates a pressure, or *static air pressure*, which is proportional to the density of the molecules. The changes in pressure due to the vibrating object are changes in this existing static air pressure. As the object vibrates, the air pressure increases above the static air pressure at any one location, then decreases below the static air pressure, and then increases again, and so on, generating a changing air pressure relative to the static air pressure. This changing air pressure moves away from the vibrating object. In other words, areas of condensation are alternating over space with areas of rarefaction. That is, molecules next to those initially moved are moved back and forth through stages of condensation and rarefaction. This pattern continues across space as the wavelike motion is propagated away from the vibrating source.

Recall that air molecules are in constant random motion, so the changes elicited by a vibrating object change the "tendency" of the motion of these molecules into the pattern of condensations and rarefactions just described. Imagine that the air molecules were photographed when the object was vibrating, freezing this pattern. Figure 3.1 represents the cartoon of what might be seen at the instant in time the picture was taken. The molecules appear to cluster at some points in space (condensation) and they are farther apart at other places (rarefaction). Although such a picture would not reveal the direction of motion of the air molecules, the molecules tend to move in the direction of the arrows shown in Figure 3.1. That is, as the object pushes out, the air molecules tend to move away from the object; and as the object moves back toward its starting point, the molecules tend to move back in the other direction. Thus, the motion at a condensation tends to be away from the source, and the motion at a rarefaction tends to be toward the source. The wave propagates out from a source in a circular manner (actually, in three dimensions the wave propagates in a spherical manner). Figure 3.2 shows con-

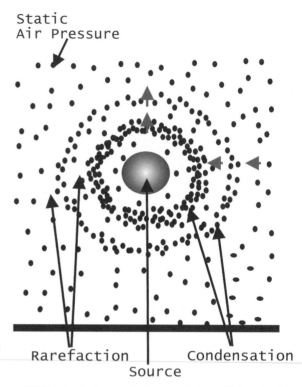

FIGURE 3.1   A diagram of what one might see if air molecules were photographed at an instant in time as a sound source vibrated. The rarefactions and condensations are shown as well as the direction (grey arrows above the source) in which the molecules were moving at the instant the picture was taken. The pressure wave moves out in a circular manner (actually as a sphere in the three-dimensional real world). As the pressure wave moves out from the source it occupies a greater area, and thus the density of molecules at rarefactions and condensations lessens. The area around the border of the figure represents the static air motion before the propagated wave reaches this area.

densations and rarefactions from an overall view. The medium-gray background represents static air pressure. Circles that radiate out from the source that are darker than the background are areas of condensations, while circles that are lighter than the background are areas of rarefaction. As the wave motion moves away from the source, the total area of any circle increases, so the density (pressure) at any one area on the circle approaches that of the background.

[handwritten annotations: "crest-con", "trough/valley", "rarefaction", "wave length"]

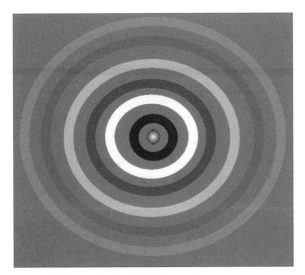

FIGURE 3.2 Another depiction of the areas of pressure condensations (darker circles, relative to the grey background representing the static air pressure) alternating with areas of pressure rarefactions (lighter circles) that radiate out from the vibrating source. The pressures in the pressure wave approach that of the static air pressure as the propagating wave moves away from the source.

Thus, at some distance from the source, areas of condensed and rarefied air pressure are no different than the background static air pressure, and as such no sound wave is propagated beyond this point. We describe this phenomenon in more detail when we discuss the inverse square law later.

Viewing waves on water provides an approximation (but only an approximation) of what happens in air when an object vibrates. If we push water (for instance, by dropping a stone in a pool), waves are formed. The water waves are similar to the air waves associated with sound propagation. The crests of the wave are the condensations, and the valleys are the rarefactions. If you have ever watched a wave "move" through the water, you have observed that the water itself does not move across the surface; rather, the wave motion is passed (propagated) along the water surface. A similar, but not identical, type of motion is associated with air molecules that are moved by a vibrating object.

The distance between each successive condensation (or rarefaction) is the *wavelength* (λ) of sound (e.g., λ is the distance between each successive dark circle or between each successive light circle in Figure 3.2). Actually, the distance between any successive identical points in the propagated wave is the wavelength (i.e., such as the distance between adjacent wave peaks in the water analogy). Wavelength is expressed in units of distance, such as meters. The more frequently an object oscillates (high frequency), the closer together the rarefactions and condensations become and the shorter the wavelength. The speed with which the wave motion is propagated through the medium (i.e., the *speed of sound*) also affects the wavelength. If the speed of sound is fast, then as the object vibrates, the first wave moves away from the object quickly and the second wave lags behind. This causes the distance between successive condensations, and, hence, the wavelength, to be long. If the speed of sound is slow, the first wave travels only a short distance before the second wave passes an identical spot, so the wavelength is short. Therefore, both frequency and the speed of sound affect wavelength. The equation relating wavelength (λ) in meters to speed of sound (c in meters per second) and to frequency (f in Hz) is

$$\lambda = c/f \qquad (3.1)$$

Wavelength is directly proportional to the speed of sound and is inversely proportional to the frequency of vibration.

The speed of sound in air is approximately 350 meters per second, although it can vary as a function of the temperature, density, and humidity of air. The speed of sound is higher in a hot, humid area at sea level than in a cold, dry place at a high altitude. As the density of the air molecules increases, so does the speed of sound.

We learn later in the book (Chapter 10) that the frequency range over which humans can detect sound is from about 20 Hz to about 20,000 Hz. If it is assumed that the speed of sound is 350 meters/sec, then according to equation (3.1) the range of wavelengths (λ) associated with these audible frequencies is from

17.5 meters (20 Hz) to 0.0175 meters (or 1.75 cm at 20,000 Hz).

Figures 3.1 and 3.2 depict the areas of condensation and rarefactions captured at a single moment (instant) in time and spread out over an area. As one can see, sound pressure varies above and below the static air pressure across space. Figure 3.3 depicts sound pressure as a function of distance for four different time points assuming there was a sinusoidal vibrating sound source. That is, Figure 3.3a (bottom panel) shows the distribution of sound pressure across space (distance from the sound source) for one moment in time, and Figures 3.3b to 3.3d show the distribution of sound pressure across distance for successive points in time after the measurement shown in

Figure 3.3a (note that the pressure peaks move from the left to the right in distance for each successive moment in time from Figure 3.3a to Figure 3.3b). Across space the pressure increases and decreases above and below the static air pressure in a sinusoidal manner (given the sinusoidal vibration of the object), and the distance between any two successive identical points on the pressure distribution is the wavelength (λ). Because sound pressure decreases as the distance from the source increases, the peak-to-peak sound pressure decreases as distance from the source increases.

Often we want to know how sound pressure at any one point in *space* changes over *time* (e.g., what the sound pressure change is at the entrance to the outer ear). In Figure 3.3 the line at a distance of 30 cm represents a point in space where one might want to calculate how sound pressure changes over time. Figure 3.4 indicates sound pressure changing over time at this distance of 30 cm. The four points in Figure 3.4 represent the four measurements taken from the four time slices shown in Figure 3.3, again assuming sinusoidal vibration of the sound source. That is, at any point the

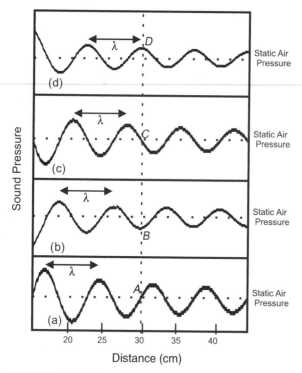

FIGURE 3.3 A depiction of the distribution of pressure over space (distance) from a vibrating source at four successive moments in time [from panel a to panel d]. The wavelength (λ) is the distance between successive identical points of pressure in the wave. As the pressure wave moves away from the source, pressure decreases.

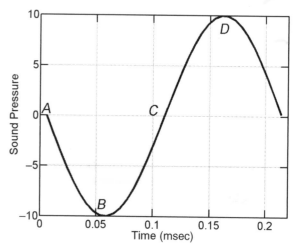

FIGURE 3.4 The pressure at one point in space (as depicted in Figure 3.3) changes over time as indicated in this figure. The points labeled *A, B, C, D* are those indicated in the four panels of Figure 3.3 representing the four successive moments in time.

TABLE 3.1 Decibel Level, in dB SPL, for Several Types of Sound Sources and Conditions

---

0 dB SPL: softest sound a person with normal hearing can hear
10 dB SPL: normal breathing
20 dB SPL: whispering
40 dB SPL: a quiet room
50 db SPL: rainfall
60 db SPL: normal conversation
110 dB SPL: shouting in an ear
120 dB SPL: thunder
140 dB SPL: immediate damage to the auditory system

---

is in terms of *sensation level* (SL). Sensation level refers to the least intense sound a particular subject can detect in a particular experimental situation (for example, at a particular frequency). Thus, 60 dB SL means a sound was 60 dB more intense than that required for detection in another experimental situation. SPL is based on the reference of 20 micropascals, whereas SL is based on the reference of the lowest level a particular subject can detect in a specific experimental context. Although many other conventions are used to define reference levels for the decibel, SPL and SL are used primarily throughout this book (we discuss other measures of level in decibels in Chapters 10 and 13). For this book, we use sound pressure level or pressure level when the magnitude of sound is expressed in decibels of amplitude (pressure or displacement) and intensity level when the magnitude is expressed in decibels of intensity (sound intensity, power, or energy). Thus, *level* refers to a decibel measure. Table 3.1 indicates the decibel level, in dB SPL, for several sound sources and conditions.

INTERFERENCE

Now that the general properties of the propagation of a sound wave through air have been described, let us consider some consequences of sound propagation in the real world. One of the more obvious properties of sound propagation is that the farther away one is

from a sound source (the vibrating object), the softer sound becomes. In terms of the situation displayed in Figures 3.2, 3.3, and 3.4, the sound source is considered a point, and sound radiates in a spherical fashion from this point source. Notice from equation (3.5), and depicted in Figures 3.2–3.4, that sound intensity (I) is proportional to pressure squared (power) divided by area. As we move away from the center of the sphere (away from the sound source), the surface area of the sphere becomes larger. Because the sound source is assumed to be producing a constant power and the area is increasing, sound intensity (I) must be decreasing as the distance between the point of measurement and the sound source increases. The area of the surface of a sphere is equal to $4\pi r^2$, where r is the radius of the sphere or, in our case, the distance from the sound source to the point of measurement.

From this relationship and the definition of sound intensity (I), we obtain the following proportionality:

$$I \propto P/4\pi r^2, \tag{3.9}$$

where $\propto$ means "proportional to," or

$$I = K(P/4\pi r^2),$$

where K is the proportionality constant, P is the power of the sound at its source, and r is the distance from the source to the point of measurement. This in turn means that sound intensity (I) is inversely proportional to distance from the sound source, squared (r^2). This is referred to as the *inverse square law*. Thus, if distance is doubled, sound intensity is decreased by a factor of 4.

Recall from equations (3.5) and (3.6) that sound intensity (I) is proportional to pressure (p) squared. Therefore,

$$p = K\sqrt{I} = K\sqrt{(P/4\pi r^2)} = k/r, \tag{3.10}$$

where k and K are constants based on the density of the sound media and the speed of sound. Equation (3.10) reveals that sound pressure is inversely proportional to distance (r). Thus, if the distance from a sound source is doubled, the sound intensity level decreases by a factor of 4, or 6 dB (10 log 4), and the sound pressure level decreases by a factor of 2, or,

Handwritten annotation at top of page: $I = \text{pressure}^2 / \text{Speed of Impedance} (Z)$

also, 6 dB (20 log 2). Thus, when expressed in decibels, level decreases by 6 dB for each doubling of the distance from the source to the point of measurement.

These relationships hold only in situations in which the sound encounters no obstacles (e.g., there can be more than or less than a 6-dB loss in sound level for each doubling of distance, depending on what obstacles the sound wave encounters). Sound waves most often do encounter obstacles. Frequently objects impede the propagation of the sound wave. This impedance to sound transmission occurs whenever there is a change in the medium through which sound must travel (e.g., from air to a wall). The term *impedance* has an exact definition, and its properties are important for an understanding of sound propagation. To discuss impedance, let us return to the mass-and-spring analogy used in Chapter 2. In general, there are two forms of impedance: *reactance* and *resistance*. The symbol Z will be used for impedance, the symbol X for reactance, and the symbol R for resistance. Both forms of impedance involve properties that oppose vibratory motion. Those properties that impede motion because of the properties of the mass and spring are the *reactance* components of impedance. There are thus two types of reactance: *mass reactance* (X_m) and *spring (or stiffness) reactance* (X_s). The amount of reactance (i.e., the amount the object's motion is impeded) depends on the frequency of vibration for both mass and spring reactance. Resistive forces that impede vibratory motion do not depend on frequency. *Friction* is one type of resistance. The following equation describes the relationship among impedance (Z), reactance (both X_m and X_s), and resistance (R):

$$Z = \sqrt{\left[R^2 + (X_m - X_s)^2\right]}. \tag{3.11}$$

In general, the impedance of any medium is called the *characteristic impedance* (Z_c) of the medium. Characteristic impedance is

$$Z_c = \rho_0 c, \tag{3.12}$$

where ρ_0 is the density of the medium and c is the speed of the sound in the medium. Notice that Z_c is the same as the denominator of the definition of sound

intensity given in equation (3.5). Therefore, we can redefine sound intensity (I) as

$$I = p^2/Z_c, \tag{3.13}$$

where p is pressure. Thus, sound intensity can also be expressed as sound pressure squared divided by the characteristic impedance of the medium through which the sound is transmitted.

Sound intensity varies according to the medium through which it is transmitted because of the characteristic impedance of the medium. If a sound wave encounters a change in media and, thus, a change in impedance, a portion of the sound wave will be reflected from the surface with the greater impedance; i.e., the sound wave bounces back from the surface. The same type of sound wave propagation as described earlier takes places for the reflected wave as it moves away from the reflective surface. The amount of sound intensity reflected depends on the difference between the characteristic impedance of the two media. The greater this characteristic impedance difference, the greater the sound intensity of the reflected wave. That portion of the sound wave not reflected away from the medium is either *transmitted* to the new medium (and the sound continues to propagate through the new medium) or *absorbed* in the new medium.

The reflected sound wave may encounter the original sound wave as it propagates away from the barrier, as shown in Figure 3.5. In this case, two types of interactions can occur between the original and reflected sound waves. Two points of condensation (or rarefactions) can occur together, resulting in an area of greater condensation (or rarefaction), called *constructive interference*. Points of condensation and rarefaction can overlap, resulting in a reduction in pressure from that of the condensation and an increase in pressure from that of the rarefaction, called *destructive interference* (Figure 3.5). That is, the net result can be the summing of two waveforms (*reinforcement*, as in constructive interference) or the subtraction of two waveforms (*cancellation*, as in destructive interference). Thus, a person sitting in front of a wall might hear a sound equal in intensity to the oncoming wave

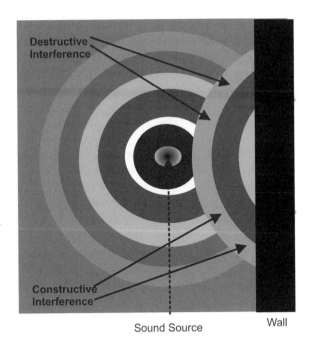

Destructive Interference

Constructive Interference

Sound Source   Wall

FIGURE 3.5 A sound wave reflects off a wall. As the sound wave returns from a reflection, it can add to the oncoming wave (*constructive interference*, in which condensation peaks meet or rarefaction valleys meet leading to an increase or decrease in pressure) or cancel the oncoming wave (*destructive interference*, in which a condensation peak meets a rarefaction valley, always leading to a decrease in pressure).

(no reflections), a more intense sound (in the case of reinforcement), or a less intense sound (cancellation).

Figure 3.5 illustrates the sound reflecting from one sound point. If sound is coming from several points or from a large area, many reinforcements and cancellations are possible. Besides the wall, anything more dense (having a greater characteristic impedance) than air will reflect sound. Determining the intensity at any one place in a room, therefore, becomes very complicated.

Notice that in Figure 3.5 there is one source producing one vibration. If two sources produce waves of different frequencies that were reflected off a wall, complex interaction patterns might result. As a consequence of these interactions, a sound of one frequency at one point in space might be easier to hear than

another frequency at that point, because its intensity is greater (reinforcement) at the point of measurement. The intensity of a sound may vary not only as a function of where in a room it is measured, but also as a function of frequency.

In summary, we must be careful in assuming that the waveform arriving at some point in a room (e.g., a person's ear) is identical to the waveform that leaves the source (e.g., a loudspeaker). The two should be nearly the same only if reflections off walls, floors, and other objects are discounted and the distance from the source is used in the calculation.

A *sound shadow* is an additional influence an object can exert on a sound wave. The sound shadow can be viewed in the context of waves on water. Imagine throwing a pebble into water and watching waves radiate from the spot of impact. As described previously, this is analogous (but not identical) to sound waves radiating from a sound source. A very large object in the water causes waves to bounce off the object, as described previously (Figure 3.5) and in Figure 3.6a, but a wave passes over a very small object with little change (Figure 3.6b). A medium-sized object produces some reflections from the object, but at some distance beyond the object the waves appear to have been unaffected (Figure 3.6c). In fact, if we look carefully at this last situation, we notice that just past the medium-sized object is an area with no waves at all or reduced wave magnitude. This area is referred to as the *sound shadow* (Figure 3.6c). At some distance beyond the sound shadow the pressure waves are unaffected by the presence of the "medium-size" object, much like the way the "small-size" object did not disturb the propagating pressure wave. What is meant by "small," "medium-sized," and "large" objects? These sizes are expressed in relation to the wavelength (recall that wavelength is measured in units of distance) of sound; objects much larger than the wavelength of sound and with a different characteristic impedance reflect sound, objects that are much smaller than the wavelength of sound do not affect wave motion, while objects whose sizes are approximately equal to the wavelength of sound may produce sound shadows. The term *diffraction* is used to

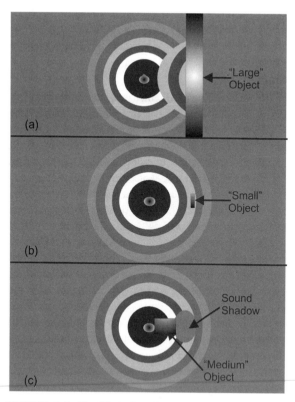

(a)

"Large"
Object

(b)

"Small"
Object

(c)

Sound
Shadow

"Medium"
Object

FIGURE 3.6 Simplified diagrams of sound waves passing objects. **(a)** Objects larger than the wavelength: most of the wave is reflected. **(b)** Objects much smaller than the wavelength: most of the wave passes the object. **(c)** Objects close in size to the wavelength: a sound shadow of reduced sound pressure is produced beyond the object.

describe the property by which sound "passes around or is scattered by" (is diffracted by) small or medium-sized objects. The area of reduced wave-motion pressure produced by a sound shadow will be at least as large as the wavelength of the oncoming sound. The average human head is about 20 cm in diameter. According to equation (3.1), the head could create a significant sound shadow (less intense sounds at the ear away from the sound source) for sounds with frequencies greater than about 1750 Hz (1750 Hz would be the frequency of sound with a wavelength of 20 cm, assuming the speed of sound is 350 meters/sec;

1750 Hz = 350 meters/sec ÷ 0.2 meters). The sound shadow produced by the head will be encountered when *binaural* (two-ear) hearing is discussed in Chapter 12.

SOUND FIELDS

Any environment that contains sound is called a *sound field*. A sound field without any reflections is called a *free field*. A truly free-field environment is almost impossible to obtain. An *anechoic room* (echo-free) is an environment in which every attempt is made to reduce reflections. This is generally accomplished by using materials and shapes that absorb rather than reflect sound. Sometimes a room with reflections is desired. Such environments are called *reverberation* (or echoic) *rooms*. One type of reverberation room or field is a *diffuse field*. In a diffuse field, an attempt is made to arrange the reflecting surfaces so that sound intensity will be as uniform as possible throughout the room. The reflecting surfaces are arranged so that constructive and destructive interference leads to constant sound intensity throughout the sound field. In any room, whether or not it is a reverberation room, measuring reflections can be useful. If the room has surfaces that reflect a large proportion of the sound, then both the original sound and the reflected sound can be heard (e.g., an echo might occur). This is usually not desirable because the echo will interfere with the ability to process the originating sound.

In a room there will be many reflections, many at some distance from the source, and the sound may be reflected multiple times by the many reflective surfaces in the room. Thus, the *reverberating* sound in the room can last a long time (often many seconds) after the originating sound is turned off. However, after a sound is terminated, the reverberation will die away over time. The primary value used in measuring this aspect of reverberation is *reverberation time*. Figure 3.7 shows a recording of a brief sound (the sound was only 0.1 msec in duration) made in a classroom. As can be seen in Figure 3.7, after the sound

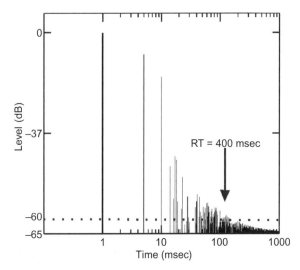

FIGURE 3.7   A depiction of a microphone recording of the sound in a room with many reflective surfaces produced by the presentation of a very brief originating sound. The early-arriving reflections can be seen as delayed versions of the originating brief sound. Later, the combined effect of the many reflections interact to produce reverberate sound, and the level of this reverberation decreased from the level of the original sound by 60 dB by about 400 msec, indicating that the reverberation time (RT) for this room is about 400 msec.

ceased there was still sound reverberating in the classroom for more than a second. Reverberation time is the time it takes for the reverberant sound pressure (due to the sound's continuing to reflect off of the many surfaces in the room) to reach some proportion (usually defined as one-thousandth, or $20 \log(1000) = 20 \times 3 = 60\,dB$) of its original pressure (in Figure 3.7, the reverberation time is 0.4 sec, or 400 msec).

Both the amount of absorption of the sound in the room and the volume of the room help determine the reverberation time. High absorption (e.g., a room with lots of thick curtains and a thick rug) and small volume leads to short reverberation time (that is, the pressure of the echo or reverberation has quickly been reduced). That is,

$$RT \propto Vol/Ab, \qquad (3.14)$$

where RT is reverberation time, Vol is room volume, Ab is total room absorption, and $\propto$ means "propor-

tional to." Sounds produced in rooms with reverberation times (RT) that exceed 1 sec are often difficult to recognize because the reverberant sound interferes with the originating sound.

As has already been discussed, sound waves and their reflections can interact in a variety of ways (as indicated in Figure 3.5). In enclosed spaces these interactions produce several effects that are of interest to acousticians, musicians, architectural designers, as well as hearing scientists. One of these interactions is the *standing wave*. The concept of a standing wave is perhaps easiest to explain in terms of a vibrating string, shown in Figure 3.8. Imagine that a string is attached to a wall and the string is vibrated by flicking it up once. A wave motion travels down the string and is reflected off the wall (Figure 3.8a). Notice that as the wave comes back from the reflecting surface (the wall), it is inverted relative to the original oncoming wave. Now imagine that you continuously "vibrate" the string. At the correct frequency, cancellations and reinforcements of the originating wave interacting with the reflecting wave will cause the entire string to move up and down without an apparent wave traveling to one end and back. In this case (Figure 3.8b), locations of minimum vibratory displacement (*nodes*) alternate over space with locations of maximal vibratory displacement (*antinodes*). If you increase the frequency of vibration of the string, you can generate a wave pattern with two antinodes, as shown in Figure 3.8c. At even higher frequencies, wave patterns with more than two antinodes can be produced. Such wave patterns with fixed locations of nodes and antinodes are called *standing waves*. Remember that the existence of a standing wave does not mean an absence of wave motion but that a wave motion does not travel left to right (transversely) along the string. The string vibrates in an up–down direction maximally at the antinode and minimally at the node.

Figure 3.9 shows how the originating wave (dashed curve, moving left to right from the source from Figure 3.9a to Figure 3.9e) and the reflected wave (dotted curve, moving right to left back from a reflective surface on the right) sum to produce a standing wave (solid curve, whose peaks do not move left to

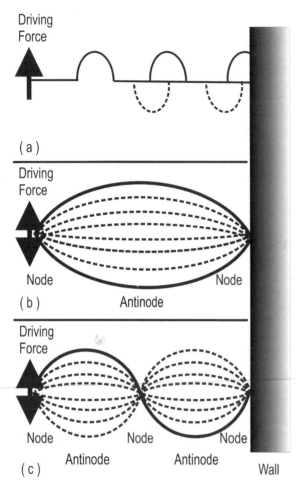

FIGURE 3.8 A diagram of the vibratory pattern of a string when it is attached at one end (e.g., to a wall) and vibrated at the other end. (a) With a single movement of the string, a wave moves to the wall and is inverted as it reflects from the wall. (b) When the string is vibrated, a standing-wave motion may exist, with a node at either end and an antinode in the middle. (c) The frequency of vibration is twice that in Figure 3.5b, yielding three nodes and two antinodes.

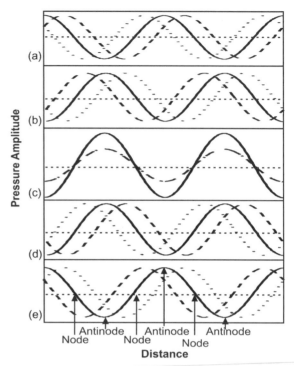

FIGURE 3.9 A sound wave (dashed curves) in a tube moves away from the source (to the right) from the time of panel a to that of panel e. The reflected wave (dotted curves) moves back (toward the left) from the reflective surface on the right over the five moments in time shown from panels a to e. In this case, the sound wave and its reflection sum to produce a standing wave (dark curves) that does not move laterally (left to right or right to left) over time, but whose pressure increases and decreases with maximal pressure changes occurring at antinodes and minimum pressure changes occurring at nodes.

right or right to left). The five panels of Figure 3.9 indicate five moments in time for the interactions that produce a standing wave. That is, the standing wave is the sum at each point in space of the original and reflective waves. As noted, the peaks of the originating waves (dashed curves) move from left to right over

the time period shown in the five panels of Figure 3.9, and the peaks of the reflected wave (dotted curves) move in the opposite direction. The peaks of the standing wave pattern (solid curves), however, occur at the same location across time, although the standing wave clearly fluctuates in displacement at each point in space over time (i.e., the standing wave at any point in space changes its amplitude over time, but the standing wave does not move left to right or right to left).

A standing wave with one antinode (Figure 3.8b) is called the *fundamental mode* of vibration. The fundamental mode occurs when the vibrating frequency has a wavelength (λ) equal to twice the length of the string. Hence,

$$f_0 = c/2L, \qquad (3.15)$$

where f_0 is the fundamental frequency of the mode, c is the speed of sound in the medium, and L is the length of the string (L and c should use the same measure of distance). Recall that $\lambda = c/f$ from equation (3.1), so the length of strength (L) required for one mode of a standing wave to occur is $\lambda_0/2$, where λ_0 is the wavelength of f_0 and $\lambda_0 = 2L$.

Thus, f_0 becomes the fundamental frequency in producing the fundamental mode of vibration. Vibrating frequencies at integer multiples of the fundamental vibrating frequency ($2f_0$, $3f_0$, $4f_0$, etc.) produce standing waves with two, three, four, and so forth, times the number of antinodes (Figure 3.8c). However, as the vibrating frequency increases above its fundamental frequency, the amplitude of the standing wave decreases (so the amplitude of the standing wave, $3f_0$, is lower than that at $2f_0$).

Standing waves are important properties of stringed instruments. Standing waves can also exist in enclosed air spaces (such as an organ pipe or a tube such as the outer ear canal) when air is forced into the space (such as occurs when sound is generated and travels down the outer ear canal). The same types of interference described earlier can generate a standing wave of air movement within the pipe or tube. If the tube is closed at both ends or opened at both ends, the standing-wave fundamental mode will occur when the wavelength of the fundamental frequency is twice the length of the tube, the same as for the string example of Figure 3.8 and equation (3.15). If the tube is closed at one end, the wavelength of the fundamental frequency is four times the length of the tube ($f_0 = c/4L$, $L = \lambda_0/4$, $\lambda_0 = 4L$). In this case, the higher modes of vibration only occur at odd-integer multiples of the fundamental frequency (i.e., at $3f_0$, $5f_0$, $7f_0$, etc.) as compared to frequencies

at all integer multiples of f_0 when the tube is open or closed at both ends.

Standing waves can exist in any environment in which a unique pattern of interference can be set up. Rooms can generate standing waves under certain conditions of vibration. These standing waves produce fixed locations of large pressure changes (antinodes) and of minimal pressure changes (nodes). In general, such standing waves are to be avoided in designing a room for acoustic purposes. Likewise, standing waves may exist in auditory structures such as the ear canal. For instance, the outer ear canal is like a tube closed at one end. As such, standing waves may be generated within the outer ear canal when sound is present; if so, the frequencies of these standing waves will influence what we hear.

SUMMARY

Sound is propagated through air from its vibrating source to a receiving object. The vibrating object causes a movement of air molecules that corresponds to the vibration of the object. The wavelength of vibration is a measure of the distance between successive pressure points (i.e., rarefactions or condensations) in the sound wave. Sound intensity is measured in units of energy or power derived from pressure. The decibel is 10 times the logarithm of the ratio of two intensities (powers or energies) and 20 times the logarithm of the ratio of two pressures. Sound waves can encounter various forms of interference. There can be cancellations and additions, standing waves can be formed, objects can create sound shadows in the sound wave field, and objects might introduce impedance to the transmission of sound. Impedance has reactance and resistive components. The intensity of sound decreases by a factor of the distance squared as a listener moves away from the sound source (inverse square law). Various sound fields can be constructed to control reflections. The frequency of a standing wave is related to the length of the space

being vibrated as well as to other properties of the space. **Reverberation time indicates the time it takes for reverberation to lose its intensity by a specified amount.**

SUPPLEMENT

In addition to the readings suggested in Chapter 2, textbooks on architectural acoustics may provide some informative discussion of topics touched on in this chapter. An excellent textbook is the classic by Beranek (1988, titled *Acoustics*, reprinted by the Acoustical Society of America from the 1954 original). The textbook by Rossing (1990), *The Science of Sound*, provides an excellent coverage of the physics of sound at an elementary level.

Although we have used the analogy of waves in water to describe sound waves in air, the reader should not assume that wave propagation is the same in both media. Caution should be used before drawing any strong parallels between waves in water (or other media) and sound waves in air.

Molecules in any gas, including air, are in constant motion, which causes the molecules to collide with one another. The gas laws describe the properties of this molecular motion. Two aspects of this motion, sometimes referred to as *Brownian motion*, relate to discussions in this chapter. The movement and collision of molecules produce a pressure called *static pressure*. The changes in pressure associated with introducing a sound source cause an additional change in this static air pressure. Temperature and humidity can also change static air pressure. The changes in air pressure due to temperature and humidity occur at a much slower rate than the air pressure changes usually associated with sound production. Therefore, it is usually easy to separate sound pressure changes from these other air pressure changes. When air molecules collide with each other, energy is given off. Some of this energy results in potential sound waves. The sound energy of this Brownian motion noise (sometimes called *thermal noise*) is very small, probably 20 or 30 db below the faintest sound a human can hear.

Thus, except for a few very sensitive humans and perhaps a few animals with greater auditory sensitivity than humans, this thermal noise is not influencing an animal's ability to detect weak sounds (see Green's *An Introduction to Hearing*, 1976, for additional information).

Frequency is a variable that is like velocity or speed, because it means cycles per second. However, frequency of vibration should not be confused with speed of sound. *Frequency* refers to the rate at which a vibrating object goes through one cycle of oscillation, while the *speed* of sound refers to the rate at which a sound wave is propagated through air (or any other elastic medium). When applying these terms to the motion of air molecules, *frequency* refers to the rate at which the air molecules at one point in space change from a particular pattern of condensation or instantaneous pressure back to this same pattern or instantaneous pressure (i.e., *frequency* refers to changes that takes place over time at one location in space). *Speed* of sound refers to the rate at which the pattern of condensation is passed from one location in space to the next location in space (i.e., *speed* of sound refers to the wave traveling across space over time).

Chapter 2 introduced the terms *velocity* and *acceleration*, and Chapter 3 has used these terms repeatedly. Velocity is a measure of change. Calculus is used to analyze such changing relationships. In calculus, velocity and acceleration are defined as $v = dx/dt$, where dx is the change in distance and dt is the change in time. Acceleration becomes $a = d^2x/d^2t$. Velocity is the first derivative of distance and acceleration is the second derivative of distance. This type of calculus nomenclature is used to describe free and damped vibrations. By using the concepts discussed in the Supplement to Chapter 2, we can describe free vibration as follows:

$$m\left[(d^2x)/(d^2t)\right] = -sx,$$

so

$$m\left[(d^2x)/(d^2t)\right] + sx = 0.$$

By solving this differential equation for x (since s and m are constant), we arrive at the equation

$$d(t) = A \sin[2\pi \sqrt{(s/m)} t + \theta],$$

which is described in the Supplement to Chapter 2. If we add the frictional forces that lead to a damped vibration, the differential equation becomes

$$m[(d^2 x)/(d^2 t)] + sx + r_f (dx/dt) = 0,$$

where r_f is the influence of friction. The solution to this differential equation yields a function with the shape shown for the damped sinusoidal vibration in Figure 2.10.

A differential equation called the *wave equation* is used to describe wave propagation in any medium:

$$\delta^2 (p/\delta^2 t) = c^2 [(\delta^2 p)/(\delta^2 x)],$$

where p is sound pressure, c is the speed of sound, x is distance, and t is time. With two independent variables, space (x) and time (t), the differential equation involves partial derivatives (δ). Solutions to the wave equation describe the type of wave motion possible in any medium. In air, solutions to the wave equation describe the propagation of sound.

There is another effect of sound transmission that has relevance to hearing, the *Doppler shift*. If you listen to the siren of an ambulance moving toward and then away from you, you will usually perceive that the pitch of the siren increases as the ambulance approaches and then decreases as the ambulance moves away. The sound of the siren itself is not changing, but the interaction of the wave motion of sound and the motion of the ambulance produces a change in the sound's wavelength at the listener's ears that is due to the Doppler shift. As a sound source (ambulance) moves toward a receiver and is producing a constant wave motion, the wavelength of the sound at the receiver decreases as the source gets closer, and, hence, the frequency (pitch) increases. The wavelength increases because at one moment in time the wave motion produces rarefaction and condensation waves that radiate out from the source at the speed of sound. But, as the source moves, the rarefaction and condensation waves will move closer together during the time of the source's motion, decreasing their wavelength (which is what happens when the frequency of

sound increases). The opposite occurs as the sound source moves away from the receiver, leading to a lengthening of the wavelength and a drop in pitch. The frequency of the perceived sound (F_{obs}) due to the Doppler shift is

$$F_{obs} = F_{source} [V_{sound}/(V_{sound} + V_{source})]$$

for approaching sources

and

$$F_{obs} = F_{source} [V_{sound}/(V_{sound} - V_{source})]$$

for retreating sources,

where F_{source} is the frequency of the sound at the source, V_{source} is the velocity (speed) of sound, and V_{source} is the velocity (speed) of the moving source.

The section "Terms, Measurements, Equations, and Conversions" following Appendix F describes the units of measurement for most of the terms defined in this chapter. In electricity, impedance, resistance, and reactance are usually measured in ohms, although from equation (3.13) acoustic impedance is defined with the following units: $(g/cm^3)(cm/sec)$. For definitions of power, energy, impedance, resistance, and reactance, there is a strong parallel between acoustic conditions and electrical conditions. In general, the definitions from one condition can be used to interpret the terms in the other condition. This must be done with some caution, however, and a careful study of physics is required to make exact comparisons. The term *voltage*, used in electrical circuits, is a pressure-like term.

As stated in Chapter 2 and in this chapter, the term *intensity* will be used for measures of sound intensity (power or energy), *amplitude* for pressure or displacement, and *level* when intensity or amplitude has been converted to decibels. However, it is common practice in the hearing sciences to use the terms *intensity* and *level* more loosely and often interchangeably.

When reinforcement and cancellation were discussed, these actions were described as addition and subtraction. Adding and subtracting sound waveforms is treated as vector addition (see Appendix A), with the amplitude of the sound wave being the vector's magnitude and the wave's starting phase representing the vector phase. It should also be emphasized that when addition and subtraction are used to determine the amount of reinforcement or cancellation, the calculation is done in units of intensity or amplitude and not in decibels (adding decibels is multiplication of intensity, and subtracting decibels is division, as explained in Appendix B).

4

Complex Sounds

COMPLEX STIMULI

Recall from Chapter 2 that Fourier's theorem states that sinusoids are the basic vibrations of sound, in that any sound is the sum of sinusoidal components. Most sounds in our everyday lives are not simple sinusoidal sounds, but are complex sounds, consisting of the sum of many sinusoids. There are various ways to describe a complex waveform. The waveforms drawn and described in Chapter 2 are defined in the *time domain*. The time-domain description relates the instantaneous amplitude or pressure of a waveform to time. When a complex waveform is described in terms of the individual sinusoids that are added to produce a sound, the waveform is being described in the *frequency domain*. In the frequency domain, the amplitude, frequency, and starting phase of each sinusoidal component in the complex waveform must be described.

Each sinusoidal component that constitutes a complex waveform is characterized by its amplitude, frequency, and starting phase. Thus, if we say that a complex sound consists of four sinusoids, we mean that four sinusoidal components with four different frequencies exist. The plot of the amplitude of each sinusoidal component as a function of its frequency is called the *amplitude spectrum* (or *power spectrum*,

depending on the measure of sound magnitude used), whereas the plot of the starting phase of each sinusoidal component is called the *phase spectrum*. When the phase and amplitude spectra of a complex waveform are completely described, the waveform has been completely defined.

Figure 4.1 demonstrates how a complex wave is portrayed in both the time and frequency domains. Figure 4.1a is a time-domain plot of a complex wave showing amplitude as a function of time. This complex wave consists of the sum of three sinusoidal components with frequencies 100 Hz, 200 Hz, and 300 Hz and all having the same amplitude and starting phase. Figures 4.1b and 4.1c show the amplitude and phase spectra of the complex sound. Figure 4.2 demonstrates how sinusoids are added to produce a complex sound. In Figure 4.2 the three sinusoids (with frequencies of 100, 200, and 300 Hz) that are summed to produce the complex wave are shown. The instantaneous amplitudes of the three sinusoids are added at each successive point in time (e.g., at points a, b, and c) to produce the complex time-domain waveform. The summed waveform at the bottom of Figure 4.2 is a perfect match to that in Figure 4.1a. Thus, this graphical application of Fourier's theorem demonstrates that the complex time-domain waveform can be created by

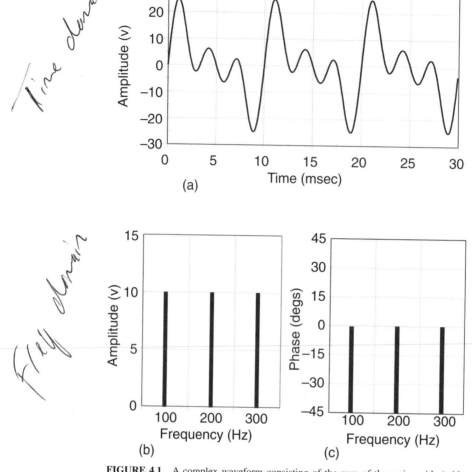

Time domain

Freq domain

FIGURE 4.1 A complex waveform consisting of the sum of three sinusoids (with frequencies of 100, 200, and 300 Hz) in (a) the time domain and the frequency domain (b: amplitude spectrum; c: phase spectrum).

adding the instantaneous amplitudes of all of the sinusoids present in the spectrum of the complex sound.

Thus, when the amplitude variation of a complex wave is displayed over time, the waveform is described in the time domain. If the frequency content of the complex wave is important, the amplitude and phase spectra are described in the frequency domain. As shown in Figures 4.1 and 4.2, it is not difficult to reconstruct the time-domain description of a wave

from the amplitude and phase spectra (i.e., by adding the instantaneous amplitudes), but deriving the frequency-domain spectra from the time-domain waveform requires the use of Fourier analysis. Although the technique of Fourier analysis is beyond the scope of this book, it is briefly described in Appendix C (see also Chapter 5).

A *line spectrum* describes a complex sound consisting of a discrete number of sinusoidal components,

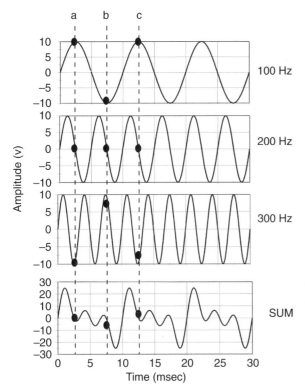

FIGURE 4.2 The time-domain representations of each sinusoid described in Figure 4.1a and 4.1b are shown at the top. The sum was constructed by adding together at each successive point in time (e.g., a, b, c) the amplitudes of the three sinusoids. The result (sum) is exactly the same as that in Figure 4.1a.

whereas a *continuous spectrum* describes a sound in which all frequencies (a continuum) between certain limits are present. For many line spectra, only integer multiples (2 times, 3 times, 4 times, etc.) of the lowest frequency exist. For instance, in Figure 4.1 the lowest frequency was 100 Hz, and its higher integer multiples existed at 200 Hz and 300 Hz. In this situation the lowest frequency (100 Hz in Figure 4.1) is called the *fundamental frequency*, and each higher integer multiple of the fundamental frequency is called a *harmonic* (200 Hz is the second harmonic and 300 Hz the third harmonic in Figure 4.1). Many complex sounds consist of a fundamental frequency and higher harmonics.

Figure 4.3 demonstrates an interesting ramification of Fourier analysis. A sinusoid turned on and off is not a simple stimulus but a complex sound consisting of the sum of many (an infinite number) sinusoidal components (it has a continuous spectrum). The shorter the sinusoid is in duration, the more noticeable these other sinusoid components in the spectrum become. Perhaps you have heard the *click* that sometimes occurs when a sound is abruptly turned on and off. The perception of a click represents the ear's sensitivity to frequencies other than that of the sound that is switched on and off. A sinusoid is perceived more like a tone and less like a click the longer it remains on. This is because the longer a sinusoid remains on, the smaller the amplitudes of the other frequency components become relative to the amplitude of the frequency component of the sinusoid. Thus, we hear only the pure tone pitch corresponding to the frequency of the sine wave and not the clicking sound from the presence of other frequencies when the duration of the pulsed sinusoid is long.

TRANSIENTS

In studying hearing, it is often useful to present a very brief acoustic signal, such as the stimulus shown in Figure 4.4a. This brief pulse is referred to as a *click* or a *transient*. The stimulus comes on at a peak value and goes off after a brief duration, D. The spectra of a click are also shown in Figure 4.4, with Figure 4.4b showing the amplitude spectrum and Figure 4.4c the phase spectrum. Notice that the amplitude spectrum is a continuous spectrum, and the amplitude goes to zero at frequencies equal to $1/D$ when D is expressed in seconds. In Figure 4.5 D is 1 msec, so the spectral amplitude goes to zero at 1000 Hz ($1/D = 1/0.001$ sec $= 1000$ Hz). Thus, if D is short, the spectrum is broad. For instance, if D is 0.0001 seconds (0.1 msec), then the spectrum has frequencies with nonzero amplitudes up to 10,000 Hz (10,000 Hz $= 1/0.0001$ sec, or 1000/0.1 msec), where the amplitude of the component at 10,000 Hz is zero. The phase spectrum is constant at 90°.

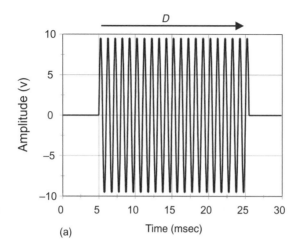

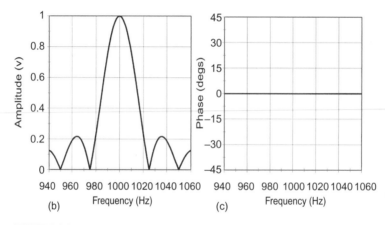

FIGURE 4.3 The amplitude spectrum, (b) and phase spectrum (c) of a sinusoid that is turned on and off with duration D (a). Note, this pulsed sinusoid is a complex sound with a continuous amplitude spectrum with zero amplitude at frequencies equal to integer multiplies of $1/2D$.

The transient may be repeated at a periodic rate (Pr = period), as shown in Figure 4.5. The spectra of this waveform are also shown in Figure 4.5. For the repeated transient the spectra are line spectra, with the lowest frequency equal to the frequency (1/Pr, Pr in sec) at which the click is repeated, with each successive harmonic present in the spectrum. The amplitudes of the harmonics change with the same function, as shown in Figure 4.4b. That is, the amplitude spectrum has a general shape (sometimes called the *spectral envelope*) determined by the duration, D, of the individual click. If the spectra in Figure 4.5 were based on a 1-msec-duration click ($D = 0.001$ sec) repeated at a 200-Hz rate (Pr = 1000/200 Hz = 5 msec), then harmonic of 200 Hz (e.g., 200 Hz, 400 Hz, 600 Hz) would be present in the spectra and the amplitudes would decrease to zero at 1000 Hz (i.e., 1000 Hz = 1/0.001 sec). Again, the phase spectrum would be flat at 90°.

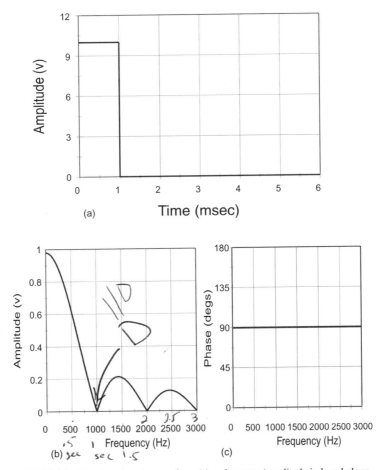

FIGURE 4.4 The time-domain waveform (a) and spectra (amplitude in b and phase in c) are shown for a single transient of duration *D*.

In Figures 4.4 and 4.5, the transients have been displayed as positive-going changes in amplitude. It is assumed that such a stimulus would produce a condensation pattern of activity in the air (see Chapter 3). Thus, this type of click is sometimes referred to as a *condensation click*. If the click were negative-going, then it could be called a *rarefaction click* (again, see Chapter 3). A rarefaction click has the same amplitude spectrum as a condensation click, but its phase spectrum contains frequency components all with 270° starting phases (an 180° phase shift relative to a condensation click).

BEATS AND AMPLITUDE MODULATION

Perhaps the most obvious way to change a simple stimulus into a complex one is to add two sinusoids of different frequencies (f_1 and f_2). Figure 4.6 shows two examples of such an addition. In the top part of the figure, the two tones are of very different frequencies (the frequencies can be seen as the time separations $1/f_1$ and $1/f_2$, shown in Figure 4.6a), whereas in the bottom of the figure the tones are very close together in frequency. In the bottom portion of Figure 4.6 the time-domain waveform appears as a single

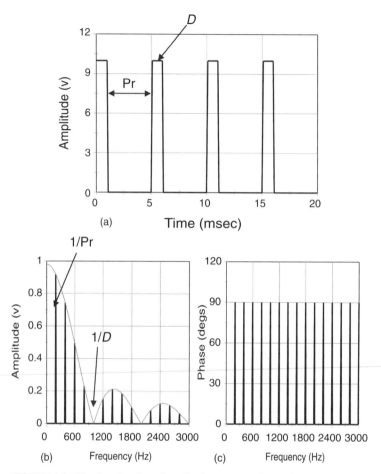

FIGURE 4.5   The time domain and amplitude spectrum of a transient with duration
D, repeated periodically with a period of Pr. (a) The time-domain plot, (b) the
amplitude-spectrum plot, and (c) the phase spectrum. The lines in the spectrum are
at the harmonics of the fundamental frequency of the repetition (1/Pr), and the
amplitudes are determined by the shape of the spectrum of a single transient of duration (see Figure 4.4b).

tone with overall amplitude that changes in a sinusoidal manner. Such a stimulus is called a *beating*
stimulus because it is perceived as a tone with a loudness that beats, or waxes and wanes (see Chapters 11
and 13). If the frequencies of the two tones that are
added are f_1 and f_2, then the frequency of the sinusoid
that appears to beat is equal to $(f_1 + f_2)/2$ and the loudness changes, or beats, appear at a rate of $f_2 - f_1$. If,

for instance, a waveform consists of 475-Hz (f_1) and
525-Hz (f_2) sinusoids of equal amplitudes and starting phases, then the sinusoid that is beating has a frequency of 500 Hz [(475 + 525)/2], and the loudness
changes would occur at the rate of 50 times per second
(525 − 475 = 50 Hz). The spectra (see Figure 4.6)
consist of two tones with equal amplitudes and starting phases.

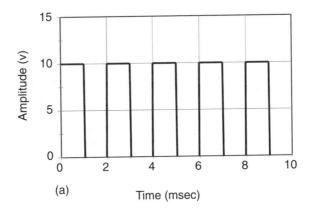

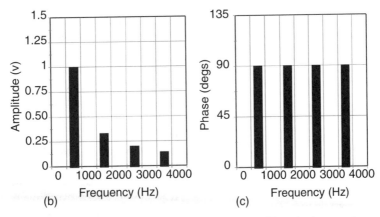

FIGURE 4.8 Time-domain (a), amplitude-spectrum, (b) and phase-spectrum (c) descriptions of a 2-msec square wave. The square wave has a spectrum with the greatest level at 500 Hz, as well as a 2-msec period.

Figure 4.5. Varying the ratio of the on to the off times changes the *duty cycle* of the square wave.

FREQUENCY MODULATION

Rather than varying the amplitude of a signal, one might wish to vary its frequency. Figure 4.9 shows two time-domain waveforms in which the frequency of the signal is changing over time. In Figure 4.9a, the frequency of the waveform decreases from high frequency (about 1000 Hz) to low frequency (about 100 Hz)

over the duration of the stimulus. In Figure 4.9b, the change in frequency over time is sinusoidal: The frequency starts high (about 525 Hz), then goes low (to about 150 Hz), then goes back to a high frequency, and so on. For sinusoidal frequency modulation, the time-domain waveform can be written as

$$A = D(t) = A\sin(2\pi F_c t).$$

Because F_c varies as a sinusoidal function of time, we write the frequency term as

$$F_c + m\sin(2\pi F_m t),$$

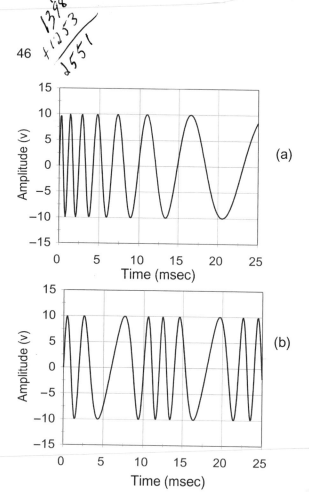

FIGURE 4.9 Two examples of frequency modulation (FM). (a) The frequency of the waveform decreases from high to low frequency from the beginning to the end. (b) The frequency of the waveform varies through two cycles of a sinusoid, starting with a high frequency and then going to lower frequencies and back to the high frequency.

where F_c is the base, or carrier, frequency described earlier and m is the magnitude of the sinusoidal change in frequency (that is, m describes the range of frequency modulation). The sinusoidal-frequency-modulated equation can then be rewritten as

$$D(t) = A\sin[(2\pi F_c t) + (m/F_m)\sin(2\pi F_m t)]. \quad (4.4)$$

In considering the spectra of such stimuli we must realize that their frequency content is changing over time. In these cases, two types of spectra can be considered: (1) the *long-term spectrum*, which is to the spec-trum of the entire waveform over its complete duration, and (2) the *short-term spectrum*, which considers the spectrum at any moment in time during the stimulus' duration. The rules for determining the long-term spectra of frequency-modulated (FM) stimuli are too complex for discussion in this text. But like amplitude modulation, frequency modulation produces sideband components spaced at the combinations of $F_c \pm nF_m$ (where $n = 1, 2, \ldots, \infty$), along with a spectral component at the carrier frequency, F_c. Such spectral considerations are crucial for understanding the sensitivity of the auditory system to frequency-modulated signals.

The changes in frequency-that occur over time for the waveforms shown in Figure 4.9 can be graphed, as shown in Figure 4.10. These are the simple descriptions of changes in frequency for these frequency-modulated signals. They display part of the information required for a short-term amplitude spectrum. Such displays do not contain any information about the amplitude of the various frequency components. For the cases shown in Figure 4.9 the amplitudes of all the frequencies components were the same, so the amplitude information may not be needed.

Suppose that the waveform shown in Figure 4.11a was displayed in some sort of short-term spectral graph. This time-domain waveform is a signal whose frequency increases over time, and the amplitude of each frequency also increases over time. Figures 4.11b and 4.11c show the changes in frequency and amplitude over time. This information can be combined into one figure, called a *spectrogram* or *spectrograph*, as shown in Figure 4.12. In Figure 4.12 time is shown on the horizontal axis, frequency on the vertical axis, and amplitude as the darkness of the plotted area. This is a type of short-term spectral display.

Many common stimuli change both in frequency and amplitude over time: They are amplitude modulated and frequency modulated. Music and speech are two such stimuli. Time-domain representations, such as those shown in Figures 4.10, 4.11a, and 4.11b, are useful means for describing these stimuli, but in many cases a spectrograph, such as that shown in Figure 4.12, provides additional information valuable in understanding auditory processing.

Music and speech are two examples of stimuli that change are am modulated and Freq modulated.

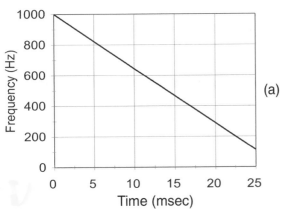

(a)

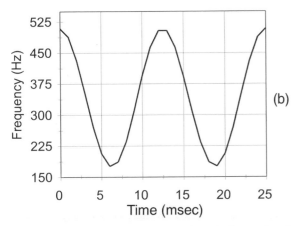

(b)

FIGURE 4.10 Two diagrams decribing how the frequencies of the waveforms shown in Figure 4.9 change over time. (a) The linear decrease in frequency displayed in Figure 4.9a. (b) The sinusoidal frequency change displayed in Figure 4.9b.

NOISE

Noise as used here means a sound with an instantaneous amplitude that varies over time in a random manner. When a noise is "Gaussian," the instantaneous amplitude varies in its probability of occurrence according to the "normal," or Gaussian, distribution. A normal distribution of amplitude fluctuations is shown in Figure 4.13. The distribution shows that the mean amplitude of Gaussian noise is zero (on the average, the instantaneous amplitude of the noise at any moment in time is zero) and that the higher or lower the amplitude, the less probable it is to occur at any moment in time.

"*White*" noise indicates that all frequencies between some limits (these frequency limits define the *bandwidth* of the noise) are present at the same average intensity or pressure; that is, white noise has a continuous and flat average power spectrum over its bandwidth. This spectrum is shown in Figure 4.14 (page 50), with *average power* for each sinusoidal component in the spectrum shown as a function of frequency for the white Gaussian noise. If this is Gaussian noise, then it has a random distribution of starting phases as a function of frequency.

There are two measures of intensity for a white noise: (1) *total power* and (2) *noise power per unit bandwidth*, often called *spectrum level*, abbreviated N_o. Most measuring instruments calculate total power. Total noise power (TP) can be viewed as the sum of the amplitudes of all the sinusoids in the spectrum of the noise (as explained in Figure 4.14; also recall that adding amplitudes is a vector addition, as explained in Appendix A). This is approximately equal to the area (height × width or equivalently bandwidth [BW] × intensity, N_o, not in dB, BW × N_o) of the spectrum shown in Figure 4.14. The energy at frequencies far away from the frequency region of interest will often have no bearing on auditory perception. In this case, the spectrum level of the noise is used. The spectrum level is the average intensity measured in a band of noise 1-Hz wide. Because the instantaneous noise intensity varies, the spectrum level is the *average* noise power in a band of noise 1-Hz wide. This can be represented by the height of the spectrum in Figure 4.14. The procedure is analogous to finding the height of a rectangle (N_o) when the area (TP) and width (BW) are known (height = area/width): N_o = TP/BW or, in decibels, N_o in dB = TP in dB minus 10log BW. (See Figure 4.13 for a description of the use of TP and N_o). For example, in Figure 4.14 the white noise has a total power of 80dB SPL and a bandwidth of 1000Hz (i.e., noise has energy in its spectrum from 500 to 1500Hz), and so N_o is 50dB SPL:

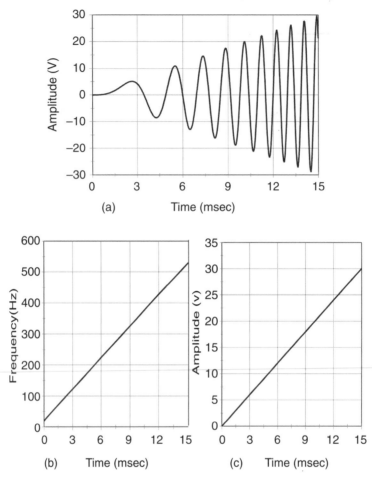

FIGURE 4.11   (a) A time-domain waveform in which both the amplitude and frequency increase over time. (b) The change in frequency as a function of time for the time-domain waveform shown in Figure 4.11a. (c) The change in amplitude for the waveform in Figure 4.11a.

$$N_o \text{ in dB} = TP \text{ in dB} - 10\log(1000).$$

So

$$N_o \text{ in dB} = 80 \text{ dB} - 30 \text{ dB} = 50 \text{ dB},$$

because $10\log(1000) = 30\,\text{dB}$ (recall that dB is simply 10 times the log of the ratio of two quantities; in this case, the quantities are frequencies).

Another type of noise, *pink noise*, with the spectrum shown in Figure 4.15 (page 50), is often used in audition. Note that the x-axis of Figure 4.15 is plotted with frequency on a logarithmic (log) scale; i.e., each equal distance long the axis is a doubling of frequency. Such log plots are used in later chapters.

For pink noise, spectrum level (N_o) decreases with increasing frequency, such that with each doubling of

Many signals can be characterized by an envelope and the *fine-structure* waveform that falls under the envelope. The SAM signal mentioned earlier in this chapter has an envelope defined by the modulator frequency and a fine structure defined by the carrier frequency. In fact most complex waveforms can be described with the following formula:

$$x(t) = e(t)f(t), \qquad (4.5)$$

where $e(t)$ is the envelope function, $f(t)$ is the fine-structure waveform, and $x(t)$ is the complex waveform. For the hearing sciences, $e(t)$ changes much more slowly than $f(t)$. Note that equation (4.3) for a SAM tone is in the same form as equation (4.5). For a SAM tone,

$$e(t) = [1 + m\sin(2\pi F_m t)] \quad \text{and} \quad f(t) = \sin(2\pi F_c t)$$

(see equation 4.3). The amplitude of other carrier stimuli, such as white noise, can also be amplitude modulated, as shown in Figure 4.17. In this case the modulator was a sinusoid, generating SAM noise, and

$$x(t) = [1 + m\sin(2\pi F_m t)]n(t), \qquad (4.6)$$

where $n(t)$ is the noise waveform [or carrier, $f(t) = n(t)$, in equation 4.5]. Thus, $[1 + m\sin(2\pi F_m t)]$, the

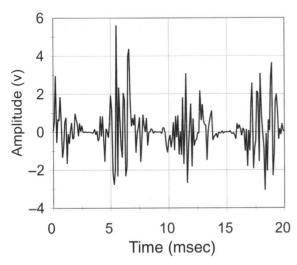

FIGURE 4.17 Sinusoidal amplitude-modulated (SAM) white Gaussian noise (rate of modulation is 200 Hz, modulation period is 5 msec).

envelope $[e(t)]$, changes more slowly than $n(t)$, the fine structure $[n(t)]$.

SUMMARY

Complex stimuli are represented in the frequency domain by their amplitude and phase spectra. These spectra can be either line or continuous spectra. White Gaussian noise, narrowband noise (with a characteristic envelope), pink noise, rarefaction and condensation clicks (transients), beating tones, amplitude-modulated signals, square waves, and frequency-modulated signals are a few of the complex stimuli used to study the auditory system. Sound spectrographs are used to display the short-term spectral information of signals with frequencies and amplitudes that change over time.

SUPPLEMENT

The ability to define any complex stimulus depends on an understanding of Fourier analysis. Appendix C introduces the student to Fourier analysis. Chapter 2 in the book by Rosen and Howell (1991) explains many of these concepts and their applications. Any serious student of hearing with a background in math, physics, or engineering should read *Signals, Sounds, and Sensation* by Hartmann (1998).

A sinusoid turned on and off does not have a single-line spectrum but rather a continuous spectrum, with the spectral shape (spectral envelope) described by the function $|(\sin x)/x|$. This is the function shown as the spectral envelope in Figure 4.3. As the duration of the pulsed sound decreases there is a greater *spread of energy* to other frequency regions, which is often audible. In many acoustic experiments a sound is turned on and off with a slowly rising and decaying amplitude, rather than abruptly, by applying a *rise-and-decay time* to the onset (rise) and offset (decay) of the sound. The spectral consequence of applying a rise–decay time is to filter the signal that is being turned on and off (see Chapter 5 for a discussion of filters), thus limiting the spread of energy (thus, a filter can also be applied to a pulsed sound to provide a rise–decay time structure).

The operations of AM and FM are well known calculations because of their use in radio and other communications broadcasting. β is sometimes used to denote the depth of frequency modulation with the ratio of m/F_m in equation (4.4) for sinusoidal-frequency-modulated tones.

The spectrum level (N_o) of noise has units of energy because it is noise power divided by frequency. Because frequency is the reciprocal of time, N_o is the same as power divided by 1 over time and will have units of energy.

The *normal equation* describes the probability of an instantaneous amplitude of a Gaussian noise: $P(a_i) = [1/\sqrt{(2\pi\sigma)}]\exp(-a_i/2\sigma^2)$, where a_i is instantaneous amplitude, $P(a_i)$ is the probability of an instantaneous amplitude, and σ^2 is the variance of the distributions of instantaneous amplitudes, such that σ^2 is proportional to the average total (rms) power of the noise. That is, the average rms power of a Gaussian noise is equal to the variance of the normal distribution of instantaneous amplitudes.

Gaussian noise may be generated by adding sinusoids with frequencies spanning the bandwidth of the noise to be generated. To obtain true Gaussian noise, the amplitudes of the sinusoids should be sampled from a *Rayleigh distribution* of amplitudes, and the starting phases for each sinusoid should be randomly sampled from a rectangular distribution of starting phases. However, if more than 20 sinusoids are being added, then a close approximation to a Gaussian noise can be obtained by adding sinusoids with amplitudes all equal to N_o and starting phases randomly sampled from a rectangular distribution of phases ($-180°$ to $180°$). The article by Hartmann (1987) describes these calculations.

In explaining the derivation of spectrum level (see Figure 4.14), a rectangle was used to approximate the shape of the noise power spectrum. However, in most situations the power spectrum of the noise does not cut off abruptly at the noise bandwidth, but, rather, noise power decreases more gradually as frequency increases above and below the spectral edges (cutoff frequencies) of the bandwidth. In these cases, the *equivalent rectangular bandwidth* (ERB) is sometimes used to define noise bandwidth. The ERB computation assumes that the noise does have a rectangular power spectrum as shown in Figure 4.14. The total power of the noise (which is easily measured) is divided by a direct estimate of spectrum level, with the resulting ERB being the bandwidth of a rectangle that would have the total power and spectrum level of the noise.

In Chapter 2, the term *rms* was defined. Its definition depends on determining the period of the sound (*PR* in equation 2.4). Some sounds, such as noise, are not periodic, and it would be difficult for a measuring instrument to determine the period of a sound before calculating its rms amplitude. Thus, rms measuring instruments usually compute the rms over a long period of time, such as 1 second. While 1 second may not be near the period of a sound, most sounds have periods that are much shorter than 1 second, so the error in calculating rms is extremely small.

Often a complex waveform can be constructed from that of two or more other complex waveforms. For instance, the complex waveform of a periodically repeating transient, such as that shown in Figure 4.5, is the combination of a transient and a harmonic series. In such cases, the amplitude spectrum of the total complex waveform is the product of the two or more complex waveforms that constitute the total waveform. So the amplitude spectrum of a periodically repeating transient is the product of the spectrum of the transient and that of a harmonic series.

The derivation of the envelope and fine structure and other aspects of narrowband stimuli are found in the book by Hartmann (1998).

5

Sound Analysis

RESONATORS

Once a sound's pressure wave has traveled from its vibrating source, it will eventually encounter the outer ear of a person or animal and the process of hearing begins. The structures of the auditory system that this sound pressure wave encounters will help in the analysis of the sound wave. Thus, we have the properties of the sound's pressure wave, along with those of the structures that will analyze the sound, to consider if we want to appreciate how the auditory system processes sound in order for hearing to occur. We have already considered many of the properties of the sound wave in Chapters 2–4; Chapter 5 deals with the analysis of sound.

In Chapter 2, *free vibration* was described as a damped sinusoidal vibration that occurred once an object was set into motion. In Chapter 3, in discussing standing waves, a continuous driving force was necessary to establish standing wave motion. The vibratory system in this second case is called *forced vibration* because the vibrating system is being forced to vibrate by some external object (for example, a hand vibrating a string). Two vibratory properties are involved: the vibration of the driving object and that of the object being vibrated. Most real-world acoustic

situations are accurately described in terms of forced vibrations.

In the simplest case, the object being vibrated has its own natural vibratory frequency, as described by its free-vibration properties. The closer the frequency of the driving force is to the natural frequency of the receiving object, the easier it is for the driving force to vibrate the receiving object. The natural vibratory frequency of the receiving object is called its *resonant frequency*. Consider a drum or a cymbal being struck by a drumstick. When the driving force provided by the drumstick forces the head of the drum or the cymbal to vibrate, the drum or cymbal vibrates (i.e., resonates) with its own pattern of vibration (at its resonant frequency). This pattern of vibration provides the distinctive sound quality of the drum or cymbal. The two have a different pattern of vibration and resulting sound quality because they are structurally different.

Chapter 3 stated that if two objects differed in their characteristic impedance, total transfer of vibratory intensity between the two objects would not occur. However, the transfer of vibration from one object to another object is as large as it can be when the driving force has a frequency at or near the resonant frequency of the receiving object. A maximal amount of amplitude transfer will occur when the frequency of the

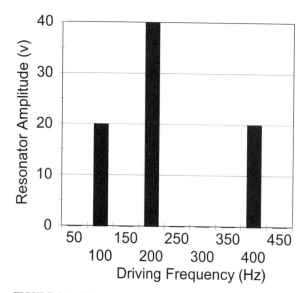

FIGURE 5.1 Relative amplitudes of a resonator driven by vibrators with different driving frequencies. The 200-Hz driving frequency provides the greatest amplitude of the resonator, most likely indicating that the resonance frequency is 200 Hz.

driving object is equal to the resonant frequency of the receiving object. If the driving frequency is less than or greater than the resonant frequency of the receiving object, the receiving, or resonating, object (called a *resonator*) will vibrate less than its maximum possible amplitude. In Figure 5.1, a resonator with a 200-Hz resonant frequency is driven by a driving object at three different driving frequencies. Notice that the maximal response occurs for the resonating object when the driving frequency is at 200 Hz (equal to the resonant frequency of the resonator). If the driving force is a complex vibration, it will consist of the sum of many sinusoidal components (see Chapter 4). As long as the spectrum of the vibrating source contains a sinusoidal component of sufficient amplitude that is at the resonant frequency of the resonator (e.g., there is a 200-Hz component for our example), the resonator is likely to vibrate (resonate) at is natural frequency. The resonator will vibrate most at its resonant frequency, not at the frequency or frequencies of the driving force.

The reactance components (both mass and spring reactance) of the characteristic impedance of simple objects determine their resonant frequencies. In general,

$$f_r = \sqrt{(s/m)}/(2\pi), \qquad (5.1)$$

where f_r is the resonant frequency, s is a measure of stiffness, and m is a measure of mass.

The resistance component of impedance also reduces the motion. The amount of resistance determines the sharpness of the peak in the resonant function (see Figure 5.1). That is, with little resistance the peak is very sharp, and thus it is difficult for driving frequencies not close to the resonant frequency to drive the resonator. The greater the resistance, the broader the resonant peak and the easier it is for drivers with different frequencies to cause significant vibrations of the resonator.

Most objects have a complex resonance pattern when they resonate (e.g., the drum or cymbal). This is because most objects can be thought of as consisting of several resonators, due to the complex structure of most real objects. Each of these *modes* of resonance has its own resonant frequencies leading to a complex resonate vibratory pattern. A tuning fork is an example of a "resonator" that has only one major resonance mode, so when a tuning fork is struck it tends to vibrate with a sinusoidal-like motion, such as the simple resonator discussed at the beginning of this chapter. The frequency at which the tuning fork resonates is largely determined by its size. Small tuning forks resonate at a high frequency (producing a high perceived pitch), while large tuning forks resonate at lower frequencies (producing lower pitches).

If a driving force creates standing waves within a closed tube (see Chapter 3), the standing wave will oscillate at the tube's resonant frequency. That is, the standing wave is a form of resonance, and the frequency of the standing wave is the tube's resonant frequency. It is possible to drive a tube with a vibration of small amplitude and produce within the tube a vibration with larger amplitude at the tube's resonant frequency. This point will become significant when we consider sound waves entering the ear canal. Does the ear canal resonate and increase the incoming sound amplitude? If so, what are the resonance frequencies of the ear canal and other parts of the auditory system?

FILTERS

Resonators may be especially designed to determine or to modify the amplitudes of the frequency components of vibrating objects; such resonators are called *filters*. We refer to those frequencies components to which the filter vibrates as the ones the filter will *pass*. If a filter passes sinusoid components with frequencies between 200 and 400 Hz and if the filter is driven with these sinusoids, the amplitudes of these sinusoids at the output of the filter will be relatively unaffected by the filter. The amplitudes of sinusoids of other frequencies will be *attenuated* (reduced) as a result of the filter. Thus, if the filter passes sinusoids with frequencies between 200 and 400 Hz with little or no attenuation, and if the driving force has a frequency of 200 to 400 Hz, these sinusoids will have amplitudes at the output of the filter that equal their driving-force amplitudes. If an object with a driving frequency of 100 Hz and a level of 80 dB SPL drives a 200- to 400-Hz filter, then at the output of the filter the 100-Hz sinusoid might have its level reduced to 20 dB SPL. Thus, a filter produces sinusoids with no reduction in amplitude or with attenuated amplitudes.

Filters need not be objects such as resonators; they can be electrical circuits or computer algorithms. That is, a sound may be "fed" to an electronic filter circuit as an electrical input, the circuit modifies the electrical signal as a filter would, and the circuit turns the electrical signal back into an output sound waveform. The result of this electrical filtering action is that the amplitudes (and starting phases) of the spectral components of the input are modified depending on the type of filtering action caused by the circuit.

There are four types of filters: *low pass*, *high pass*, *bandpass*, and *band reject*. A low-pass filter will pass all sinusoidal components with frequencies below a particular value; sinusoidal components with frequencies above that value will have their amplitudes attenuated. A high-pass filter passes sinusoidal components with frequencies above a particular value. A bandpass filter passes all sinusoidal components with frequencies between two particular values (the frequency region that a bandpass filter passes sinusoidal components unattenuated is called the *pass band* of the filter). The frequency values above, below, or between which the filter passes the sinusoidal components without reducing their amplitudes are called the *cutoff frequencies* of the filter. A band-reject filter attenuates the amplitudes of all sinusoidal components with frequencies between its cutoff frequencies (i.e., a band-reject filter is the opposite of a bandpass filter). The frequency region over which a band-reject filter provides attenuation is called the *reject band* of the filter. Thus, a low-pass filter with a cutoff of 2000 Hz will pass all sinusoidal components with frequencies below 2000 Hz and will attenuate the amplitudes of all sinusoidal components with frequencies above 2000 Hz. A 2000-Hz cutoff, high-pass filter will do just the opposite, attenuating the amplitudes of all components with frequencies below 2000 Hz. A bandpass filter with cutoffs at 1000 Hz and 4000 Hz (a 3000-Hz pass band) will pass only sinusoids with frequencies between 1000 and 4000 Hz, while a band-reject filter with these same cutoff frequencies (a 3000-Hz reject band) does the opposite; i.e., it will attenuate the amplitudes of all sinusoidal components with frequencies between 1000 and 4000 Hz and will pass all components with frequencies less than 1000 Hz and greater than 4000 Hz. Figure 5.2 shows the four types of filters (for the bandpass filter, notice the similarity to the resonance curve shown in Figure 5.1).

The amount of attenuation beyond the cutoff frequency is expressed in decibels of attenuation per *octave* of frequency. An octave indicates a doubling of frequency. The octave is expressed relative to the cutoff frequency of the filter. The first octave of 200 Hz is 400 Hz; the second octave is another doubling, or 800 Hz; the third octave is 1600 Hz, and so on. Table 5.1 shows the harmonics and octaves of a 1000-Hz sinusoid. Octaves should not be confused with harmonics; octaves express a ratio scale, with the ratio being 2 to 1, and harmonics represent integer

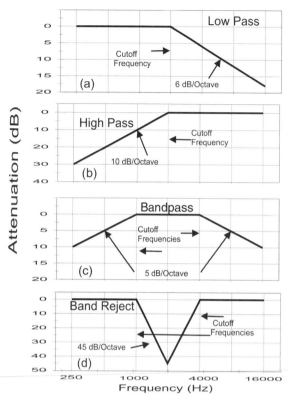

TABLE 5.1   Harmonic and Octave Relations of a 1000-Hz Fundamental Frequency Tone

Tone	Harmonics	Octaves
Fundamental frequency	1000 Hz	1000 Hz
2nd harmonic and 1st octave	2000 Hz	2000 Hz
3rd harmonic	3000 Hz	
4th harmonic and 2nd octave	4000 Hz	4000 Hz
5th harmonic	5000 Hz	
6th harmonic	6000 Hz	
7th harmonic	7000 Hz	
8th harmonic and 3rd octave	8000 Hz	8000 Hz

FIGURE 5.2   Four filters. (a) Low-pass filter with 2000-Hz cutoff and 6 dB/octave roll-off; (b) high-pass filter with 2000-Hz cutoff and 10 dB/octave roll-off; (c) bandpass filter with 1000-Hz and 4000-Hz cutoffs and 5 dB/octave roll-off; (d) band-reject filter with 1000-Hz and 4000-Hz cutoffs and 45 dB/octave roll-off. The amount the filter attenuates the sound is shown as a function of frequency, which is plotted on a log axis. The frequency axis is a log axis.

multiples. If a low-pass filter has a 2000-Hz cutoff and an attenuation rate of 6 dB per octave, then the filter passes all sinusoids with frequencies below 2000 Hz, and the amplitudes of sinusoids with frequencies above 2000 Hz are attenuated at the rate of 6 dB for each doubling of the cutoff frequency, 2000 Hz. Thus, the amplitude of a 4000-Hz sinusoid would be attenuated 6 dB below its amplitude at the input, an 8000-Hz sinusoid is attenuated 12 dB, a 16,000-Hz sinusoid is attenuated 18 dB, and so forth. In Figure

5.2a the *roll-off*, or rate of attenuation, for the various filters is 6 dB per octave; in Figure 5.2b it is 10 dB per octave; in Figure 5.2c it is 5 dB per octave; and in Figure 5.2d it is 45 dB per octave.

Filters may be used to determine the frequency spectra of unknown signals. That is, filters can be used to perform a type of spectral analysis of a complex waveform. Chapter 4 described how to compute the time-domain waveform from the amplitude and phase spectra, but not how to determine the spectra from the time-domain waveform. To estimate the amplitudes of the spectral components of a waveform, a series (a *filter bank*) of bandpass filters can be established. A bank of four bandpass filters might have the following cutoff frequencies (see Figure 5.3): 95–105 Hz, 195–205 Hz, 295–305 Hz, and 395–405 Hz. If we found, after analyzing an input waveform with these filters, that the total power of the waveform at the output of the first filter (95–105 Hz) and third filter (295–305 Hz) was greater than that for the other two filters, then the input waveform must have a greater power in the 100-Hz and 300-Hz regions of the spectrum than in the 200-Hz and 400-Hz regions (100, 200, 300, and 400 Hz are the centers of the pass bands for each of the four filters). The actual power at the output of each filter can be used to estimate a power spectrum for the unknown input waveform. In this case, we plot the power at the output of each filter as a function of the center frequency of each bandpass filter, and this plot forms an estimate of the waveform's power spectrum. The accuracy with which such

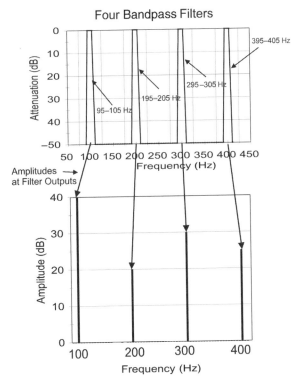

FIGURE 5.3   A stimulus with an unknown amplitude spectrum is analyzed by four bandpass filters: 95–105 Hz, 195–205 Hz, 295–305 Hz, and 395–405 Hz. The amplitudes of the outputs of these filters can be used to form an estimate of the sound's power spectrum.

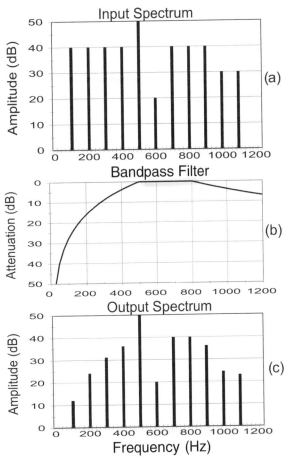

FIGURE 5.4   An input stimulus with the amplitude spectrum shown in (a) is passed through the filter described in (b); the output stimulus has the amplitude spectrum shown in (c). The output spectrum is obtained by subtracting the attenuations (dB) shown in panel (b) from the input amplitudes in decibels (panel a).

a bank of bandpass filters can estimate the spectrum of a sound depends on the number of filters, the width of the pass band of each filter, and the steepness of the roll-off of each filter. The more filters, the narrower the pass bands, and the steeper the roll-off, the better the filter bank will be in estimating a sound's spectrum.

Another use of filters involves "shaping" the spectra of signals. Imagine that a complex waveform with the amplitude spectrum shown Figure 5.4a is passed through the filter shown in Figure 5.4b. The complex wave will have at the output of the filter the amplitude spectrum shown in Figure 5.4c. Because the filter is a bandpass filter, the amplitudes of the sinusoids within the band of frequencies passed by the

filter (the pass band) have not been attenuated, whereas those outside the pass band have been attenuated by 12 dB per octave. If the amplitude spectrum and attenuation of the filter are expressed in decibels, then the amplitudes in decibels in the output spectrum are obtained by subtracting the attenuation values introduced by the filter from the amplitudes in the input spectrum. Thus, a filter has been used to alter the amplitude spectrum of a complex waveform.

Filters also introduce a phase delay to signals that pass through them. To describe a filter fully we must indicate not only the type of filter, the cutoff frequencies, and the roll-off rate, but also how the phase of each sinusoid is altered. Although the phase shift introduced by a filter is not as easy to describe as the attenuation rate, both of these values must be known if the waveform at the output of the filter is to be determined. The phase shifts introduced by the filters mean that certain frequencies relative to other frequencies may be delayed in reaching the output of the filter. For instance, if a filter introduces a 180° phase shift to a 1000-Hz tone, then a sound passing through that filter will have its 1000-Hz component delayed by 0.5 msec (a 1000-Hz tone has a 1-msec period and 180° is one-half of that period, or 0.5 msec) relative to the time delay introduced to other frequency components.

As described in Chapter 4, if the amplitude or the phase spectrum of a complex wave is modified, then the time waveform representing the complex wave will also be altered. Because filters modify spectra, they will also alter time-domain waveforms. Thus, a filter will change the time-domain representation as well as the spectrum of a signal. An example is shown in Figure 5.5.

Any object that has mass and is moved by a driving force acts as a low-pass filter. The cone of a loudspeaker, fluids, and the eardrum all act as filters. When the driving force pushes on the loudspeaker cone, the cone moves outward. When the driving force draws in, the speaker cone does likewise. When the frequency of the driving force is low, the speaker cone can follow the driving vibration with no loss in amplitude. As the driving frequency increases, the loudspeaker cone cannot follow the driving force and the amplitude of the speaker cone movement will be reduced. This happens because the cone has mass, and it takes some time to move an object with mass (a property of inertia). When the driving force has a high frequency, the speaker cone responds to the outward push after a small time delay due to the force attempting to move some mass. Thus, by the time the speaker cone begins to move outward, the high-frequency driving force is already moving inward, so the speaker

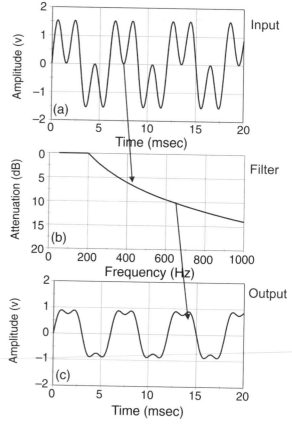

FIGURE 5.5 A complex sound (a) is passed through a low-pass filter with a 200-Hz cutoff and a 6-dB-per-octave roll-off (b). As can be seen, the complex time-domain waveform at the filter's output is different from that at the input because of the attenuation of the level of sinusoids with frequencies greater than 200 Hz (c).

cone also tries to move inward. As a result, the cone does not move as far outward as it did at lower frequencies, creating low output amplitude at this high frequency. The speaker cone thus acts as a low-pass filter. The eardrum and other structures within the ear have mass. They can react as low-pass filters. The greater the mass, the greater the inertia for movement and the lower the cutoff frequency for the low-pass filtering operation performed by the object. Thus, if one does not want an object to alter the driving sound, it is best if the object is very light. These effects are discussed in greater detail in the next few chapters.

NONLINEARITIES

So far we have discussed situations in which the sound input to some object, such as a filter, has been modified by a decrease in the magnitude of the input value *passively*. If a waveform consisting of 100, 200, and 300 Hz is the input to a filter, the filter will alter only the amplitudes and phases of these sinusoids. There are, however, objects and systems that not only modify the values of the input but also add sinusoids at other frequencies. For instance, a complex input waveform to a system might have frequency components of 100, 200, and 300 Hz, but at the output of the system the measured frequency components might consist of the original components of 100, 200, and 300 Hz, and perhaps the additional components with frequencies of 400, 500, and 600 Hz. That is, spectral components are present in the output of this system that were not present in the input. A passive system that adds sinusoids to the input waveform is called a *nonlinear system*, whereas a system that changes only the amplitudes and phases of the frequency components of the input signal is referred to as a *linear system*.

For instructive purposes, the interaction of a nonlinear system and waveforms will be discussed in terms of two waveforms: one, a simple waveform consisting of only one frequency, f_1; the other, a complex waveform consisting of the sum of two sinusoidal components with frequencies f_1 and f_2. If one sinusoid (f_1) is an input to a linear device, then its output is a single sinusoidal component with a frequency of f_1, and the amplitude and starting phase of this one component may be altered relative to their values at the input. If one sinusoidal component (f_1) is an input to a nonlinear device, then the output contains a sinusoidal component with frequency f_1 and it may contain its higher *harmonics*: $2f_1$, $3f_1$, $4f_1$, and so on. Thus, if f_1 is 1000 Hz, the nonlinear device could yield the following nonlinear frequency components: 2000 Hz, 3000 Hz, 4000 Hz, and so on.

If the two sinusoidal components with frequencies, f_1 and f_2, are inputs, then linear outputs would be only at f_1 and f_2, but nonlinear outputs consist of frequency components at the harmonics of each frequency ($2f_1$, $2f_2$, $3f_1$, $3f_2$, and so on) as well as frequency components made up of the combinations of f_1 and f_2. These frequencies, called *combination tones*, consist of both *summation tones* and *difference tones*. Typical summation tones are $f_1 + f_2$, $2f_1 + f_2$, $f_1 + 2f_2$, and typical difference tones are $f_1 - f_2$, $2f_1 - f_2$, $2f_2 - f_1$. If the input frequency components were 100 and 250 Hz, the nonlinear combination tones could be 350 Hz, 450 Hz, and 600 Hz (summation tones), and 150, 50, and 500 Hz (difference tones). Thus, the total nonlinear output contains such harmonics and combination tones as 350, 200, 150, 50, 450, and so on. In general, a nonlinear device produces harmonics and combination tones according to this equation:

$$mf_1 \pm nf_2,$$

where

$$m = 0, 1, 2, 3, \ldots, n = 0, 1, 2, 3, \ldots \quad (5.2)$$

Table 5.2 displays combination tones for sinusoids with input frequencies of 100 and 250 Hz. The amplitudes and phases of the nonlinear components present in the output depend on the frequencies, amplitudes, and phases of the input *and* on the nature or type of nonlinearity.

So far, a nonlinear device has been discussed in terms of spectral changes in the frequency domain. Time-domain waveforms are also changed by nonlinear devices, as shown in Figure 5.6. The change in the time-domain representation resulting from a nonlinear device is sometimes called *distortion*. Thus, the output time waveform of a nonlinear device is distorted and differs from the input time waveform. A linear system, such as a filter, also modifies the input time-domain waveform, as shown in Figure 5.5. That is, for both a linear and a nonlinear system the spectra of the sound can be altered. If the frequency-domain spectra are altered, so is the time-domain waveform (see Chapter 4). Therefore, we cannot simply note that an output time-domain waveform is different from the input waveform to decide whether a system is nonlinear; it is best if we investigate changes in the frequency domain. If there are frequency components present in the output spectrum that are not present in the input spectrum, then a passive system is nonlinear. One question of great interest to hearing

TABLE 5.2 Some (for n = m = 3) Combination (Summation and Difference) Tones and Harmonics Resulting from Two Input Frequencies, 100 Hz (f_1) and 250 Hz (f_2)

Symbol	Harmonic tones	Combination tones Summation tones	Difference tones
f_1	100 Hz		
f_2	250 Hz		
$2f_1$	200 Hz		
$3f_1$	300 Hz		
$2f_2$	500 Hz		
$3f_2$	750 Hz		
$f_1 + f_2$		350 Hz	
$f_1 + 2f_2$		600 Hz	
$f_1 + 3f_2$		850 Hz	
$2f_1 + f_2$		450 Hz	
$3f_1 + f_2$		550 Hz	
$2f_1 + 2f_2$		700 Hz	
$2f_1 + 3f_2$		950 Hz	
$3f_1 + 2f_2$		800 Hz	
$f_1 - f_2$			150 Hz
$f_1 - 2f_2$			400 Hz
$f_1 - 3f_2$			650 Hz
$2f_1 - f_2$			50 Hz
$3f_1 - f_2$			50 Hz
$2f_1 - 2f_2$			300 Hz
$2f_1 - 3f_2$			550 Hz
$3f_1 - 2f_2$			200 Hz

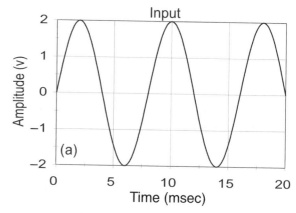

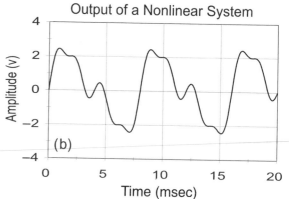

FIGURE 5.6 A nonlinear system changes (*distorts*) a time-domain waveform. A simple sinusoid (a) becomes a complex sound (b) when a nonlinear system adds harmonics. Panel (b) is a complex wave because the nonlinearity added tones of other frequencies to the original sinusoid. Note that both a filter (Figure 5.5) and a nonlinear system (this figure) change a time-domain waveform.

scientists is whether the auditory system is linear or nonlinear. If it is a nonlinear, what types of nonlinearities (i.e., which harmonics, summation tones, and difference tones) are produced? If such nonlinear components are produced, do we perceive them?

A linear system is one in which the output of the system (out) is a *linear function* of the input (in), i.e., out = a(in) + b, where a and b are constants and in and out are time-domain descriptions. An equation of the form $y = ax + b$ is a linear equation and is defined by a straight-line relationship between x (in) and y (out). A nonlinear relationship can be defined as out = a(in) + b(in)^2 + c(in)^3 + d(in)^4 + etc. This equation represents a nonlinear, or curvilinear, relationship between in and out. The presence of the terms with a power greater than 1 (e.g., in^2) produces harmonics and combinations tones in such a nonlinear system (see Appendix A).

A particular form of a nonlinear equation applies to the auditory processing performed by the inner ear. Figure 5.7 shows the output as a *compressive nonlinear* function of the input. A compressive nonlinearity means that as the input increases there is less and less change in the output (i.e., the output curve "flattens out" at high values of the input). Note that the same change in the input at a low value of the input (on the left of Figure 5.7) leads to a much larger change in the

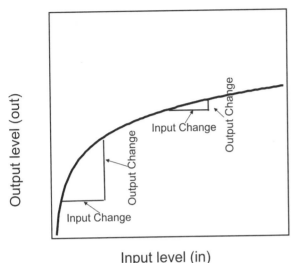

FIGURE 5.7 A compressive nonlinear relationship between an input (in) and an output (out). A compressive nonlinearity means that as the value of the input increases, the same change in the input generates a smaller and smaller change in the output, as indicated in the figure.

output than when this same change in the input is applied at a higher value of the input (on the right of Figure 5.7). Such a compressive nonlinearity when applied to complex sound will produce nonlinear spectral components consisting of harmonics and combination tones of a complex sound input.

SOUND AND ITS ANALYSIS

Sounds can be described by the frequencies, amplitudes, and phases of sinusoidal components. Thus, to describe hearing we need to describe how the auditory system determines the frequencies, amplitudes, and starting phases of the various sinusoids that make up any sound. We will use the analogy of bandpass filters (similar to Figure 5.3) as a way in which the auditory system determines the "neural" spectrum of a sound and from such a neural spectrum how the auditory system estimates frequency and amplitude.

Our everyday hearing experience reveals that we often perceive sound in terms of its frequency-domain representation. For instance, when yo͟͟u you often hear the many pitches that ͟r musical sound. The perception of the͟s you are sensitive to the frequencies that make up the complex musical sound. As such, your auditory system has analyzed the musical sound in terms of the frequency domain.

Thus, we will show that the auditory system determines the frequencies and amplitudes of sound with processes that are analogous to bandpass filters. As indicated earlier, the many structures of the auditory system alter sound and its analysis (often in a nonlinear manner). The physical concepts of resonance, filtering, and nonlinearity are used to describe these alterations.

SUMMARY

In a forced vibration system, the receiving, or resonant, object has a resonant frequency that depends on its characteristic impedance. Filters are resonators that can be used to determine the amplitude spectrum of an unknown waveform. There are four types of filters (low pass, high pass, bandpass, and band reject), and each is characterized by its cutoff frequency and the attenuation roll-off in decibels per octave. A linear system changes only the phase and amplitude of an input waveform, whereas a nonlinear system adds sinusoidal components to the input. These nonlinear additional sinusoids are harmonics and combination tones (summation and difference tones) of the input sinusoids. Although filters and nonlinear devices are usually described in terms of altering the frequency domain of waveforms, both types of systems also alter the time domain of the waveform. Resonance, filtering, and nonlinearity are concepts that will be used when we describe how the auditory system processes sound.

SUPPLEMENT

Filtering and nonlinearity are independent aspects of any system that analyzes sound. These concepts are described in any introductory physics or electrical engineering textbook. The book by Rosen and Howell (1991, Chapters. 6, 7, and 8) presents the material at a slightly more advanced level. The more advanced reader should consult the book by Hartmann (1998).

Earlier, the example of a cymbal, drum, or tuning fork being struck with a drumstick or something like a drumstick was used to explain resonance. In this case, a single strike of a drumstick can be thought of as a very brief transient driving source. As such, the spectrum of this transient driving source will be broadband, containing a continuum of spectral components (see Figure 4.4), and it is highly likely that several of these components are at the resonant frequencies of the drum or cymbal or tuning fork.

The cutoff frequency of a filter is usually defined as that frequency at which the power of the signal has been attenuated by half its maximal power. Because decreasing the power by one-half yields 3 dB of attenuation, the cutoff frequency is determined at that frequency for which the intensity of the sound has been decreased by 3 dB from that existing in the *pass band* of the filter. This definition of the cutoff frequency is referred to as the *half-power* or the *3-dB cutoff*. The bandwidth of a bandpass filter is usually computed as the frequency difference between the half-power cutoff frequencies. When comparing the bandwidths from one filter to another, a term called the Q of the filter is used:

$$Q = (\text{center frequency of the filter})/$$
$$(\text{bandwidth of the filter}).$$

An equal Q set of filters is a filter set in which, as the center frequencies of the bandpass filters increase, the pass band increases in direct proportion to the center frequency. For instance, if Q for a set of filters is 2 and the pass band of a filter centered at 1000 Hz is 500 Hz, then the pass band of a filter centered at 5000 Hz is 2500 Hz. Although the Q of a filter can be determined at the 3-dB cutoff frequencies, it can also be determined at other cutoff frequencies, for instance, at the 10-dB cutoff frequencies. The Q of such a filter is often referred to as Q_{10}.

Attenuation in decibels (Atten_{dB}) for any particular frequency (f), cutoff frequency (cut), and roll-off rate (roll) is

$$\text{Atten}_{dB} = \text{roll} \times \log_2(\text{cut}/f) \quad \text{for} \quad f < \text{cut},$$

and is

$$\text{Atten}_{dB} = \text{roll} \times \log_2(f/\text{cut}) \quad \text{for} \quad f > \text{cut},$$

and $\log_2$ is the logarithm to the base 2 ($\log_2 = 3.3219 \times \log_{10}$). So if roll = 6 dB/octave, cut = 3000 Hz, and f = 7000 Hz, then the attenuation of the component at 7000 Hz is

$$6 \times \log_2(7000/3000) = 6 \times 3.3219 \log_{10}(2.33)$$
$$= 19.93 \times 0.367 = 7.31 \text{ dB}.$$

The chapter used a two-tone complex (f_1 and f_2) to describe nonlinearly produced harmonics and combination tones. If the sound input contains many frequencies, then a nonlinear system may produce nonlinear components at harmonics of all of the input components and combination tones among all of the input components. Thus, the output spectrum of a nonlinear device may be extremely complex if the input sound is itself complex.

A more general description of a linear system involves the relationship between the input to and the output from the system. The change the stimulus undergoes while "passing through" the system can be described by some function, $F[x(t)]$. If $x(t)$ is the input, then the output, $y(t)$, can be expressed as

$$y(t) = F[x(t)].$$

For the system to be linear, the function F must meet certain requirements. The major property is *superposition*. If the function F meets the concept of superposition, then the following equation would hold true for a situation involving more than one input [$x_1(t)$, $x_2(t)$, $x_3(t)$, and so on]:

$$y(t) = F[x_1(t) + x_2(t) + x_3(t) + \text{etc.}].$$

Then, if superposition holds,

$$y(t) = F[x_1(t)] + F[x_2(t)] + F[x_3(t)] + \text{etc.}$$

The equations state that the function F can be distributed across the various inputs treated separately. This, in turn, means that once we know the function F, we can always predict how the system will act when a new, but unknown, input $[x(t)]$ is presented. Notice, for instance, that superposition does not allow for more output relationships to occur than there were input relationships. This was the primary concept we used in defining linear and nonlinear systems. A linear system produces the same frequency components at the output as were in the input, whereas a nonlinear system produces a waveform with more spectral components at the output than were in the input.

In the chapter, we referred to a *passive* system terms of linearity or nonlinearity. A passive system contrast to an *active* system. A passive system is one that does not have some additional source of energy that can cause it to change an input. For instance, an electrical circuit could accept a sound input and then add additional components to the sound by creating another sound and adding the two sounds together. The fact that the circuit generates another sound makes it an active system. Active systems can create almost any type of output imaginable, and these outputs could have all sorts of spectral components that were not in the input. Only a nonlinear *passive* system can produce spectral components at its output that were not in the input.

6

The Outer and Middle Ears

The previous chapters discussed the nature, transmission, and analysis of sound. Chapters 6–9 investigate how acoustic energy is collected by the outer ear and transmitted to the fluids of the inner ear; how the inner ear transforms this energy into neural impulses; and how these neural impulses code for or analyze the basic acoustic information dealing with sound, most especially amplitude, frequency, and time/phase information.

Figure 6.1 summarizes the structure, mode of operation, and function of four general divisions of the auditory system: *outer ear*, *middle ear*, *inner ear*, and *central auditory nervous system*. The central auditory nervous system includes all of the complex interconnections in the auditory nervous system, from the *auditory branch* of the *eighth cranial* (VIIIth) *nerve* to the several brainstem nuclei and the *auditory cortex*. The complex central auditory nervous system is not diagramed in Figure 6.1 but will be discussed in more detail in Chapter 15. Chapter 6 deals with the outer and middle ears, and Chapters 7–9 deal with the inner ear.

Acoustic pressure is transmitted to the fluids of the inner ear via the outer and middle ears in a variety of ways. The neural process of hearing begins within the inner ear. The outer and middle ears help overcome middle and inner ear impedances (Chapter 3) due to bone, tissue, and fluids in the inner ear and, thus, allow for a very efficient transmission of the acoustic stimulus to the inner ear. The outer and middle ears also provide protection for the inner ear against excessive changes in the environment.

Appendices E and F will assist the reader in understanding the general areas of anatomy (the structure of the body and the interrelation of its parts) and physiology (the function of an anatomical system).

STRUCTURE OF THE OUTER EAR

The changing acoustic pressures that constantly impinge on us from sound sources are collected by the outer ear. The outer ear consists of the visible part of the ear (*pinna*) and a canal (*external auditory canal*) leading to the eardrum. The human pinna (illustrated in Figure 6.1) is formed primarily of cartilage without useful muscles, and it has many small superficial bumps and grooves. The human pinna is unique from person to person, in that the shape and location of the various bumps and grooves differ considerably across the population. The deep center portion of the pinna is called the bowl, or *concha* (cave). In adult humans

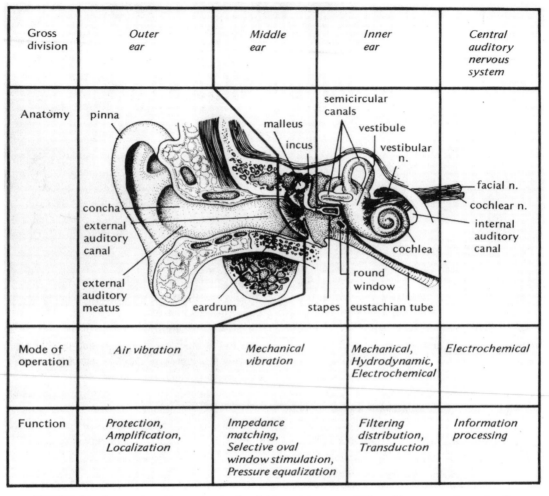

Gross division	Outer ear	Middle ear	Inner ear	Central auditory nervous system
Anatomy				
Mode of operation	Air vibration	Mechanical vibration	Mechanical, Hydrodynamic, Electrochemical	Electrochemical
Function	Protection, Amplification, Localization	Impedance matching, Selective oval window stimulation, Pressure equalization	Filtering distribution, Transduction	Information processing

FIGURE 6.1 Cross section of human ear showing divisions of the outer, middle, and inner ears and central auditory nervous system. Below are listed the predominant modes of operation of each division and its suggested function. Adapted with permission from Ades and Engstrom (1974) and Dallos (1973).

the concha has a diameter of 1 to 2 cm (1 inch = 2.54 cm = 25.4 mm) and leads to an opening with a diameter of about 5 to 7 mm. This opening (or *meatus*) is called the *external auditory meatus*; it leads into a canal 2 to 3 cm in length called the external auditory canal (*outer ear canal*). The lateral (toward the pinna) third of the canal consists of cartilage containing glands and lined with hairs; the rest of the canal is bony, with a tight skin lining close to the *eardrum*, or *tympanic membrane*.

STRUCTURE OF THE MIDDLE EAR

The tympanic membrane is held in place by fibers and cartilage situated in a bony groove between the bone called the *footplate* (the overall shape of the stapes is like that of a stirrup, and the stapes is sometimes referred as the stirrup). The footplate is implanted in the *oval window* (part of the inner ear). The stapes' footplate is surrounded at its rim by a ring-shaped ligament situated along the edge of the oval window, which is a thin membrane leading to the inner ear. This ligament, called an *annular ligament*, assists in supporting the footplate in the oval window. Thus, the tympanic membrane is directly joined, or "coupled," to the inner ear by the three ossicles (malleus, incus, and stapes).

The three ossicles are suspended in the tympanic cavity by means of the *axial ligaments*, which consist of the *posterior ligaments* of the incus and the *anterior ligaments* of the malleus, as shown in Figure 6.4. Also shown in Figure 6.4 are the middle ear muscles that control the actions of the ossicles. One of the middle ear muscles is the *tensor tympani muscle*, which in adult humans is about 25 mm in length. Most

of this muscle is enclosed within a bony canal that runs parallel to and above the eustachian tube. A tendon emerges from the bony canal to connect the muscle to the upper part of the manubrium of the malleus. The other middle ear muscle, the *stapedial muscle*, also originates within a bony canal. Only about 6 mm in total length, it is the smallest muscle in the body. The tendon of the stapedial muscle completes the attachment to the head of the stapes.

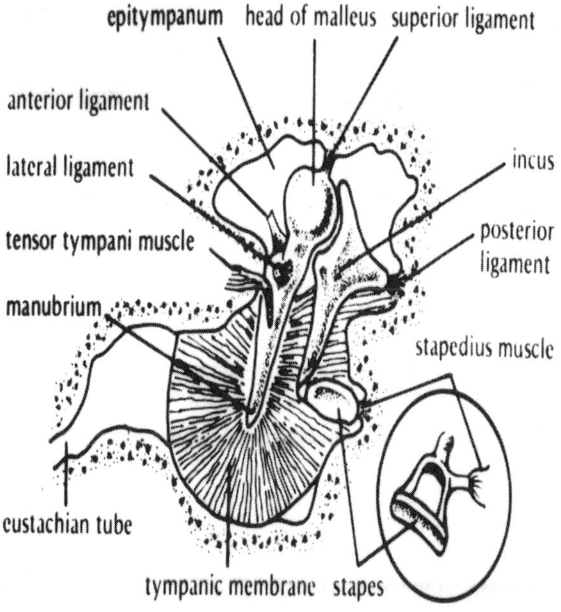

Thus, the inner ear communicates with the acoustic environment outside of the body by means of a funnel (the pinna), a short tube (the external auditory canal), a thin membrane (the tympanic membrane), and three small bones (the ossicles). All of these structure are very small, thin, and light (often the smallest structures in the body), to ensure that they vibrate maximally when stimulated with sound. We now consider in more detail the functions served by the pinna, external canal of the outer ear, tympanic membrane, and the ossicles of the middle ear.

FIGURE 6.4 Schematic drawing of the human middle ear indicating the ossicular chain and other prominent parts of middle-ear anatomy. From Moller (1970), with permission.

FUNCTION OF THE OUTER EAR

TORSO, HEAD, AND PINNA

As sound travels from its source to the outer ear, it passes over the torso and head (including the pinna). These parts of the body provide obstacles to sound transmission and thus change the sound before it reaches the outer ear. That is, the parts of the body slow down and attenuate sound as it travels from its source to the outer ear canal. One way to describe the changes to sound transmission that take place across the torso and head is to measure the spectral changes in the amplitude and phases of the spectral components of the sound due to the influences of the various parts of the body and outer ear and middle ears. The structures of the torso and head attenuate and slow sound in a frequency-dependent manner (due to the interaction among the structures' size, the location of the sound source relative to the head, and sound wavelength; see Chapter 3) as sound travels from its source to the outer ear. To measure these spectral changes, the spectrum of the sound source (input spectrum) is first determined, and then the spectrum of the sound in the outer ear (output spectrum) is measured. The difference between the input and output spectrum describes how the structures of the torso and head alter the amplitudes and phases of the sinusoidal components that make up the input stimulus. Sound-pressure measurements in the outer ear can be accomplished by inserting either very small microphones into the outer ear canal or by placing a tube into the outer ear canal and measuring the sound pressure in the tube. The combination of the amplitude and phase spectra that describe sound pressure changes due to the intervening structures is called a *transfer function* (i.e., the attenuation and phase shifts provided by a filter describe the filter's transfer function). This measurement process is sometimes called *real-ear measurement*.

Figure 6.5 portrays the amplitude spectra of the outer ear transfer function for one human listener. That is, Figure 6.5 shows how the amplitudes of the spectral components of a sound from a source are attenuated by the structures of the torso and head. In this case, the sound source was a single, very brief acoustic transient, and as such it has an amplitude spectrum with all frequency components up to 20,000 Hz that are about equal in amplitude (see Chapter 4). Thus the spectral changes seen in Figure 6.5 are entirely due to the torso, head, and pinna. Note that the high-frequency components are greatly attenuated relative to the low-frequency components and that the amplitude differences between the two ears are small at the low frequencies. The amplitudes in the high-frequency regions at the right ear (the ear away from the sound source) are much lower than those at the left ear. Most of this *interaural* (between ears) amplitude difference is due to the head's providing a sound shadow (see Chapter 3). Because most of the structures of the pinna that the sound wave encounters are small, it will only be the short wavelengths (high frequencies) of the originating sound that will be altered (see Chapter 3).

These transfer functions (spectra) describing changes between the source and the outer ear are called *head-related transfer functions* (HRTFs). Thus, HRTF describes how the torso, head, and pinna change the amplitudes (attenuate the amplitudes of the spectral components of the originating sound) and phases (adds phase shifts to those of the spectral components of the originating sound). The phase spectrum of the HRTF is discussed in Chapter 12 of a sound as it travels from a source toward the outer ear. The HRTF has important consequences for sound localization (see Chapter 12).

Many of the spectral changes noticed in the HRTFs at high frequencies are due to the pinnae. Only mammals have pinnae, but among mammals there is great diversity in their form. In general, only animals with relatively high-frequency hearing have mobile pinnae. Because the pinnae of humans and other primates have no useful muscles, they are relatively immobile. Mobile, and to some extent immobile, pinnae help in processing high-frequency sounds by funneling them toward the external canal, in distinguishing sounds originating in front of the head from

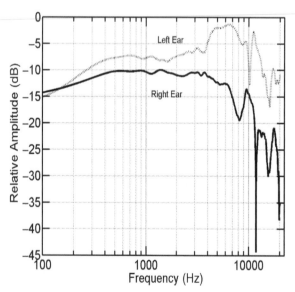

FIGURE 6.5 The Head-Related Transfer Functions, HRTFs, for an adult human when presented a brief transient source directly opposite the left ear. The HRTF shows the amplitude spectra at each ear (measured within the ear canal) on an arbitrary decibel scale. The sound at the right ear is attenuated relative to that at the left, especially at high frequencies.

those behind the head, and in providing other types of filtering of an incoming sound wave.

OUTER EAR

In addition to the spectral changes, such as those shown in Figure 6.5, the outer ear causes an increase in level of about 10 to 15 dB in a frequency range from roughly 1.5 kHz to 7 kHz (kHz means 1000 Hz; thus, 7 kHz is 7000 Hz). Experiments have shown that this frequency-dependent increase in sound-pressure level between the measurements made at the sound source (*free-field measurements*) and measurements at the tympanic membrane is due mainly to the effects of the concha and the external auditory canal, as shown in the transfer functions of Figure 6.6. In Chapters 3 and 5 we discussed the concept of resonance and resonances that can occur in tubes like the concha and external auditory canal. Given the sizes of the concha and external auditory canal (especially their lengths; see Chapter 3), the resonant frequency of the external

auditory canal is about 2.5 kHz and the resonance frequency of the concha is closer to 5 kHz. The resonance of the concha and external canal complement each other to produce a gain in acoustic pressure within the outer ear for frequency components in the range from 1.5 to 7 kHz.

Thus, the sound from a source is significantly altered by the torso, head, pinna, and external auditory canal before it reaches the tympanic membrane. In general, the sound pressure level in the frequency range from 1.5 to 7 kHz is increased due to resonance properties of the pinna and external auditory canal, and the sound pressure is decreased at higher frequencies due to properties of the HRTF. The only other known function of the external ear is that of protection of the middle ear from foreign bodies and changes in humidity and temperature. Because it seals off the external auditory canal from the middle ear cavity, the tympanic membrane provides some protection for the middle ear against foreign bodies.

TYMPANIC MEMBRANE

The tympanic membrane vibrates as a result of sound waves traveling in the external auditory canal, and this vibration is passed along to the ossicular chain. The vibratory pattern of the tympanic membrane has been the subject of much research since Helmholtz published his first experiments in 1868. Figure 6.7 shows that the membrane vibrates maximally at a point below the umbo and directly about the fold (see Figure 6.7, point 15). Modern investigative methods show the complicated vibratory patterns illustrated on the bottom of Figure 6.7. In Figure 6.7, the lines with numerical labels indicate areas of the membrane that are moving the same distance, and each line represents a different amount of displacement. In the top figure, the maximal displace is 15 times greater in the lower middle of the membrane near the umbo than it is toward the top. In the lower figure, the displacement varies over a factor of 8.2 to 1 as a function of the location within the tympanic membrane. The bottom figure is oriented at a different

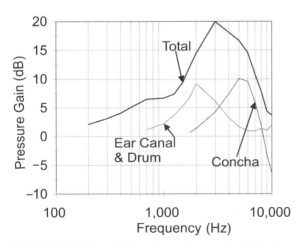

FIGURE 6.6 Estimated change in sound pressure level from free field to site of measurement—concha and combined ear canal and eardrum—and the total transfer function, including the concha, ear canal, and eardrum from the free field to the tympanic membrane (Total). The Total curve is essentially the sum of the other two curves. Adapted from Shaw (1974), with permission.

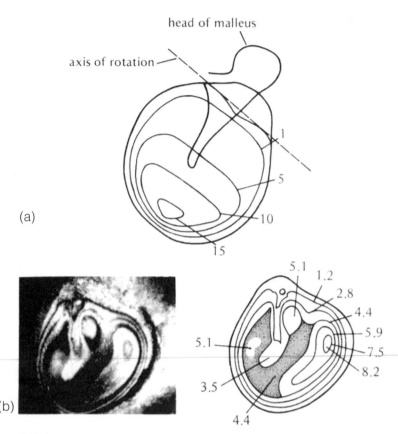

FIGURE 6.7 **(a)** The vibratory pattern of the right tympanic membrane to a 2-kHz tone. The closed curves represent contours of equal displacement amplitude on a relative scale; 15 is the maximum amplitude. This is von Bekesy's 1941 stiff-plate model. **(b)** Tonndorf and Khanna's 1972 time-averaged holograph of the left tympanic membrane vibration. The stimulus was a 525-Hz, 121-dB SPL tone. In the explanatory drawing, each isoamplitude contour must be multiplied by 10^{-5} cm to obtain the actual displacement. Thus, the maximum displacement of 8.2 is actually 8.2×10^{-5} cm, the minimum displacement is 1.2×10^{-5} cm, etc. Adapted from Tonndorf and Khanna (1972), with permission.

angle than the top figure, in that the umbo where maximum displacement occurs is located toward the right in the bottom figure and toward the bottom in the top figure. It is generally agreed that the vibratory pattern of the tympanic membrane is the most complicated at higher frequencies and higher levels. The complicated vibratory response illustrated by time-averaged holography (bottom of Figure 6.7) shows variations with frequency of the stimulus. At the low frequency used in Figure 6.7b, the point of maximum displacement is in the superior posterior (top rear, the 8.2 contour) section of the membrane. The vibratory pattern of the tympanic membrane, although complicated, allows for an efficient transfer of the acoustic stimulus from the outer ear to the middle ear and the middle ear structures.

FUNCTION OF THE MIDDLE EAR

The major function of the middle ear is to provide an effective and efficient means to deliver sound to the inner ear, where the neural process of hearing begins. If the ossicles of the middle ear were missing in humans, then one would experience about a 60-dB hearing loss because sound was not being delivered to the inner ear effectively. Once the acoustic stimulus reaches the tympanic membrane, it can be transmitted through the middle ear to the inner ear via three methods: (1) bone conduction (i.e., sound could travel via direct vibration of the bones of the skull, bypassing the middle ear, going directly to the inner ear), (2) air pressure changes in the middle ear cavity (i.e., the sound wave would travel through the middle ear without encountering the ossicles and stimulate the oval window directly), and (3) across the middle ear cavity by means of the ossicular chain (the malleus, incus, and stapes) to the inner ear. The ossicular chain, which vibrates in response to tympanic membrane vibration and passes this vibration onto the fluids and structures of the inner ear, is the most effective and normal method of transmitting sound to the inner ear. For the time being, we will consider this the normal way that sound is transmitted through the middle ear.

For the ossicular chain to vibrate efficiently, the middle ear must not be a closed cavity. If the middle ear cavity were closed, then changes in atmospheric pressure (not related to sound) would cause air pressure to build up or to be reduced within the middle ear without any release. That is, in the absence of any sound, the pressure in the middle ear cavity would be fixed if the middle ear were a closed cavity. If the tympanic membrane pushed in, the size of the middle ear cavity would decrease and the pressure inside the middle ear would increase (same number of air molecules in a smaller space). The opposite would happen if the tympanic membrane moved out from its normal resting position. Thus, changes in air pressure that occur frequently in rising and falling elevators, traveling up and down mountains, in airplanes, or under water would cause the tympanic membrane to move either in or out, and as a consequence the pressure in

the middle ear cavity would increase or decrease, even when no sound was present. If the tympanic membrane is already stretched due to unequal pressure between the middle ears and the outside air pressure, then pressure changes caused by a sound wave will not be very successful in vibrating the tympanic membrane, and one would experience a hearing loss. The eustachian tube allows for equalization of pressure in the middle ear, by providing another path for the pressure, via the nasal passages. The eustachian tube allows the tympanic membrane to operate efficiently in a variety of atmospheric pressures because the pressure on its outside (in the outer ear connected to outside air pressures) is the same as that on the inside of the middle ear. That is because the middle ear is connected to the outside air pressures via the eustachian tube's connection to the nasal passages and the nasal passages' connection to outside air pressure via the nose and mouth. When the eustachian tube or nasal cavity is blocked, sound transmission is not very efficient because the air pressure within the middle ear cavity can now change (i.e., the middle ear becomes a closed cavity). In these conditions, one can experience a hearing loss and perhaps pain (due to stretching of the tympanic membrane and the tissues around it). The pain and loss of hearing one suffers (especially children with middle ear disease, or *otitis media*; see Chapter 16) with a cold or other forms of nasal congestion can be a result of a blocked eustachian tube.

The ossicular chain vibrates a membrane (*oval window membrane*) of the inner ear, which causes the fluids of the inner ear to move and the neural process of hearing to begin. If this oval window membrane were pushed or driven by air alone, then air pressure would be the driving force (the second option listed earlier for how the inner ear could be vibrated by actions in the middle ear) for hearing. Because inner ear fluids and tissue are denser than air, air would not be very efficient in moving the fluids and tissue (i.e., fluids and tissue have much higher characteristic impedance than air). Thus, the auditory system would lose some of its sensitivity (about 35 dB, although the loss is frequency dependent) due to the impedance

Ossicular chain provides compensation for impedance mismatch.

(see Chapter 3) of the fluids and structures of the inner ear. The difference in impedance between air and the fluids and tissues of the inner ear is referred to as an *impedance mismatch*, meaning that more pressure is required for a stimulus to be propagated in the inner ear than in air. Nature has compensated for this mismatch by having sound transmitted to the inner ear via the ossicular chain. It is principally the size difference between the areas of the tympanic membrane and the stapes footplate and, to a limited extent, the lever action of the ossicular chain and the shape of the tympanic membrane that overcome the impedance mismatch.

When stimulated by high sound pressure levels, the tympanic membrane operates as a stretched membrane, and only part of the pressures acting on it is transferred to the manubrium of the malleus. Measurements show that only about two-thirds of a total area of $85\,mm^2$ of the tympanic membrane is stiffly connected to the manubrium and, thus, vibrates at high levels. Therefore, the effective surface area of the tympanic membrane in adult humans is approximately $55\,mm^2$. The stapes, which is the last part of the middle ear chain, makes contact with the oval window and the fluids of the inner ear. The area of the stapes footplate in adult humans is about $3.2\,mm^2$, which is considerably smaller than the effective area of the tympanic membrane. This difference in surface area between the effective area of the tympanic membrane and the stapes footplate acts to increase the pressure exerted on the tympanic membrane. Consider that if all of the force that impinges on the tympanic membrane is transferred to the stapes footplate, then the force per unit of area ($p = F/A$; see Chapter 3) must be greater at the footplate because it is smaller in area than the tympanic membrane. The increase in pressure can be expressed as the ratio of the effective area of the tympanic membrane to that of the stapes footplate; that is, $55\,mm^2/3.2\,mm^2 = 17$. Thus, the pressure at the footplate is 17 times greater (i.e., greater by $20 \log 17 = 25\,dB$) than at the tympanic membrane, and, therefore, this increased pressure can partially overcome the impedance mismatch, and the fluid- and tissue-filled inner ear can be effectively stimulated.

The transfer of the force from the tympanic membrane to the stapes footplate also depends on the action of the ossicles. The ossicles work as a lever system because the lengths of the manubrium and neck of the malleus are longer than the long process of the incus (see Figure 6.3). The lever action of this system is 1.3 to 1; i.e., the force at the tympanic membrane is increased by a factor of 1.3 at the stapes. In addition, the tympanic membrane tends to buckle as it moves, due to its conical shape, causing the malleus to move with about twice the force. Thus, the pressure increase of a factor of 17 due to the area difference of the tympanic membrane and stapes footplate is multiplied by 1.3 due to the lever action, and then the buckling action causes an additional multiplication by 2. These calculations result in a theoretical maximum total pressure increase of $17 \times 1.3 \times 2$, or 44.2 dB (a pressure increase of 44 to 1 corresponds to $20 \log 44 = 33$ dB at the stapes footplate). The actual pressure transformation depends on the frequency of the acoustic stimulus, because the structures of the middle and inner ears offer both resistive and reactance impedance (see Chapter 3). Figure 6.8 shows that the increase of pressure between the eardrum and the

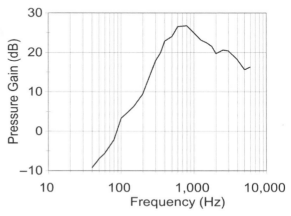

FIGURE 6.8 Transfer function for the middle ear showing that the pressure in the fluids of the inner ear is increased over that at the tympanic membrane by the decibel value shown as a function of the frequency of the stimulus. Adapted from Nedzelnitsky (1980), with permission.

our ears are less sensitive to low and high freq, because of

inner ear is 30 dB or more in the region of 2500 Hz. Above this frequency, the ratio decreases. In addition, as showed earlier, the resonances of the concha and external canal are in the 2-kHz range. The total increase in pressure due to the outer and middle ears is about 60 dB in a frequency range centered at about 2 kHz. Thus, most of the 60-dB impedance mismatch is counteracted by the acoustic and vibratory properties of the outer and middle ears. Nature has designed an ingenious system to match the impedance of air to that of the inner ear fluids and tissues. The combination of the resonance of the external auditory canal and the increases due to the ossicular chain causes a significant pressure increase across a wide frequency range, which is important for the perception of sounds such as speech. Thus, to a first approximation and over a considerable frequency range, a pressure change in air results in an equivalent pressure change in the inner ear, which means that there is not a loss of sensitivity due to an impedance mismatch. The fact that this does not occur at all frequencies is one of the reasons we have a lower sensitivity to sound at low and high frequencies, as we discuss in Chapter 10.

Previously we described the suspension system of the ossicles and stated that there were several ligaments and muscles that performed this function. The muscles are normally in a state of tension, but when the ear is excited by sound, they exert an increased pull, which is a reflex action that makes it more difficult for the ossicles to move. The sound that elicits the reflex must be about 80 dB SL. Contraction of the middle ear muscles reduces the transmission of pressure through the ossicular chain. The reduction in transmission of sound due the middle ear muscle contraction has a maximum value of about 0.6 to 0.7 dB per decibel increase in stimulus level above the threshold of the reflex (approximately 80 dB SL). The reduction amounts to approximately 10 to 30 dB for loud sounds and is frequency-dependent, having more effect for low frequencies below 2 kHz. The time for the reflex action to occur is a minimum of 10 msec for high-intensity sounds and can be as long as 150 msec for relatively low-intensity sounds (near 80 dB SL). Therefore, loud sounds cause a reflex that pulls the

ossicular chair, and as a result the ossicular chain exerts less force on the inner ear. The muscles, thus, can provide a type of protection because they can reduce the amount of fatigue and damage that might exist in the inner ear from exposure to high-intensity, low-frequency, steady sound. However, such protection is probably limited for low-intensity, high-frequency, and/or abrupt-onset sounds.

Another possible function of the middle ear muscles is to limit distortion (nonlinearities). If the contact pressure between two vibrating bodies is smaller than the driving pressure acting during the vibration, the two bodies (such as the ossicular bones) will separate, and as a result of the separation a distortion of the transmitted signal could easily occur at the joint. In the middle ear when the vibrations are small, the elastic ligaments can exert a pressure sufficiently great that the ossicular bones do not separate. For larger vibrations, however, the pressure of the ligaments may not be sufficient. The middle ear muscles assist in reducing the distortion at high levels, in that they work against one another to press the stapes against the incus, thus limiting the separation and therefore distortion. Anatomically, it is also interesting that each of the middle ear muscles is enclosed throughout its length in a long, narrow canal. This permits the muscles to produce only a pull based on normal muscle action and not to be set into vibration by sound pressure in the middle ear, because the canal isolates the muscles from sound waves in the middle ear. If the muscles did vibrate due to acoustic stimulation, they would produce harmonics (nonlinearities) that could be translated to the fluids of the inner ear and could become audible. Thus, the middle ear muscles and the way in which the muscles are encased in canals reduce the chance that the acoustic signal is significantly distorted by the middle ear processes.

At moderate intensities the ossicular chain moves so that the footplate of the stapes swings about an imaginary axis drawn vertically through the posterior crus, much like a swinging door pivoting about its hinges. The anterior portion of the footplate pushes into and out of the inner ear at the oval window like a piston. This piston-like action is possible because of the asymmetric fiber length of the annular ligament. At very low frequencies (below 150 Hz) and at extremely high intensities this rotation of the footplate is thought to change dramatically. Under these conditions the axis of rotation is through the crura, becoming perpendicular to the previous vertical axis. The motion of the stapes becomes a rocking motion around the axis, much like that of a seesaw. Because of this complex form of rotation, further increases in level result in very little motion of the oval window and, hence, very little vibration of the fluids and tissue of the inner ear. This complex motion is thought to help protect the inner ear from being overstimulated at very high levels.

Despite claims that the middle ear reflexes and stapes footplate motion may provide protection, hearing loss caused by exposure to manmade environmental noises (see Chapter 16), such as some industrial noises and loud music, might be positive evidence that the ear does not have an adequate protective mechanism against our present levels of acoustic stimulation.

MIDDLE EAR AND INNER EAR IMPEDANCES

IMPEDANCE

The membranes, fluids, bones, muscles, and ligaments of the middle and inner ears all contribute to impedance, and the differences in the impedance of various tissues and fluids lead to most of the pressure changes described in this chapter. Remember from Chapter 3 that impedance is composed of resistance and reactance. The main resistive component of the middle ear is the friction of the inner ear fluid against the motion of the stapes footplate. Friction caused by the moving parts of the middle ear also contributes to the resistance, but to a lesser degree. This resistive component of the impedance does not vary with the frequency of stimulation, as the reactive components do. Two types of reactance are involved in middle ear

impedance. One is the mass reactance that is due to the mass of the middle ear structures (e.g., the ossicles). This mass reactance affects high frequencies more than low frequencies, so the impedance due to mass reactance increases with increasing frequency of stimulation. The other reactance of the middle ear is the springlike property of the ligaments and muscles. When we are referring to the ease with which a spring can be stretched, we speak of its *compliance*; but if we are speaking of the difficulty with which we can stretch a spring, we refer to its *stiffness*. Thus, stiffness and compliance are reciprocally related. In the middle ear the springlike properties affect low frequencies of stimulation (below 1 kHz) and the springlike reactance dominates impedance at low frequencies. In the middle frequencies (about 1–2 kHz) these two reactive components (mass and spring) partially cancel each other, and the resistive component dominates the middle ear impedance.

One tool used to measure the impedance of the middle ear is the *electroacoustic impedance bridge*, or just *impedance bridge*, and the measurement is often referred to as *tympanometry*. The outer ear cavity must be sealed for this measurement, and the air pressure in the outer ear is increased or decreased as the measurements are made. A very small loudspeaker presents a low-frequency tone (usually 220 Hz) into this sealed outer ear cavity. A small microphone (probe microphone) is used to record the sound pressure created by the small stimulating loudspeaker in the sealed outer ear cavity. If the middle ear is stiff, the pressure in the cavity will be higher than if the middle ear is compliant (that is, sound would be absorbed at the tympanic membrane for a compliant middle ear). Thus, the sound pressure recorded by the probe microphone can be used to measure the springlike-impedance qualities of the middle ear.

Often the middle ear impedance measured with the electroacoustic bridge is expressed in terms of compliance. This is because the impedance is usually measured at low frequency (220 Hz), and most often only the springlike quality of the middle ear is being measured. The higher the compliance, the lower the impedance and the easier the system works. The electroacoustic bridge provides a convenient method for measuring abnormal function of the tympanic membrane and middle ear (especially the ossicles) as a way to diagnose the extent to which a hearing loss may be due to abnormalities of the middle ear.

When the middle ear muscles reflexively contract due to a loud sound, the middle ear becomes less compliant (stiffer). This increased stiffness due to the middle ear muscle's contraction, or *acoustic reflex*, as it is often called, can be measured by the electroacoustic bridge. Measuring the acoustic reflex is useful for measuring the action of the middle ear muscles. That is, when the muscles contract, the compliance lessens, leading to a sudden increase in the sound level at the recording microphone of the electroacoustic bridge. The acoustic reflex is a neural reflex involving the processing of sound by the inner ear, auditory nerve, and parts of the central nervous system. Then the central nervous system sends a neural signal to the middle ear muscles to contract. Thus, acoustic reflex measurements indicate the function of all of these parts of the auditory system.

NONOSSICULAR FUNCTION OF THE MIDDLE EAR

From the point of view of evolution it is not surprising that as animals developed from living in water to living on land, a middle ear system evolved that matched the high impedance of the fluid-filled inner ear with airborne stimulation. What about those pathways to the inner ear other than the middle ear ossicle—i.e., direct air conduction and bone conduction (the first and second options listed earlier for how the inner ear could be stimulated by actions of the middle ear)? If the middle ear ossicles were missing, the inner ear could be stimulated directly by air pressure variations in the middle ear cavity. Again, because the impedance difference between air and the structures and fluids of the inner ear are so great, the inner ear fluids are driven by negligible amounts by the direct influence of sound pressure changes in the middle ear.

There is another reason why air pressure alone is not an efficient way to vibrate the fluids and structures of the inner ear. We will see in the next chapter that the *round* and *oval windows* lead to the inner ear on opposite sides of the *basilar membrane* (an important structure for the proper function of the inner ear). Positive pressure on the round window will cause the basilar membrane to move in one direction, and positive pressure on the oval window will cause it to move in the same direction. Thus, with only air pressure changes in the middle ear, both the oval and round windows would be stimulated simultaneously and in the same direction. Applying the same pressure to both windows simultaneously results in a very inefficient system because the basilar membrane would not move very much, and its movement is crucial for hearing. Thus, another function of the middle ear system is to direct the stimulation to the oval window only, allowing the round window to move according to pressure vibrations within the inner ear.

The final way the inner ear can be stimulated is by bone conduction, in which acoustic pressure changes impinging on the body cause the bones of the head (primarily the *temporal* bone, the bone on the side of the head that encases the inner ear) to vibrate, and this vibration is passed directly to the inner ear fluids. Because of the enormous difference in characteristic impedance between air and bone, stimulation of the inner ear by bone conduction does not occur as an important part of normal auditory function. If, however, a vibrator is applied to the skull, the inner ear can be stimulated (vibrated) via direct conduction of the vibration through the bones of the skull. The impedance difference between the skull and the fluids of the inner ear is small enough to allow for some of the vibration to be transmitted to the inner ear. Stimulation of the skull by a vibrator can be used during hearing diagnosis to test the viability of the middle and inner ears (see Supplement to Chapter 10). If a patient can detect bone-conducted sound normally via a vibrator placed on the mastoid but cannot detect sound delivered via air to the middle ear within the normal range, then this implies that the middle ear structures are not working properly. That is, the bone-conducted sound bypassed the middle ear to stimulate the inner ear and the person detected the sound/vibration within the normal limits, indicating that the inner ear is working normally. Because the sound that traveled through the middle ear to the inner ear was not detected within the normal range, this indicates that the middle ear may be abnormal. As discussed earlier, tympanometry is also used to asses the function of the middle ear, and tympanometry provides a more detailed description than bone-conduction measures of the abnormalities that may exist in middle ear function. Thus, the most effective way to stimulate the inner ear so that hearing sensitivity is maximized is via the interaction of tympanic-membrane and ossicular-chain motion.

SUMMARY

The outer ear consists of the pinna and the external auditory canal and ends at the lateral border of the tympanic membrane. The three ossicles (malleus, incus, and stapes) in the middle ear couple the tympanic membrane to the inner ear. Two muscles and several ligaments help support these ossicles. Transfer functions, such as the head-related transfer function, describe the spectral changes that take place as a sound travels from its source to the external auditory canal. The resonance of the external auditory canal and the tympanic membrane, along with the lever action of the ossicular chain and the area difference between the tympanic membrane and oval window membrane, help increase the air pressure at the external auditory meatus so that air pressure can drive the dense fluids of the inner ear to overcome the impedance mismatch due to the fluids and tissues of the inner ear. The transduction of sound to the inner ear via the middle ear and the ossicles is the most effective and efficient of the three ways to stimulate the inner ear. In some limited fashion, the ossicular muscles may help protect the auditory system. The structures of the middle ear provide sources of impedance for the transmission of sound to the inner ear.

SUPPLEMENT

Chapter 2 in the book by Pickles (1988) covers many of the topics of this chapter. The early research on the function of the external ear was conducted by von Bekesy (1941, 1989/**1960**), Wiener (1947), and Wiener and Ross (1946). The vibratory pattern of the tympanic membrane and of the middle ear ossicles has been the subject of research ever since 1868, when Helmholtz published his work (see Warren and Warren, 1968). Tonndorf and Khanna (1972) were among the first to suggest the complicated vibratory pattern shown in Figure 6.7b. Their results are consistent with those of Helmholtz. See also the recent work of Rosowski and colleagues (e.g., Rosowski et al., 2003). Those interested in the use of the middle ear impedance measurements in the clinic as a diagnostic tool should read Jerger and Hayes (1980) or the work by Margolis and Hunter (2000). The books by Geisler (1998) and Moller (2003) should also be consulted for a description of outer and middle ear structure and function.

It is often stated that the middle ear muscles protect against high-intensity stimulation. The middle ear reflex has a threshold of 80 dB SL and a minimum latency of 10 msec. It attenuates primarily stimulation below 2 kHz and probably not by more than about 10 dB. Thus, it protects only against gradual-onset low-frequency sounds. Von Bekesy (1989/1960) first suggested that the middle ear muscles may reduce distortion by tightening the joint between the malleus and stapes at high levels. The middle ear muscles might also help reduce sounds produced by one's own speech and mouth movements, because these actions stimulate the muscles. Guinan and Peake's (1967) work suggests, however, that a stimulus of 150 dB SPL is needed before a rocking motion occurs. Therefore, we can conclude that while the external and middle ears collect, amplify, and transmit acoustic information to the inner ear, the high incidences of deafness due to overstimulation of the inner ear make it evident that none of the suggested protective mechanisms can defend us completely against present levels of stimulation. Rosowski (1991) discusses the changes that

7

Structure of the Inner Ear and Its Mechanical Response

In Chapter 6 we considered the course of the acoustic stimulus as it traveled from the environment toward the inner ear. This chapter describes the remaining anatomy of the inner ear and how this anatomy relates to the vibratory stimulation it receives from the stapes.

In general, the motion of the stapes moves the fluid and other structures of the inner ear. This motion causes the *hair cells* of the inner ear to be stimulated and to elicit neural discharges in the auditory nerve. Thus, the mechanical energy of sound vibration is changed into neural information within the inner ear. This process is called *mechanical-to-neural transduction*. The inner ear provides the nervous system with information about the frequency, intensity, and temporal content of acoustic stimulation. Part of the spectral analysis of sound is provided by the mechanics of the inner ear in a way that can be described as *filtering*.

STRUCTURE OF THE INNER EAR

The inner ear can be divided into three parts: the *semicircular canals*, the *vestibule*, and the *cochlea*, all of which are located in the *temporal bone* region of

the skull. Three semicircular canals—*superior, posterior, and lateral*—open into the vestibule as well as the *utricle* and *saccule*. These structures affect the sense of balance (the *vestibular system*) rather than hearing. They are, however, part of the total inner ear system to which acoustic disturbances are delivered. The sensory receptor cells of the vestibular system, as in the auditory system, are *hair cells*, and the two systems (hearing and vestibular) are often discussed together. However, we will not cover the structure and function of the vestibular system (the semicircular canals, utricle, and saccule).

The vestibule is the central inner ear cavity (see Figure 7.1). In adult humans it is about 5 mm front to back and top to bottom and about 3 mm wide. The vestibule is bounded on its lateral side by the oval window, which is located in its wall facing the middle ear cavity (*tympanic wall*). The footplate of the stapes connects to the oval window. As just mentioned, the vestibule contains the utricle and the saccule, which are sense organs of the vestibular system.

The cochlea, a small shell-shaped part of the bony labyrinth shown in Figure 7.2 and illustrated schematically in Figure 7.1, contains the primary auditory organ of the inner ear. The cochlea resembles a tube of decreasing diameter, which is coiled increasingly

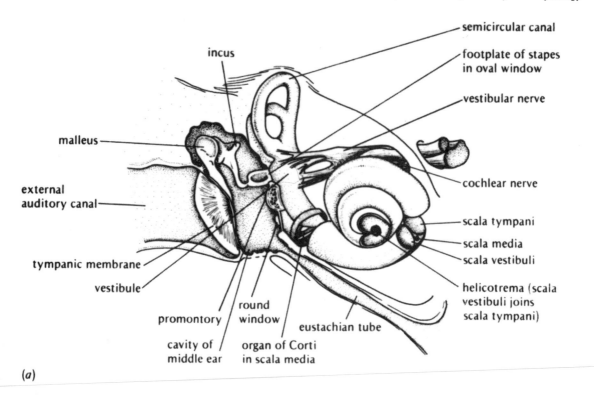

incus

semicircular canal

footplate of stapes
in oval window

vestibular nerve

malleus

external
auditory canal

cochlear nerve

scala tympani

scala media

scala vestibuli

tympanic membrane

vestibule

helicotrema (scala
vestibuli joins
scala tympani)

promontory

round
window

eustachian tube

cavity of
middle ear

organ of Corti
in scala media

(a)

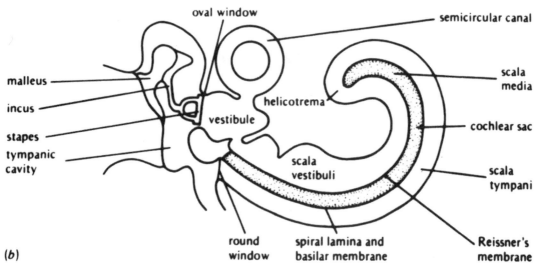

oval window

semicircular canal

malleus

scala
media

incus

helicotrema

stapes

vestibule

cochlear sac

tympanic
cavity

scala
vestibuli

scala
tympani

round
window

spiral lamina and
basilar membrane

Reissner's
membrane

(b)

FIGURE 7.1 (a) Main components of the inner ear in relation to the other structures of the ear. Adapted from Dorland (1965). (b) Schematic diagram of the middle ear and partially uncoiled cochlea, showing the relationship of the various scalae. Adapted from Zemlin (1981), with permission.

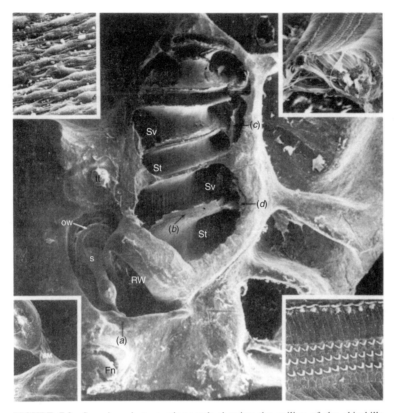

FIGURE 7.2 Scanning electron micrograph showing the coiling of the chinchilla cochlea ($3^3/_4$ turns). Also shown: S = stapes; OW = oval window; RW = round window. The insets show details at the points indicated on the central photograph (a = lower left, b = upper left, c = upper right, and d = lower right. **(a, lower left)** SM = stapedial muscle. **(b, upper left)** Tympanic layer below the basilar membrane. **(c, upper right)** Cross section of the organ of Corti. **(d, lower right)** Cilia of the inner and outer hair cells. Sv = scala vestibuli; St = scala tympani; tt = attachment of tensor tympani; Fn = facial nerve. Photograph courtesy of Dr. Ivan Hunter-Duvar, Hospital for Sick Children, Toronto.

sharply on itself, approximately $2^5/_8$ times in humans. The cochlea terminates blindly in its third turn at the *apex*. Its central axis is called the *modiolus*, which acts as an inner wall. The spiraled canal of the cochlea is about 35 mm long and is partially divided throughout its length by a thin spiral shelf of bone, known as the *osseous spiral lamina*, projecting from the modiolus (Figures 7.2 and 7.3). Across this shelf, the basilar membrane connects to the outer wall of the bony cochlea at the *spiral ligament* and completes the division of the canal into two passages (tubes or ducts), except for a small opening at the apex called the *helicotrema*. The lower passage of the canal (*scala tympani*) has an opening, known as the *round window*, which is covered with a thin membrane (*round window membrane*) that connects back to the tympanic (middle ear) cavity and separates scala tympani from the tympanic cavity. The upper passage of the canal (scala vestibule) is connected to the tympanic cavity via the footplate of the stapes and oval

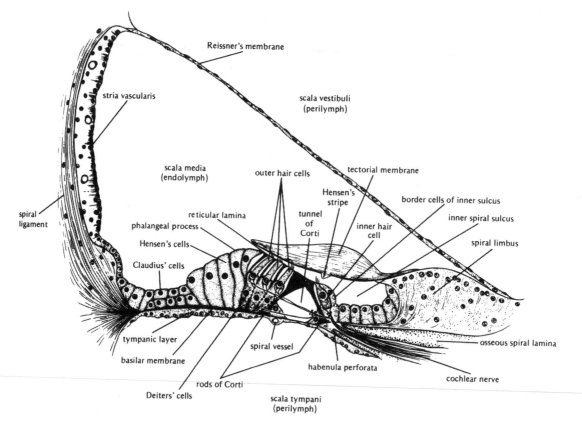

FIGURE 7.3 Drawing of a cross section of the cochlea showing the organ of Corti situated in the scala media on the basilar membrane. Drawing by Sara Crenshaw McQueen, Henry Ford Hospital, Detroit.

window and separates scala vestibule from the upper part of the tympanic cavity. A delicate membrane, *Reissner's membrane*, extends upward diagonally from the osseous spiral lamina to a region of the outer wall slightly above the *basilar membrane*; it extends the length of the cochlea to the apex, where it joins the basilar membrane at the helicotrema. Thus, there is a completely sealed sac within the middle of the cochlea, called the *cochlear sac* (or *cochlear duct*), which runs the length of the cochlea except for a small portion at the apex (at the helicotrema). The cochlear sac is bounded "above" by Reissner's membrane, "below" by the basilar membrane, and on its one "side" by the *stria vascularis*; surrounded by a watery

fluid called *perilymph*, it contains its own fluid, called *endolymph*. The stapes pushes on the oval window, causing perilymph to move through the scala vestibuli around the helicotrema to the scala tympani and then to push on the round window.

Cross sections of the cochlea, as in Figure 7.3, show the entire canal divided into three parts, ducts, or scala. These three ducts (*scala*) are the *scala vestibuli, scala tympani*, and *scala media*. The scala vestibuli extends from the oval window in the vestibule to the helicotrema. In cross sections (see Figure 7.3) of the cochlea it is usually shown as the upper scala. The scala tympani extends from the round window to the helicotrema. In cross sections it is often shown at the bottom. The scala media is the central (middle) duct, which is bounded by the basilar membrane (on the bottom), a portion of the outer wall of the cochlea, and Reissner's membrane (on the top). It is easy to remember the names of the different scalae, because the scala vestibuli lies opposite the vestibule, the scala tympani communicates with the tympanic cavity via the round window, and the scala media lies in the middle.

Almost the entire outer wall of the scala media is covered by the *stria vascularis*, which has a dense layer of blood capillaries and specialized cells. The stria vascularis has three cell layers and it produces *endolymph*, one of the cochlear fluids. The rich blood supply within the stria vascularis provides the oxygen required for the basic metabolic control of the cochlea. The great sensitivity of the cochlea requires a high level of metabolic energy. Cutting off the blood supply to the stria vascularis will quickly result in the loss of sensitive cochlear function.

The scala vestibuli and scala tympani contain the fluid perilymph, and the scala media contains the fluid endolymph (which is generated in the stria vascularis). Perilymph is primarily sodium ions (Na^+) with some potassium ions (K^+), while endolymph contains more potassium than sodium ions. Endolymph has a more positive ionic voltage (+80 mV) than does perilymph, which is near-zero ionic volts. The apical surfaces of the hair cells are bathed in endolymph, while the base, near the auditory nerve, is in perilymph. This produces a large electrochemical potential difference across the hair cells (i.e., from the scala media to the scala tympani), which is crucial for the generation of neural activity in the hair cells and then in the auditory nerve (see Appendixes E and F and Chapter 8). This biochemistry allows for the cochlea's very high sensitivity to sound.

Whereas the bony cochlea becomes smaller and smaller in cross-sectional area as the apex is approached, the basilar membrane lying within the cochlea becomes progressively wider as it approaches the apex, as shown in Figure 7.4. The osseous spiral lamina is broadest at the vestibular (basal) end, where the basilar membrane is about 0.16 mm wide; near the

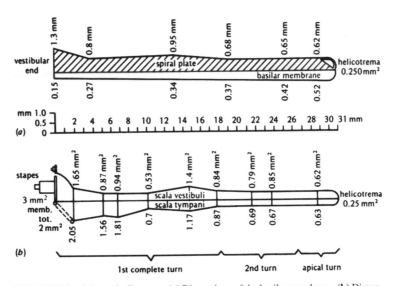

FIGURE 7.4 Schematic diagrams. **(a)** Dimensions of the basilar membrane. **(b)** Dimensions of the scalae of the human cochlea. The basilar membrane is wider at the apical end than at the basal end, but the scalae are smaller at the apex than at the base. Adapted with permission from Fletcher (1953); data are from Wrightson and Keith (1918).

helicotrema the basilar membrane has broadened to 0.52 mm. Measuring the various characteristics of the basilar membrane was of primary interest to von Bekesy, who later built models of the membrane and described its complicated pattern of motion. Current models of the cochlea and its function depend on accurate measurement of the size, shape, and weight of these cochlear structures.

From von Bekesy's and later work it can be concluded that the human basilar membrane is a stout layer of closely attached fibers about 34 mm long from base to helicotrema. It is wider, more flaccid, and under no tension at the apical end. The base end is narrower and stiffer than the apical end and may be under a small amount of tension. These facts become important in considering the vibratory pattern of the membrane in response to acoustic stimulation.

On the scala media surface of the basilar membrane lies the *organ of Corti* (see Figures 7.3 and 7.5). The organ of Corti is divided into inner and outer portions by the *pillars,* or *rods, of Corti* that lie in the approximate middle of the organ of Corti. The rods of Corti form a tunnel that is almost triangular in cross section and runs the length of the cochlear sac. The space between the rods, called the *inner tunnel of Corti,* contains a fluid called *cortilymph.* The inner portion of the organ of Corti is on the modiolar side (inside) of the rods, and the outer portion lies toward the bony cochlear wall (toward the stria vascularis).

On the inner side of the inner rods is a single row of hair cells, called the *inner hair cells,* and on the outer side of the outer rods are three or four rows of smaller hair cells, called the *outer hair cells,* with various supporting cells. The inner and outer hair cells slant toward each other and are held in place in three ways. First, cells of *Deiters* and *Hensen* serve as lateral buttresses for the outer hair cells, and the *border cells* of the inner sulcus serve the same purpose for the inner hair cells. Second, a *reticular membrane* (or *lamina*) holds the upper ends of the hair cells and assists in maintaining their alignment. Third, the Deiters cells are found below the hair cells, with one Deiters cell per hair cell. The upper end of the cylindrical Deiters cell is a cup-shaped

structure that encloses the base of the hair cell. From the cupped end of the cylindrically shaped Deiters cell a slender process passes to the surface of the organ of Corti, forming a *phalangeal process* and a part of the reticular membrane (see Figures 7.5 and 7.6). These Deiters cells and phalangeal processes form the main vertical supportive mechanism for the hair cells.

Figure 7.7 shows the detailed structure of the inner and outer hair cells and the difference in their shape. The upper surface of each inner hair cell consists of a membrane with a cuticle into which the bases of the *stereocilia* (cilia, or tiny hairs) are rooted. On each inner hair cell are about 40 cilia, arranged in two or more parallel rows that form a very shallow "U" (Figures 7.8 and 7.9a). One small area of the surface of the hair cell is cuticle free, and in this area a basal body or modified *kinocilium* is usually found. A kinocilium is an extremely long cilium found in other hair cell receptor systems. During embryonic life, the human cochlea hair cells also have a long, coarse kinocilium. After birth the kinocilium generally disappears, and only a basal body remains, although a rudiment of the kinocilium may also remain. The basal body of the inner hair cell is located on the outer edge of the cell, that is, away from the modiolus, toward the inner rods of Corti.

The upper surface of the outer hair cell contains about 150 stereocilia arranged in three or more rows on each cell in the shape of a "V" or "W" (Figures 7.8 and 7.9b). The basal body lies at the bottom of the W, toward the stria vascularis. The tips of the tallest row of cilia of each outer hair cell are in contact with a structure of colorless fibers, known as the *tectorial membrane* (Figure 7.10), while the stereocilia of the inner hair cells do not appear to contact the tectorial membrane, or, if they are in contact, it is different than that of the outer hair cell stereocilia. The tectorial membrane is a soft, ribbon-like structure attached along one edge to the spiral limbus and perhaps attached along the other edge to the outer border of the organ of Corti (near the supporting cells).

The stereocilia are arranged in an elegant geometrical form that provides a great deal of strength. Figure

FIGURE 7.5 (a) Light micrograph of a cross section of a chinchilla organ of Corti. Clearly shown are: IHC = inner hair cells; OHC = the three rows of outer hair cells; OP, IP = outer and inner pillars of Corti; TC = tunnel of Corti; TL = tympanic layer of cells below BM; D, H = supporting cells of Deiters and Hensen; Tm = tectorial membrane; HS = Hensen's stripe; ISC = inner sulcus cells; TR = a tunnel radial nerve fiber. (b) Scanning electron micrograph of a cross section of a chinchilla organ of Corti. Many of the same parts of the organ of Corti are shown, but with the advantage of added dimensionality. This view also shows the head of the IP cells between the stereocilia (Sc) of the inner and outer hair cells. BM is the basilar membrane. The Tm is pulled back to expose the stereocilia. Photographs courtesy of Dr. Ivan Hunter-Duvar, Hospital for Sick Children, Toronto.

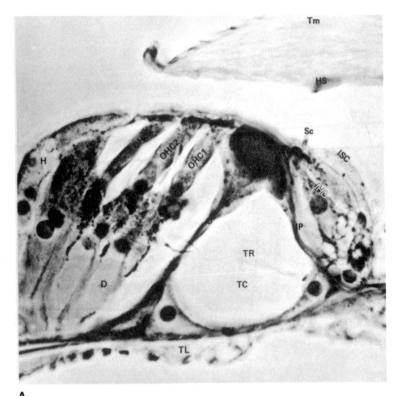

A

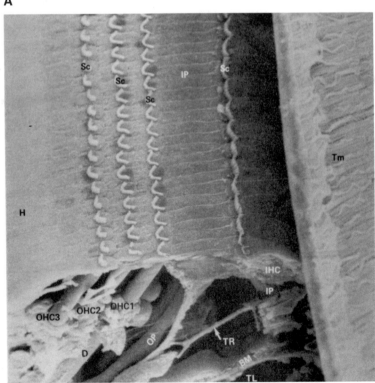

B

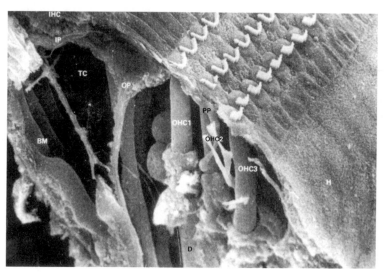

FIGURE 7.6 Scanning electron micrograph showing the supporting structure of the organ of Corti provided by Deiters cells (D) and their phalangeal processes (PP) in relation to the hair cells (OHC1, OHC 2, OHC3). The phalangeal processes arise from the top of the Deiters cells and form part of the reticular lamina at the top of the hair cells. The stereocilia are above the reticular lamina; the body of each hair cell sits in the cup-shaped top of a Deiters cell. BM = basilar membrane; H = supporting cells of Hensen; IHC = inner hair cells; IP = inner pillars of Corti. Chinchilla photograph courtesy of Dr. Ivan Hunter-Duvar, Hospital for Sick Children, Toronto.

7.11 shows the detailed structure of the stereocilia, with the strength-enhancing *cross bridges,* or *tip links.* These cross bridges help strengthen the stereocilia, and they play a crucial role in the transduction of the movement of the stereocilia into the chain of chemical events that take place within the hair cells that eventually leads to neural impulses in the auditory nerve (see Chapter 8).

The hair cells and supporting cells contain many proteins that are crucial for the function of the cochlea and especially in maintaining the high sensitivity of the cochlear structures to vibration. *Actin* and *myosin* are two proteins found within the organ of Corti, as seen in Figure 7.12. As we describe in Chapter 8, these two proteins might allow for the motile action of the outer hair cells and could play a roll in the transduction of neural potentials in the hair cells, especially in the stereocilia and tip links connecting the stereocilia. The protein *prestin* is also a candidate protein important for the motile action of the outer hair cells.

MECHANICAL RESPONSE OF THE INNER EAR

The vibratory patterns representing the acoustic message reach the inner ear via the stapes. As we have seen, the stapes moves the oval window, which causes the fluid-filled cochlea that contains the cochlear sac to vibrate. These vibratory undulations contain the information that must be coded into neural information. One key factor in this process is the mechanical response of the basilar membrane and the organ of Corti. Here we will refer to the basilar membrane instead of the whole cochlear sac, because its vibratory patterns are more easily illustrated. However, it is crucial to note that it is the biomechanical motion of the entire organ of Corti that is important for the eventual actions of the hair cells.

The general function of the cochlea, and hence of the basilar membrane, is to translate the mechanical vibrations of the stapes and the inner ear fluids into

FIGURE 7.7 (a) Transmission electron micrograph showing the detailed structure of an inner hair cell (IHC) and an outer hair cell (OHC1). The stereocilia (Sc) of the hair cell project into the scala media (Sm) and are rooted in the cuticular plate (CP). The nucleus (N) of the inner hair cell is clearly seen. At the base of the hair cell, nerve fibers of the inner spiral bundle (IS) are visible. Also shown: inner and outer pillars (IP, OP) of the tunnel of Corti (TC). (b) Transmission electron micrograph of the outer hair cells (OHC). Note the difference in shape between the IHC and the OHC. The OHC are seen sitting in the cup-shaped Deiters cell (D). At the base of the OHC, an efferent nerve fiber (E) is also seen. The space between the OHC is the space of Nuel (SN); within the SN, parts of the phalangeal processes (PP) are seen. The tops of the PP form part of the reticular lamina and separate and hold in place the hair cells. Chinchilla photographs courtesy of Dr. Ivan Hunter-Duvar, Hospital for Sick Children, Toronto.

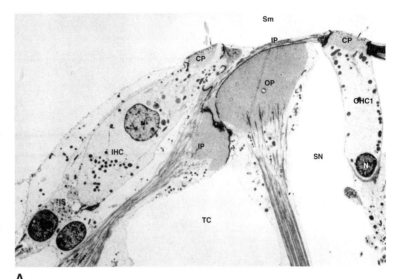

A

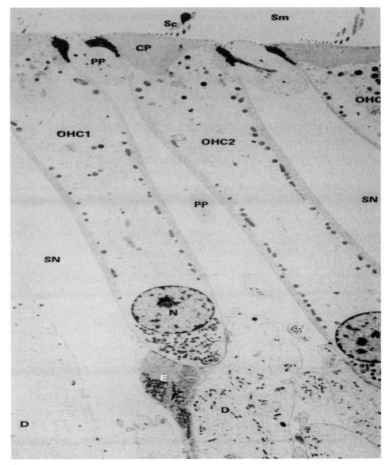

B

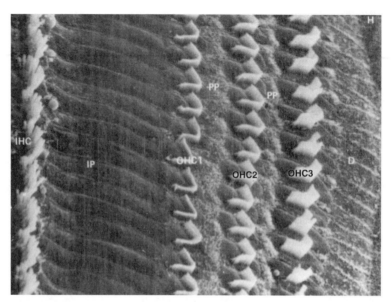

FIGURE 7.8 Scanning electron micrograph of the top of the organ of Corti, with the tectorial membrane removed to expose the stereocilia of the inner (IHC) and outer (OHC1, OHC2, OHC3) hair cells. One row of inner hair cells and three rows of outer hair cells are clearly seen. Between the inner and outer hair cells, the heads of the inner pillar cells (IP) are seen. Between the tops of the rows of outer hair cells, the tops of the phalangeal processes (PP) are seen. The supporting cells of Deiters (D) and Hensen (H) are at the outer edge. Note that the "W" formation of the stereocilia of the outer hair cells is slanted in relation to the inner hair cells and is slightly different for each row. Chinchilla photograph courtesy of Dr. Ivan Hunter-Duvar, Hospital for Sick Children, Toronto.

neural responses in the auditory branch of the VIIIth cranial nerve. The auditory nerve interacts with the hair cells by way of synaptic junctions (see Appendix E), and the hair cells are attached to the basilar membrane by the supporting cells. Thus, the vibration of the fluids causes the basilar membrane to vibrate, which in turn causes the cilia of the hair cells to bend. The bending of the cilia causes the hair cell to start the initiation of a neural potential, which is sent along the auditory nerve. Thus the hair cells, in connection with the basilar membrane, translate (*transduce*) mechanical information into neural information (the inner hair cells are the actual biological transducers).

Most of the early work that demonstrated the importance of the vibration of the basilar membrane was done by von Bekesy, using both direct observa-
tion of the cochlea and cochlear models. These early measures have been confirmed and refined by several modern methods (see Appendix F). Changing the elasticity of the round window or the length of the cochlear canals does not affect the vibratory pattern of the basilar membrane. Even altering the position of the stapes and changing the fluid does not affect the vibratory pattern of the basilar membrane. Thus, the vibratory pattern of the basilar membrane remains very stable under many conditions. This implies that the vibratory pattern must depend heavily on the characteristics of the basilar membrane itself—that is, the changes in elasticity and width discussed previously, as well as the other structures of the organ of Corti. The exact nature of the vibratory pattern of the entire cochlea (not just the basilar membrane) depends on

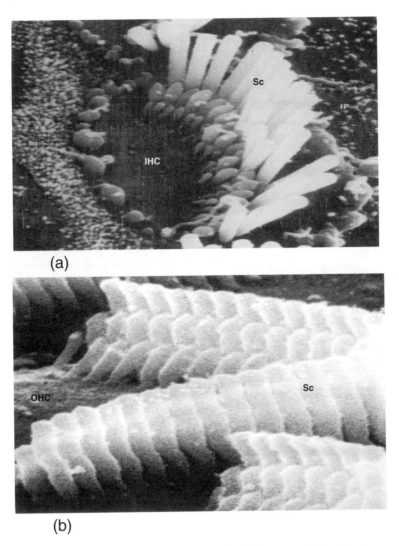

FIGURE 7.9 **(a)** Scanning electron micrograph showing the stereocilia (Sc) of an inner hair cell (IHC) in detail. Also shown: the head of an inner pillar cell (IP) and some small cilia, called *microcilia* (m). **(b)** Scanning electron micrograph showing the stereocilia (Sc) of an outer hair cell (OHC) in detail. In both photographs, the gradation in size of the stereocilia is clearly seen. Chinchilla photographs courtesy of Dr. Ivan Hunter-Duvar, Hospital for Sick Children, Toronto.

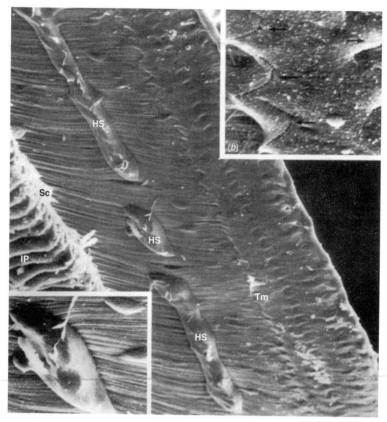

FIGURE 7.10 Scanning electron micrograph of the under side of the tectorial membrane (Tm). The inner pillar cells (IP) of the tunnel of Corti and the stereocilia (Sc) of the inner hair cells are shown at left for reference. The inserts, further magnified, show: **(a)** Hensen's stripe (HS); **(b)** the "W" imprint of the tallest row of stereocilia for each outer hair cell (arrows). These imprints are evidence that the stereocilia of the outer hair cells are in contact with the tectorial membrane. There are no imprints in the tectorial membrane corresponding to the stereocilia of the inner hair cells. Chinchilla photograph courtesy of Dr. Ivan Hunter-Duvar, Hospital for Sick Children, Toronto.

the condition of the inner ear. Even moderate damage or alterations of the inner ear can cause significant abnormal changes in the biomechanics of the cochlea.

Each point along the basilar membrane that is set in motion vibrates at the same frequency as the stimulus. However, the amplitude of the membrane vibration is different at different locations along the organ of Corti, depending on the frequency and level of the input stimulus. In a sense, a wave motion is set up

along the membrane as the fluids in the inner ear are driven by the stapes.

The basilar membrane becomes wider as the distance from the stapes to the helicotrema increases, and its flaccidity also increases toward the helicotrema; thus, the natural frequency of vibration of the basilar membrane decreases toward the helicotrema (i.e., larger, flexible membranes have lower resonant frequencies than smaller, stiffer membranes, see Chapter

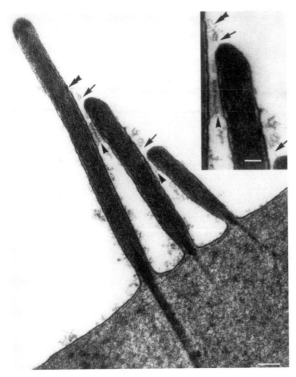

FIGURE 7.11 A high magnification of the stereocilia and the cross bridges, or tip links, shown at the arrows. The inset is a view of the tip links at higher magnification. From Osborne et al. (1988), with permission.

5). Because of the variation in width and stiffness, different frequencies will cause maximum vibration amplitude at different points along the membrane. If two different frequencies are received by the cochlea simultaneously, they will each create maximum displacement at different points along the basilar membrane. This separation of a complex signal into different maximal points of displacement along the basilar membrane, corresponding to the sinusoidal components of which the complex signal is composed, means that the basilar membrane is performing a type of spectral analysis (see Chapters 3 and 5 and Appendix C), which is often described as a type of bandpass filtering action.

The vibratory wave-motion of the basilar membrane is a *traveling wave*. A traveling wave is a wave, unlike a standing wave (see Chapter 3) that moves longitudinally. A standing wave can be generated by vibrating a string at one end when the string is attached at its other end (see Chapter 3). The attachment causes the wave motion to be reflected back to the string. To create a traveling wave, the string is vibrated at one end, but the string is not attached to anything at the other end. When the string is vibrated, it will "travel" away from the end that is vibrated and no reflections occur. The traveling wave motion of the membrane appears to travel toward the helicotrema away from the stapes. The pressure of the sound is distributed immediately throughout the cochlea because the stapes is transmitting the pressure variations to a relatively incompressible fluid environment (perilymph and endolymph). An example of the vibratory pattern along the membrane that is "frozen" or stopped at an instant in time is called an *instantaneous waveform of the traveling wave* (or *basilar membrane vibratory pattern*).

Figure 7.13 shows a representation of two instantaneous patterns of the traveling wave along the basilar membrane. The bottom figure presents a more realistic representation than the usual display (top of Figure 7.13) because the basilar membrane is shown attached at its two edges and is displaced or bent in response to sound in a transverse (medial or crosswise) direction as well as in the longitudinal direction. Most instantaneous patterns of basilar membrane displacement are shown as if Figure 7.13a were viewed from the side, the basilar membrane being represented by a single line (see Figure 7.14). Keep in mind that the condition shown in the bottom of Figure 7.13 is more accurate. Figure 7.14 shows several instantaneous patterns in successive temporal order (1–4) for a sinusoidal input. That is, curve 1 shows the basilar membrane displacement for the first instant in time, curve 2 shows the next instant in time, and so on. These instantaneous patterns indicate that one part of the basilar membrane may be displaced toward the scala tympani, while at the same time an adjacent part may be deflected in the opposite direction. This is also obvious in Figure 7.13. This difference in direction of displacement can be viewed as a local phase differ-

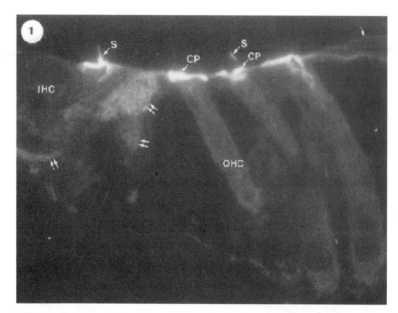

FIGURE 7.12 Autoradiograph of the organ of Corti of a guinea pig injected with an antibody against actin. The light areas on the top of the hair cells (OHC and IHC) show the areas where actin is found near the stereocilia (S) and cuticular plate (CP). The double arrows indicate regions where actin is present near the supporting cells. From Slepecky and Ulfendahl (1992), with permission.

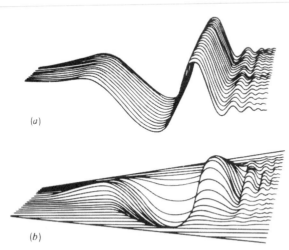

FIGURE 7.13 Instantaneous pattern of a traveling wave along the basilar membrane. **(a)** The pattern that would result if the membrane were ribbon-like. **(b)** The membrane vibration illustrated more realistically; since the basilar membrane is attached along both edges, it must vibrate in a radial or transverse direction, as in Figure 7.11. Adapted from Tonndorf (1960), with permission.

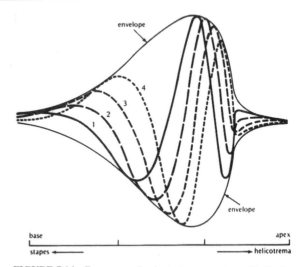

FIGURE 7.14 Four successive instantaneous patterns (1–4) of a traveling wave. The envelope (solid line) of the traveling wave formed by connecting all the points of maximum amplitude along the membrane is also shown. Adapted from Ranke (1942), with permission.

ence between the vibratory patterns of two adjacent portions of the membrane. This local phase difference is greater in the apical portion (ahead of the peak of the displacement pattern) of the wave than in the basal portion. The membrane displacement increases in magnitude as the level of the sound increases, so the greater the input sound level, the greater the amount of displacement at all locations along the membrane.

If a line is drawn through the points of maximum displacement for a specific traveling wave, the resulting curve is the *envelope of the traveling wave*. The envelope of the maximum points of positive and negative displacement of the traveling wave of Figure 7.14 is illustrated as the solid line; some illustrations of the envelope of the traveling wave show only the positive envelope. Figure 7.15 is a schematic representation of the cochlea and the envelope of the traveling wave that would occur for stimuli of three different frequencies. One instantaneous waveform is also shown for each frequency. Notice that the maximum point of the envelope is different for each frequency. For the lowest frequency (60 Hz), the maximum displacement of the envelope is near the apical end; for the highest frequency (2 kHz), the maximum displacement is near the base; and the intermediate frequency has its maximum between the other two. Figure 7.15 illustrates another important point—that is, lower-frequency stimulation will stimulate not only the basal end of the membrane but also the apical end, where the point of maximum displacement occurs. Higher frequencies, however, stimulate only the basal end of the cochlea. As shown by the envelopes of the traveling waves created by high-frequency stimulation, the amount of displacement apical to the point of maximum displacement is reduced rapidly. In contrast, the amount of displacement basal to the point of maximum displacement is reduced slowly in a basal direction for all frequencies and extends completely to the base. The traveling wave always travels from the base toward the apex. How far toward the apex it travels depends on the frequency of stimulation; lower frequencies travel farther. Figure 7.16 depicts traveling wave motion for a complex sound input consisting of two tones. The two peaks in

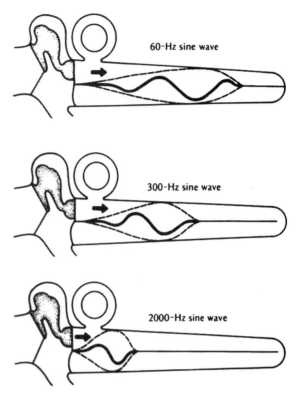

FIGURE 7.15 Instantaneous patterns and envelopes of traveling waves of three different frequencies shown on a schematic diagram of the cochlea. Note that the point of maximum displacement, as shown by the high point of the envelope, is near the apex for low frequencies and near the base for higher frequencies. Also note that low frequencies stimulate the apical end as well as the basal end but that displacement from higher frequencies is confined to the base. Adapted from Zemlin (1981), with permission.

the basilar membrane vibratory pattern are caused by the two different stimulating frequencies.

If we measure the phase relationship between the vibration of stapes and that at locations along the basilar membrane for different frequencies of stimulation, we can calculate the time it takes for the traveling wave to "travel" to a particular location on the membrane. Figure 7.17 shows the phase shift between a point on the membrane (horizontal axis) and the motion of the stapes. For instance, a 200-Hz tone will set up a vibration that moves in phase with stapedial

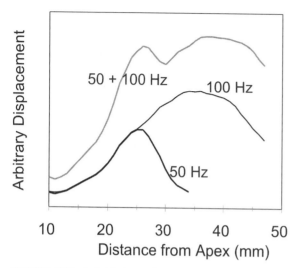

FIGURE 7.16 Individual traveling wave envelopes to a 50-Hz and a 100-Hz tone, and the envelope to a complex sound consisting of the sum of the two tones, showing two displacement peaks. Adapted from Tonndorf (1962), with permission.

motion at 20 mm from the stapes. At about 27 mm from the stapes the vibration from the 200-Hz tone is 180° out of phase with stapes vibration. Because a 200-Hz tone has a 5-msec period, the 180° phase shift indicates that the vibration at 27 mm from the stapes occurs 2.5 msec (that is, one-half period) after the stapes moves. That is, the time delay between displacement at the base (or stapes) and that at the apex results in a phase shift along the cochlear partition. Because the time delay from base to apex is relatively constant, the phase shift depends on the frequency of stimulation.

In trying to visualize these traveling wave patterns, we should keep in mind some basic characteristics of the basilar membrane motion. First, the basal end of the basilar membrane responds best to high-frequency stimulation, but it can also respond to low-frequency stimulation. The apical end of the basilar membrane vibrates only to low-frequency stimulation. Furthermore, there is a time lag between the stapes movement and the movement of the apical end of the basilar

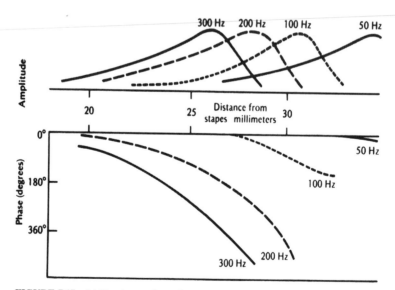

FIGURE 7.17 (a) Envelopes of traveling waves of four different frequencies. (b) The phase shift, in degrees, between the motion of the stapes and a point on the basilar membrane. By calculating the period of the sinusoid and the amount of phase shift, one can calculate the time for the traveling wave to "travel" to a particular point on the membrane. See text for an example. Adapted from von Bekesy, 1947, with permission.

membrane. Thus, high-frequency stimulation causes maximum displacement in the basal end of the membrane. Low-frequency stimulation causes the basal end to vibrate first, with a small displacement; while high frequencies cause the base to vibrate with the greatest amplitude and there is essentially no vibration at the apex. The greater the stimulus level, the greater the amount of basilar membrane displacement. And finally, the temporal pattern of basilar membrane displacement at any point along the membrane follows the temporal vibratory pattern of the stimulating sound. That is, the membrane moves up and down in synchrony with the vibrating stimulus, more at one point than at others due to the traveling wave properties. Basilar membrane displacement provides information about the frequency, level, and temporal pattern of acoustic stimulation, i.e., about the key physical parameters of any sound.

With a constant, moderately intense input, a particular location along the basilar membrane will be displaced maximally by only one frequency. It is also true that for that particular location, the basilar membrane will be displaced by frequencies lower than the one that displaces it maximally. In contrast, higher frequencies will displace that location on the membrane only a little, if at all, even at high levels. From our discussion of filters in Chapter 5, it can be seen that a given location along the basilar membrane acts as a filter with a sharp high-frequency roll-off. That is, a location along the basilar membrane will pass (or vibrate best) to only certain frequencies. Higher frequencies cause very little displacement at that place, and because lower frequencies progressively displace the membrane less and less at that location, that location also has a gradual low-frequency roll-off. Thus, a particular location along the basilar membrane acts as a bandpass filter of the vibrating motion. This filter has a sharp high-frequency roll-off for a constant, moderately intense input. We might expect that the neural output of the cochlea would reflect this filtering characteristic of the basilar membrane. This neural output and the bandpass filtering characteristics described earlier will be seen in the discharges of the individual nerves that leave the cochlea (Chapter 9).

Measurements made with the *Mossbauer* technique and with the technique of *laser inferometry* (see Appendix F) allow one to study the details of basilar membrane displacement to acoustic stimulation. Recall that the structures of the inner ear are very small and that the amount of displacement is also extremely small. Thus, inner ear structures are not easily accessible for measurement, so special techniques are required to actually measure the motion of the inner ear structures, such as the organ of Corti. Figure 7.18 shows the results of basilar membrane motion using the Mossbauer technique. These data were collected by presenting tones with different frequencies to the inner ear and measuring the level for each tone required to displace the basilar membrane a fixed but extremely small amount (1.9×10^{-8} cm). Thus, at the point of measurement along the cochlear partition of the chinchilla, an 8350-Hz (8.35-kHz) tone required the least level to displace the basilar membrane. This curve, therefore, represents the

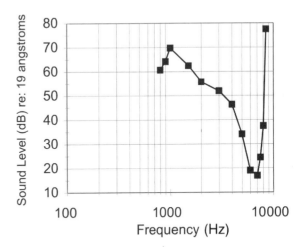

FIGURE 7.18 The amplitude required to maintain the basilar membrane at a constant displacement (1.9×10^{-8} cm) as a function of the frequency of the tonal input is shown for the Mossbauer technique for measuring basilar membrane motion in the chinchilla. The particular location at which the measurement was made had its maximum displacement when the frequency of the input was approximately 8350 Hz (8.35 kHz). Based on data from Robles, Ruggero, and Rich (1986), with permission.

responsiveness of the basilar membrane at this point (near the base) of the cochlear partition. As a result, an 8.35-kHz tone would cause the most vibration at this place along the basilar membrane, and as such this tonal frequency is called the *critical* or *center frequency* (CF). For this location along the basilar membrane, tones with frequencies higher and lower than 8.35 kHz had to have higher levels in order to vibrate the basilar membrane with the same amount of displacement as that caused by the 8.35-kHz CF tone, as is consistent with the traveling wave motion described earlier.

The measure of the biomechanical response of the inner ear can take on a variety of forms. Displacements at different points along the basilar membrane can be measured for a <u>fixed stimulus</u>, as was done in Figures 7.13 through 7.17. In Figure 7.18 the tonal level required to <u>displace the membrane a fixed distance</u> (the *isosensitivity* measure) was measured as a function of varying the tone's frequency and level. The displacement at one point along the membrane for tones of different frequencies but of constant level could also be measured.

The motion of the basilar membrane is often nonlinear. A consequence of the nonlinear motion (see Chapter 5) is that basilar membrane displacement may not be linearly related to stimulus level. Figure 7.19 shows *input–output* functions for basilar membrane velocity as a function of stimulus level for tones of different frequencies. The amount of basilar membrane velocity was measured at one point along the membrane for a 9000-Hz and a 1000-Hz tone presented at different levels. A tone with a frequency of 9000 Hz causes maximal displacement at the point along the basilar membrane where the measurements were made (i.e., 9000 Hz is the CF for this basilar membrane location). The 9000-Hz CF tone leads to a nonlinear input–output relationship between stimulus level and basilar membrane velocity, whereas the 1000-Hz tone produces a nearly linear input–output relationship (compare the data curves with the light straight—linear—line). The form of the nonlinearity for CF tones is <u>compressive</u>, in that, from about 30 to 80 dB SPL, increases in tonal level input produce less

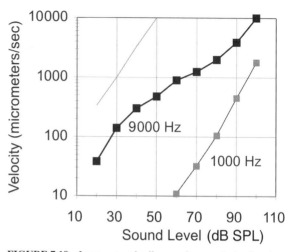

FIGURE 7.19 Input–output basilar membrane velocity functions showing basilar membrane velocity as a function of sound level for a 9000-Hz and a 1000-Hz tone. The CF for this place is 9000 Hz. The response shows a compressive nonlinearity for 9000 Hz and is linear at 1000 Hz. A straight line in the upper left of the figure is also shown for comparison. Based on data from Ruggero, Rich, and Recio (1996), with permission.

and less change in output membrane velocity as the input level increases (see Chapter 5). At very low (below 30 dB SPL) and, perhaps, at very high (above 90 dB SPL) levels the relationship appears more linear. Tones above and below the CF (e.g., the 1000-Hz tone in Figure 7.19) produce nearly linear relationships between tonal input level and output membrane velocity.

There are several consequences of this nonlinearity near the CF. First, the range over which the membrane moves is less than the range over which stimulus level varies, leading to a compression of the *dynamic range of basilar membrane motion* near the CF. Thus, <u>changes</u> in low-level sounds cause a greater <u>change</u> in basilar membrane motion than <u>changes</u> at higher stimulus levels. Note that for the 9000-Hz tone a change in sound level from 20 to 30 dB (at a low level) resulted in a change of about a factor of 4–5 in membrane velocity, while a change from 50 to 60 dB (at a higher level) resulted in a change of only about a factor of 2–3 in velocity. Second, the nonlinearity can produce distortion products such as harmonics and difference tones (see Chapter 5). As we will learn in Chapters 11, 13, and 14, listeners' perceptions are influenced by the compressive nonlinear actions of cochlear motion and listeners can detect nonlinear harmonic and difference tones.

In discussing measurements of the basilar membrane vibration, both displacement and velocity have been used. As previously mentioned, the chain of events that leads to a neural discharge in the auditory nerve starts with the bending of the stereocilia of the hair cells. The key property of this stereocilia bending may be the displacement or the velocity (displacement per unit time) or the acceleration (velocity per unit time) of the stereocilia. This factor is discussed in more detail in the next chapter. When considering the vibration of inner ear structures, the indices of level must take into account the transfer function of the outer and middle ears, in that the level of the sound (vibration) that arrives at the inner ear is different from that at the sound source in a frequency-dependent manner as determined by the various transfer functions of the torso, head, pinna, outer ear, and middle ear (see Chapter 6).

Knowing the exact motion of the organ of Corti is crucial for understanding how the neural response in the auditory nerve relates to the biomechanical response of the cochlea. If the neural response is substantially different from the biomedical response, another mechanism that helps transform the biomechanical response into the neural response must be present. If the biomechanical and neural responses are similar, then the neural response is probably reflecting faithfully the biomechanical responses of the organ of Corti. In addition, any damage to these inner ear structures will have dire consequences for how well the auditory nervous system can process sound (see Chapter 16).

This chapter described the differences in the size and shape of the basilar membrane from base to apex as these differences influence the traveling wave motion. There are other important changes in the structures of the cochlea that change from base to apex that also influence the motion of the organ of Corti and how this motion effects the bending of the stereocilia of the hair cells.

SUMMARY

The auditory part of the three major inner ear structures is the cochlea, which is divided by the basilar membrane and Reissner's membrane into three sections: scala vestibuli, scala media, and scala tympani. The scala vestibuli and scala tympani contain the fluid perilymph, and the scala media contains endolymph. The basilar membrane is supported on the modiolar side by the osseous spiral lamina and on the stria vascularis side by the spiral ligament. The basilar membrane is wider, more flaccid, and under no tension at the apical end. The base end is narrower and stiffer than the apical end and may be under a small amount of tension. In the scala media is the organ of Corti. On the inner (modiolar) side of the tunnel of Corti are the inner hair cells. On the outer side of the tunnel of Corti are the three rows of outer hair cells; their cilia are in contact with the tectorial membrane. The hair cells and nerve fibers are held in place by supporting cells. The basilar membrane has a traveling wave motion when excited by the stapes. The traveling wave yields maximal displacement, after a time delay, at the apex for low-frequency stimulation and at the base for high-frequency stimulation. Level variations cause variations in the amount of displacement of the basilar membrane, and the temporal pattern of vibration at any place along the membrane follows that of the stimulus. The motion of the basilar membrane is nonlinear, especially near the CF, where it is compressively nonlinear.

SUPPLEMENT

Chapter 3 in the textbook by Pickles (1988) covers most of the topics of this chapter. In addition, the books edited by Altschuler et al. (1989), Popper and Fay (2005), Dallos, Popper, and Fay (1996), and Jahn and Santos-Sacchi (2001) provide an in-depth overview of the anatomy and physiology of the inner ear. The books by Geisler (1998) and Moller (2003) also cover the inner ear in considerable detail. Von Bekesy pioneered our understanding of the vibratory characteristics of the basilar membrane. Much of his work is summarized in his book *Experiments in Hearing* (reprinted by the Acoustical Society of America, 1989). The work of Zheng et al. (2000) revealed the potential of Prestin to help explain the motile action of the outer hair cell. The work of Hudspeth (2005) should also be consulted regarding the structure and function of the hair cells.

To study the micromechanics of the cochlea, we must know as much as possible about the organ of Corti. However, because it is small, inaccessible, and fragile, the organ of Corti is extremely hard to investigate systematically. As we will learn in Chapter 16, the responses of the organ of Corti vary significantly if the inner ear is damaged. Thus, much of the original biomechanical work of von Bekesy does not agree in detail with that obtained with modern measures. It is now known that most of the differences are because von Bekesy worked with damaged inner ears.

Modern measurements also suggest that the responses of the auditory nerve fairly faithfully represent basilar membrane motion. Thus, the inner hair cells appear to behave as true biological transducers, changing basilar membrane vibration into neural impulses without significantly altering the information about sound provided by basilar membrane motion.

The primary distortion product generated by nonlinear basilar membrane motion is the cubic difference tone. That is, if two tones with frequencies f_1 and f_2 are presented with frequencies near the CF, then the basilar membrane will vibrate at frequencies of f_1 and f_2 and at a frequency equal to the cubic difference tone of $2f_1 - f_2$ (see Chapter 5) although the magnitude of vibration at the frequency of $2f_1 - f_2$ is less than that occurring at f_1 and f_2 (see Ruggero et al., 1992).

Some scientists have taken a comparative (studying a variety of different animals) approach to understanding the inner ear in an attempt to relate structure with function. This work demonstrates that less complex hair cell sensory systems of some nonmammalian animals can be very useful in drawing conclusions about the more complex mammalian cochlea (see Fay and Popper, 1994).

See the section on Anatomical and Physiological Measurements following the appendixes at the end of the book for data describing the sizes and weights of several of the inner ear structures.

8

Peripheral Auditory Nervous System and Hair Cells

In Chapter 7 the biomechanical, traveling wave vibration of the cochlea was described. This vibration causes the stereocilia of the hair cells to undergo a form of bending (*shearing*). The shearing of the stereocilia in turn triggers a neural response in the auditory nerve, and the neural process of hearing begins. This chapter presents some of the details on how the hair cells transduce the biomechanical vibrations of the cochlea into neural responses. Because the auditory system is extremely sensitive to sound pressure and is able to discern very small differences in frequency, the hair cells' ability to transduce vibrations into neural responses must be very effective and efficient. In addition, the transduction processes are nonlinear, and this chapter describes some of these cochlear nonlinearities. This chapter also describes the basic anatomy of the auditory nerve, in preparation for Chapter 9, in which the function of the auditory nerve is discussed.

COCHLEAR POTENTIALS

As described in Chapter 7, the cochlea contains endolymph and perilymph that produce a $+80\,mV$ potential difference. The hair cells and the auditory nerve generate biochemical-electrical potentials based on a flow of potassium and sodium into and out of these neural cells (see Appendix E). As a consequence, the intricate motions and interactions of the motions of the various cochlear structures generate several different types of electric potentials that are relatively easy to measure. Whether or not all of these potentials actually play an important role in the transduction process is an unanswered question. Even if they are nonfunctional by-products of the mechanics of the inner ear, they are of interest because they yield information about the cochlear transduction process. These potential differences can be *dc (direct current) potentials*, which are baseline potential changes that do not vary once they occur. Or these cochlear potentials are *ac (alternating current) potentials*, which change as a function of the tissue vibrations within the cochlea. Four potentials can be recorded from the cochlea:

1. *Resting potentials*, which are dc potentials that exist without acoustic stimulation.
2. The *summating potential*, which is also a dc potential but appears only during acoustic stimulation.
3. The *cochlear microphonic*, which is an ac potential difference that appears only during acoustic stimulation.
4. The *auditory action potential*, which is also an ac potential difference but is generated by the auditory nerve rather than in the structures of the cochlea.

In general, the potentials in the cochlea as well as those of the auditory nerve are measured with very small wire or glass micropipettes, as shown in Figure 8.1. The electrode measures the electric potential at the site of its penetrations relative to some reference site. The reference site might be another part of the auditory system or, more often, a neutral location, such as a neck muscle. Thus the potentials are the differences in electrical (ionic) charge between two points, for instance, between points *A* and *B* in Figure 8.1. Note that the potential differences are due to a difference in concentrations between ions in the fluids that flow in the cochlea (see Appendix E.)

RESTING POTENTIALS

Three dc potentials can be observed in the resting and responding cochlea. The one of greatest significance is the *endocochlear* or *endolymphatic potential*

(EP). The EP is located in the endolymph of the scala media. The EP is about +80 millivolts (mV); that is, the electrical charge in the scala media of a normal resting cochlea is 80 mV above 0 mV. This is the highest positive resting potential found in the body, and it is not found in the endolymph of the vestibular system despite the fact that the endolymph is continuous in both structures. This can be explained if the source of the EP is the stria vascularis, which is located on the wall of the cochlear duct but is not present in the other endolymphatic spaces (e.g., vestibular system) of the inner ear. Because the hair cells have an *intercellular* resting potential of about −70 mV, the +80 mV of the external endolymph makes the potential difference across the top of the hair cells between the inside and outside of the hair cell about 150 mV, an extremely high potential difference to be found in the body. Because of this large potential difference, it is thought that the EP could serve to increase the size of the electrical response of the hair

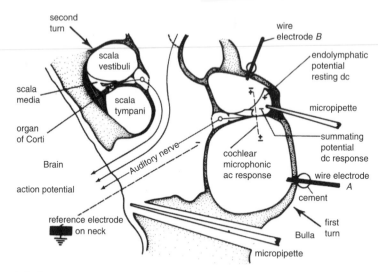

FIGURE 8.1 Drawing of a mid-modiolar section (see also Figure 8.15) of the first and second turns of the guinea pig cochlea showing where most of cochlear potentials are measured. The wire electrodes introduced into the scala vestibuli and scala tympani produce differential recordings of the cochlear microphonic (CM), action potential (AP), and summating potential (SP) from the first turn. One glass micropipette records the endocochlear potential (EP), CM, and SP from the scala media of the first turn; the other records single neurons of the auditory nerve as they exit from the modiolus. Adapted from Davis (1956), used with permission.

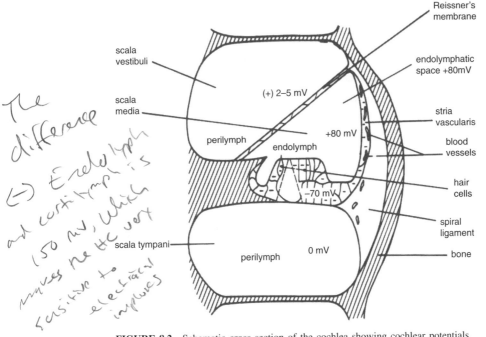

Handwritten annotation (left margin): The difference (−) Endolymph and cortilymph is 150 mv, which makes the HC very sensitive to electrical impulses

Handwritten annotation (right margin): w/o endolymph the inner ear cannot function as a mech-to-elec transducer and hearing loss will occur.

FIGURE 8.2 Schematic cross section of the cochlea showing cochlear potentials. The scala vestibuli is 2–5 mV more positive than the scala tympani. The scala media has a +80 mV potential called the endocochlear or endolymphatic potential (EP). In sharp contrast to the EP, the intracellular potentials of the hair cells are about −70 mV. Thus the potential difference across the top of the hair cells is about 150 mV. Adapted from Tasaki, Davis, and Eldredge (1954), with permission.

cells, making it a more effective and sensitive biological transducer. Damage to the stria vascularis will result in the loss, or decrease, of the EP, and without the EP, the inner ear will not perform the mechanical-to-electrical transduction process. Figure 8.2 shows the resting potentials of the three scalae of the cochlea.

SUMMATING POTENTIAL

The summating potential (SP) is a stimulus-related dc electrical response recorded from the cochlea. There is a baseline shift in the potentials recorded from the cochlea whenever a stimulus is present, as shown in Figure 8.3. This baseline shift can be either in the positive or negative (voltage) direction (it is

shown as negative going in Figure 8.3). Experimenters who have attempted to quantify the SP have found it to be composed of different potentials, which interact in a complicated manner. There have been as many as six sources suggested for the generation of the SP.

COCHLEAR MICROPHONIC

The cochlear microphonic (CM) is an ac potential that occurs only during the presentation of an acoustic stimulus. For instance, if the ear is stimulated with a 500-Hz pure tone of moderate level, the CM will appear as a 500-Hz electrical sine wave that is recorded within the cochlea. In other words, the electrical potential difference measured in the cochlea, the CM, oscillates in

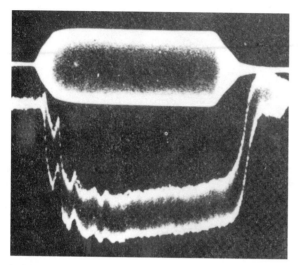

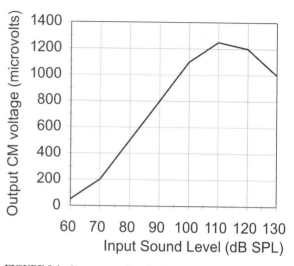

FIGURE 8.3 The upper trace records the stimulus, a 21.5-kHz tone burst. The lower trace is a round-window electrode recording the response to the stimulus. The downward dc shift of the trace during the presentation of the stimulus is the summating potential (SP). The section of the recording that replicates the input signal is the cochlear microphonic (CM). The wiggle at the beginning of the response as it begins its downward shift is the action potential (AP). The round-window recording technique, therefore, yields a composite response composed of SP, CM, and AP. From Pestalozza and Davis (1956), used with permission.

FIGURE 8.4 Input–output function (or intensity function) for the cochlear microphonic (CM) response recorded differentially from the first turn of the guinea pig cochlea (see Figure 8.1 for electrode placements) to an 8-kHz tone burst. As the sound pressure level (SPL) increases to 90 dB, the CM increases linearly. From 90 to about 100 dB SPL, the CM increases at a slower rate (the function is compressively nonlinear). For this stimulus the CM is largest at about 100 dB SPL and then decreases as the input intensity increases beyond 100 dB SPL.

the same manner as the driving stimulus. From observations of the level of the CM and its temporal oscillatory shape, it appears that over a fairly wide range of sound levels the CM faithfully reflects the intensity and frequency components of the sound input. If the sound intensity becomes too high, however, the voltage level of the CM stabilizes and then decreases in magnitude. Figure 8.4 is one example of the growth of the level of the CM output as a function of the level of the input sinusoid. Such intensity curves are sometimes called *input–output functions*. Repeated or lengthy stimulation at extreme sound levels results in either temporary or permanent impairment of hair cell function (see Chapter 16), which is clearly manifest in a decline in CM level. Consequently, understanding the decline in the CM input–output function at high levels may provide clues to preventing impairment of hair cell function caused by overstimulation.

The source of the CM is thought to be the cilia-bearing end of the outer hair cells. This can be inferred when a recording electrode approaches the top of a hair cell. The CM becomes larger and then reverses its electrical signal phase as the electrode passes through the organ of Corti. That is, if in the scala tympani the CM potential was positive, the CM becomes negative when the electrode enters the scala media. The growth in CM level and CM polarity reversal indicates that its generation is at the boundary of the hair cells and the scala media, near the level of the reticular lamina and the roots of the cilia of the hair cells.

The level of the CM is proportional to the displacement of the basilar membrane. This fact, together with the ability to record from small areas along the cochlear partition by the differential electrode technique (recording the CM with a technique that allows for the cancellation of the SP and the ability to record from local regions of the organ of Corti), led to the electrophysiological investigation of the motion of the basilar membrane by means of the CM. That is, the CM has been used to measure the displacement action of the basilar membrane. The level of the CM measured at each of several cochlear locations for different stimulating frequencies reveals a traveling wave that moves toward the apex to a location dependent on the frequency of the stimulus. This pattern agrees well with the mechanical movement observed by von Bekesy in his models. That is, the apical end of the cochlea responds to only low frequencies, but the basal end responds to all frequencies. Figure 8.5 shows that a low-frequency (500-Hz) tone generates a CM in all turns of the cochlea, along the entire basilar membrane. However, the amplitude of the CM is greatest at the apex (third turn), and a phase shift occurs (180° at 500 Hz) between the first-turn (base) recording and the third-turn recording. A high-frequency tone (8000 Hz), however, generates a CM only in the first turn (base) of the cochlea. This agrees exactly with the characteristics of the traveling wave discussed in Chapter 7. Thus, even with the recent developments of laser light and Mossbauer techniques, the CM remains (with certain limitations) a useful tool for studying the traveling wave motion of the cochlear sac to a wide range of levels and frequencies of stimulation. The CM also has the advantage that it can be measured using noninvasive or nearly noninvasive techniques, whereas most other measures of cochlear function are highly invasive. Thus, even though the CM is an indirect measure of cochlear function, it is relatively easy to measure in a wide variety of conditions.

AUDITORY ACTION POTENTIAL

The whole auditory nerve action potential (AP), unlike the other potentials discussed, is not a true cochlear potential, although it can be recorded from the cochlea. The AP is the sum of the action potentials of many individual auditory neurons that are firing nearly simultaneously within the bundle of auditory nerves (see Chapter 9. Because stimulation of the individual neurons depends on the displacement of the basilar membrane, neurons that innervate the base of the cochlea will be stimulated at an earlier point in time than those at the apex. The time difference is the length of time it takes the traveling wave to move from the base to the apex (i.e., 2.5 to 4 msec, depending on the animal species tested and the measuring technique). This situation creates a general asynchrony of discharge among the individual neurons, which terminate at different points along the cochlea. Because each neuronal discharge consists of potentials with both positive and negative values that vary in time (see Appendix E), the potentials tend to cancel each other or to sum only partially. However, at the onset of a click or of a high-frequency tone burst with a sudden

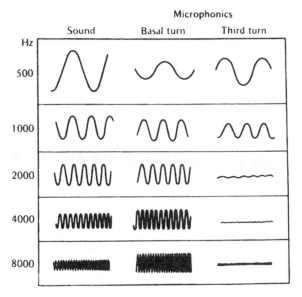

FIGURE 8.5 Cochlear microphonics (CMs) recorded differentially from the first and third turns of the guinea pig cochlea. Rows: responses to the various frequencies. Column 1: acoustic stimulus. Columns 2 and 3: CM from turns 1 and 3. For 500 Hz, the CM is larger in turn 3 than in turn 1. Also, the 500-Hz CM shifts 180° out of phase between turns 1 and 3 because of the time taken by the traveling wave of displacement to reach turn 3. For the highest-frequency stimulus used (8000 Hz), the response only in turn 1 indicates that the traveling wave does not reach turn 3. See Figure 7.17 for a similar set of responses from the traveling wave. Adapted from Davis (1960), used with permission.

onset, only the basal end of the cochlea is stimulated initially. The near-simultaneous discharge of a large number of neurons in the base is then followed by less-synchronous nerve impulses from more apical locations of the cochlear partition. The sum of the initial synchronous discharges of nerve impulses from many basal fibers to an abrupt high-frequency tone burst or click produces a fairly large potential, which is the major part of the AP. AP is at first negative and then positive, and it is usually followed by a later negative component arising from the nerves that innervate more apical portions of the cochlea and possibly other, more central, sources of potentials. Figure 8.3 shows the waveform of an AP superimposed on the CM at the beginning of the recording (the part of the recording as it first goes negative toward its SP baseline). The most widely used stimulus for AP studies is the click (Chapter 4) because a click has a sudden onset and a broadband amplitude spectrum.

Within the limitations we have mentioned (i.e., the overwhelming contribution of auditory nerve fibers in the basal turn), the AP reflects grossly the neural output of the cochlea as information is being sent along the auditory nerve bundle. The input–output function and waveshape of the AP from a normal cochlea are known, and so deviations from normative data can be used as indications of cochlear dysfunction. This is particularly important because the AP can be recorded for humans, and as a consequence the AP can be used to access human cochlear function.

HAIR CELLS, STEREOCILIA, OUTER HAIR CELL MOTILITY, AND NEURAL TRANSDUCTION

The hair cells stimulate a neural response that is sent to the auditory nerve via the bending of the hair cells' stereocilia. Recall that the hair cells and their stereocilia are located between the tectorial membrane and the basilar membrane. When the basilar membrane vibrates, the tectorial membrane must also move, but there is an important difference in the motion of the two membranes due to differences in

their support. As shown in Figure 8.6, the tectorial membrane is hinged on one end at the spiral limbus, whereas the modiolar edge of the basilar membrane is thought to be hinged on the osseous spiral lamina. As the basilar and tectorial membranes are displaced, they pivot about the two hinging points, and the indicated shearing forces are created. The actual method of shearing is probably different for inner and outer hair cells, because the stereocilia of outer hair cells appear firmly attached to the tectorial membrane, while the stereocilia of inner hair cells are probably not attached to tectorial membrane. For the inner hair cells, the fluids trapped between the stereocilia and tectorial membrane probably cause inner hair cell stereocilia shearing. Shearing is a particular form of bending in which the top of the stereocilia moves more than the bottom.

Thus, mechanical energy is transduced into electrochemical activity in the hair cell by the shearing of the hair cell's stereocilia. In order to function well over a long period of time and to provide a connection between the hair cell and the tectorial membrane, the stereocilia need to be strong and resilient to breakage. The stereocilia are arranged in an elegant geometrical form that provides a great deal of strength (see Figure 7.9). It is believed that the transduction of neural information in the hair cell takes place near the top of the hair cells in the region of the stereocilia. In experiments in which a hair cell is excised from the organ of Corti (see Appendix F) and the stereocilia are carefully displaced small amounts with a micropipette, recordings of electrical changes either within the hair cell (*intercellular recordings*, again see Appendix E) or near the hair cell (*extracellular recordings*) implicate the top of the hair cell and a region near the bottom of the shortest stereocilia as the sites where neural transduction is most likely occurring.

In order for the hair cell to transduce stereocilia shearing into a neural response, the permeability of the hair cell membrane must change to allow for neural transduction of sodium and potassium ions into and out of the hair cell (see Appendix E). It is believed that the tip links (see Figure 7.11) aid in causing *"ion channels"* to open and close near the top of the hair

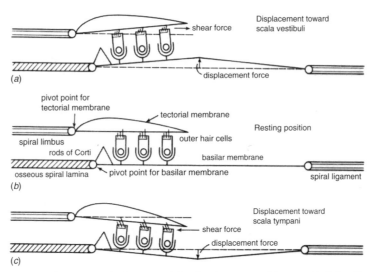

FIGURE 8.6   Schematic diagrams of shearing forces created between the hair cells and the tectorial membrane as a result of basilar membrane displacement. **(a)** Shearing force that results from displacement of the basilar membrane toward the scala vestibuli. **(b)** Relationship between hair cells and the tectorial membrane with no stimulation. **(c)** Shearing forces in the direction opposite to that in panel (a) for displacement in the opposite direct. Note how the stereocilia bend (shear) in each panel. Adapted from Zemlin (1981), used with permission.

cell. These channels allow for ionic transport into and out of the hair cell that is necessary for neural transduction. As the tip links stretch and contract during the shearing of the stereocilia, they may act to open and close a type of trapdoor on the stereocilia, and the trapdoor allows for ions to flow in and out of the hair cell, starting the neural transduction process.

There are two types of hair cells—inner and outer—and they differ in several important ways. The next section explains additional differences between the two types of hair cells that lead to a theory as to how the two types of hair cells work together allowing for the exquisite sensitivity and frequency-resolving capacity of the inner ear. These interactions also account for the nonlinear properties of cochlear function. In general, the inner hair cells act as the actual biological transducers that start the neural process of hearing. The outer hair cells serve a very different function, allowing for the highly sensitive biomechanical vibrations that occur within the cochlea based on the cycle-by-cycle changes in the stimulating sound.

OUTER HAIR CELLS AND MOTILITY

So far we have described the changes that occur within the organ of Corti when sound is present in terms of the passive reaction of the tissue to vibration. The outer hair cells exhibit a type of active response, in that they change their size in response to acoustic stimulation. That is, when stimulated, the outer hair cells expand and contract. The outer hair cells' stereocilia shearing and the transduction that occurs during the motion of the tip links trigger a motile change in the size of the outer hair cells. Inner hair cells do not exhibit this *motility*.

The changes in hair cell size, primarily length, appear to take place on two different time scales. There is a fast motility (changes that occur within 0.15 to 0.2 msec after stimulation) that probably can take place on a cycle-by-cycle basis for all frequencies of stimulation. The slower change that takes place in hair cell length after stimulation (changes that take place after several seconds) might reflect some slower biochemical action, such as that which occurs when muscles contract. The ability of the outer hair cells to change size at the rate of the change in sound pressure requires that the outer hair cell is responding as fast as 20,000 times per second (20,000 Hz is the upper limit of audible frequencies; see Chapter 10). Such rapid changes require special mechanisms since normal neural processes cannot change this fast. It is known that the outer hair cells contain some of the crucial proteins (actins) for muscle-like contractions and, therefore, might contract and expand based on similar principles. The protein prestin is especially important in allowing for the fast motile response of outer hair cells. Figure 8.7 shows changes in outer hair cell length as a function of changing the voltage on the excised hair cell in a patch-clamp experiment (see Appendix F). Note that the length decreases with increasing voltage (*depolarization*; see Appendix E) more than it increases with decreasing voltage (*hyperpolarization*; see Appendix E). Not only do the outer hair cells themselves change, but because they are attached to the tectorial membrane by means of the stereocilia, such changes affect the connection between the basilar and tectorial membranes. Thus, changes in the length of the outer hair cells causes a change in the biomechanical vibratory pattern of the cochlea during the time of sound stimulation. Such changes might allow for the high sensitivity of cochlear responses, the ability of the cochlea to respond differently to different sound frequencies, and the nonlinear cochlear function.

Outer hair cell motility is also influenced by efferent fibers that come from the brainstem (the *olivocochlear bundle*; see below) and directly synapse on the outer hair cell. This efferent control of outer hair cells is a slow process because of the time it takes for a neural signal to be sensed, travel to the brainstem, and then travel back down to the outer hair cell. Because the innervation pattern of the olivocochlear bundle fibers comes from brainstem nuclei on both sides of the brain, efferent control of outer hair cell function is bilateral. The exact role of efferent control of outer hair cell function is not well understood.

INNER HAIR CELLS, THE AUDITORY BIOLOGICAL TRANSDUCER

Most of the fibers in the auditory nerve connect with the inner hair cells. Thus, the inner hair cells are the biological transducers for sound. When the stereocilia of the outer hair cells are sheared and the tip links open and close ion channels, a neural signal is generated in the inner hair cell. This neural action of the inner hair cell causes a neural spike to be generated in the auditory nerve fiber that innervates the hair cell at its base. The greater the displacement of the organ of Corti, the more shear that is imparted to the stereocilia and the more likely it is that the inner hair cell will cause a neural discharge in the auditory nerve. The stereocilia shear in phase with the vibratory pattern of the organ of Corti, so the neural response can also follow the vibratory pattern of sound (at least up to some frequency limit). Thus, the inner hair cell can somewhat faithfully code for the stimulus properties of sound as it is relayed to the inner hair cell via the biomechanical traveling wave motion of the inner ear.

THE ROLES OF INNER AND OUTER HAIR CELLS

The general theory is that the stereocilia of the outer hair cells senses the vibrations within the cochlea that cause a change in the length (and width) of the outer hair cell. This motility affects a change in the mechanical coupling between the basilar and tectorial membranes. Presumably this coupling is chang-

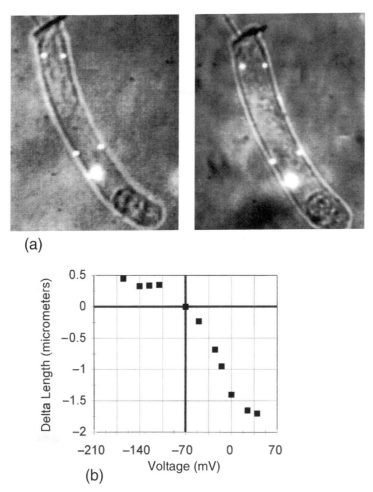

FIGURE 8.7 **(a)** An example of the change in the length of an outer hair cell due to electrical stimulation. The hair cell was excised from the cochlea in an in vitro experiment. The picture on the left shows the hair cell before chemical stimulation with potassium, and the picture on the right show the decrease in length and increase in width after stimulation. From Zajic and Schacht (1991), with permission. **(b)** Change in the length of an outer hair cell as a function of applying hyperpolarizing and depolarizing voltages to the hair cell. From Ruggero and Santos-Sacchi (1997), used with permission.

ing in synchrony with the vibrations within the cochlea, even when these vibrations occur at very high frequencies. In so doing, the changes in the coupling make the vibratory pattern of the cochlear partition very sensitive to small vibrations and highly fre-

quency selective. This vibratory pattern also reflects significant nonlinear responses, which are crucial for the proper functioning of the inner ear. The stereocilia of the inner hair cells are sheared in response to the sensitive cochlear vibrations, and the neural response generated within the inner hair cell is transmitted to the auditory nerve fibers that innervate the inner hair cell and sends a neural signal up the auditory nerve bundle to the brainstem. Thus, the outer hair cells seem to *feed back* energy into the cochlea via its motility, and as a consequence the sensitivity of the cochlea is amplified, making it easier for the inner hair cells to respond. This leads to the concept that the outer hair cells help provide a *cochlear amplifier* for transducing small vibrations into neural impulses.

In addition to frequency tuning caused by the traveling wave (i.e., the fact that one place along the basilar membrane responds selectively to tones of different frequencies), the hair cells themselves are also most likely frequency tuned. This is certainly true in many amphibians. The hair cells and their stereocilia can be tuned either mechanically or electrically or both. *Mechanical tuning* means that the shearing of the stereocilia is frequency specific, in that, independent of the traveling wave, the stereocilia shear more to some frequencies than to others. *Electrical tuning* means that in the generation of a neural response via the movement of ions into and out of the hair cell, the properties of this ion exchanges causes the cell's biochemical voltages to be dependent on the frequency of stimulation. The extent to which hair cell tuning occurs in mammalian systems and whether such tuning has a significant influence on frequency resolution are still subject to debate.

Thus, the loss of outer and/or inner hair cells can lead to several different forms of hearing abnormalities. As Chapter 16 explains in more detail, the ability of the inner ear to efficiently transduce vibration into a neural response is seriously compromised when either the inner or outer hair cells are damaged. Outer hair cell damage causes a significant loss in sensitivity and frequency resolution, in that the outer hair cells help provide for the high sensitivity and high-frequency resolution of the cochlea so that inner hair cell transduction will also be highly sensitive and exhibit high-frequency resolution. As is also discussed in Chapter 16, hair cells in mammalian species do not regenerate after they are damaged, but hair cells in birds and fish do appear to regenerate.

COCHLEAR EMISSIONS

If a click is delivered to the outer ear canal, then approximately 5 to 10 msec after the click has ceased, sound may be recorded within the sealed outer ear canal as if there were an echo from the inner ear to the click. Although there is no evidence that this "echo" is a cochlear potential, the data show that the echo comes from the cochlea and not from the middle ear or from neural activity in the central nervous system. And, as we discuss later in the chapter, the source of the "echo" is related to the motility of the outer hair cells. In addition to the recording of an acoustic echo in the outer ear, there is also evidence of tonal-like emissions measurable within the outer ear that appear to originate from the cochlea in the absence of any external acoustic stimulation. Both the *acoustic echo* (usually referred to as an *otoacoustic emission*, OAE, or *evoked otoacoustic emission*, EOAE) and the *cochlear emission* (usually referred to as *spontaneous otoacoustic emissions*, SOAEs) are very low in level (near or below the thresholds of hearing), and the nature of the phenomenon varies from person to person and from animal to animal. However, almost every person with normal hearing shows evidence of some form of otoacoustic emission (people with abnormal functioning of the inner ear usually do not have otoacoustic emissions), although the variability from person to person (and even ear to ear) can be large.

Three types of evoked emissions, or echoes, are typically measured: *transiently evoked otoacoustic emission* (TEOAEs), *distortion-product otoacoustic emissions* (DPOAEs), and *single-frequency otoacoustic emissions* (SFOAEs). The TEOAE is evoked by a click and the SFOAE by a short-duration sinusoidal sound delivered to the outer-ear canal, and the echo's time-domain waveform and its amplitude spectrum are measured in the sealed outer ear cavity. If tonal stimuli (SFOAE) are used, the emission contains frequencies near that of the stimulating tone. If a click is used (TEOAE), then the spectrum of the emissions often have several narrow spectral peaks that are not directly related to the frequency content of the

[handwritten margin note: Outer / spiral fibers (type II) innervate 10 OH cells.]

AFFERENT FIBERS

There are two types of auditory afferent fibers: (1) *radial fibers* (R), or *Type I fibers*, and (2) *outer spiral fibers* (OS), or *Type II fibers*. The radial fibers comprise about 85% to 95% of the afferent fibers. As illustrated in Figure 8.9, Type I fibers innervate the inner hair cells exclusively, each fiber innervating the base of only one or two inner hair cells and then leaving the organ of Corti through an opening in the osseous spiral lamina called *habenula perforata* to travel to the modiolus. Figure 8.10 is a transmission electron micrograph showing the path taken by the radial fibers. There are about 45,000 or 50,000 afferent fibers in the cat, and 95% of them are thought to innervate the 2600 inner hair cells. Thus, each inner hair cell may be innervated by 16 to 20 radial fibers, as shown schematically in Figure 8.9. Similar calculations for the human cochlea estimate that an average of eight radial fibers would innervate one or two inner hair cells. Thus, the radial, or Type I, fibers are said to have a many-to-one connection to the inner hair cells. The Type I fibers tend to be thicker than the Type II fibers.

The Type I radial fibers may also differ in how they innervate the inner hair cells.

The other 5% to 15% of the afferent fibers are the outer spiral, or Type II, fibers and are said to have a one-to-many connection, as shown in Figure 8.9. In the basal area the outer spiral fibers innervate the outside row of the outer hair cells. As they move in an apical direction they innervate the middle and finally the innermost row of outer hair cells. They then travel further in an apical direction for about 0.6 mm, finally crossing along the floor of the tunnel of Corti between the pillar cells and through the habenula perforata to the modiolus. The involved course of the outer spiral fibers along the base of the first row of outer hair cells is shown in Figure 8.11. Figure 8.12 shows endings of a number of outer spiral fibers at the base of an outer hair cell. On the average each outer spiral fiber innervates about 10 outer hair cells. Thus, the afferent fibers in the auditory nerve innervate either one or a small number of hair cells.

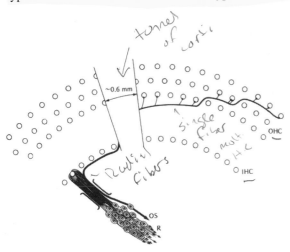

FIGURE 8.9 Horizontal schema of the afferent innervation of the organ of Corti. OS is an outer-spiral, Type II fiber that crosses the tunnel of Corti in the middle and innervates 10 or so outer hair cells (OHCs). R are the radial, Type I fibers going to one or two inner hair cells (IHCs). From Spoendlin (1978) in Naunton and Fernandez (1978), used with permission.

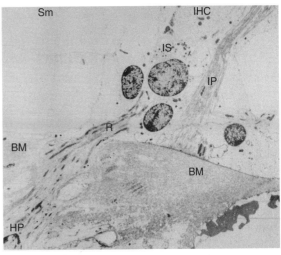

FIGURE 8.10 Transmission electron micrograph showing the radial fibers (R) entering the habenula perforata (HP) and going toward the base of the inner hair cell (IHC). The fibers of the inner spiral bundle (IS) are also seen in their path below the base of the IHC. For orientation, the following are also labeled: BM = basilar membrane; IP = inner pillar cell; Sm = scala media. Chinchilla photograph courtesy of Dr. Ivan Hunter-Duvar, Hospital for Sick Children, Toronto.

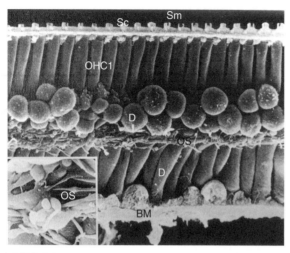

FIGURE 8.11 Scanning electron micrograph of the first row of outer hair cells (OHC1) and supporting Deiters cells (D), as seen from the tunnel of Corti with the outer pillar cells removed. At the base of the outer hair cells the fibers of the outer spiral bundle (OS) are seen. The inset shows their interwoven pattern in detail. Note that the Deiters cells at the base of the first row of hair cells have bulges rather than the phalangeal processes shown arising from the Deiters cells beneath the third row of outer hair cells as in Figure 7.6. BM = basilar membrane; Sm = scala media. Chinchilla photographs courtesy of Dr. Ivan Hunter-Duvar, Hospital for Sick Children, Toronto.

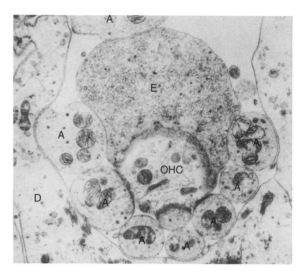

FIGURE 8.12 Transmission electron micrograph showing many afferent nerve fibers (A) coming from the outer spiral bundle surrounding the base of an outer hair cell. A large efferent nerve ending (E) is also seen. D = Deiters cells. (The inset shows the location of the section, in the area of the middle outer hair cell; see Figure 7.5.) Chinchilla photograph courtesy of Dr. Ivan Hunter-Duvar, Hospital for Sick Children, Toronto.

EFFERENT FIBERS

The efferent innervation of the hair cells is by the *olivocochlear bundle* (OCB), which is series of nerves that come from the *olivary complex* (*olive*) in the auditory brainstem to the hair cells in the organ of Corti (see Chapter 15 for a discussion of the auditory brain stem). The efferent fibers that come to the inner ear from the olivary region of the brain stem (Figure 8.13) on the same side are called the *uncrossed olivocochlear bundle*, or UCOCB. That is, UCOCB fibers come from the olivary region on one side of the head to the cochlea on that same side (*ipsilateral side*). The bundle of efferent fibers that arises from the olive on the opposite side is called the *crossed olivocochlear bundle*, or COCB. That is, COCB fibers come from the olivary region on one side of the head to the

cochlea on the other side of the head (*contralateral side*). The OCB fibers can originate from a location that is lateral within the olivary complex (the *lateral olivary complex*, LOC) or from locations that are medial within the olive (the *medial olivary complex*, MOC). The LOC fibers project predominantly to the inner hair cells and the MOC fibers to the outer hair cells. Figure 8.13 shows the distribution and innervation of OCB fibers for the cat. The LOC fibers synapse on the afferent nerves leaving the inner hair cells, while the MOC fibers synapse directly on the outer hair cells. Figure 8.14 shows the synapse of an MOC efferent fiber on an outer hair cell.

ORGANIZATION OF THE AUDITORY NERVE BUNDLE

The auditory nerve fiber anatomy may be outlined as follows:

[Handwritten annotations at top of page: "both efferent and afferent fibers do not have myelin from OC to ? perforate"]

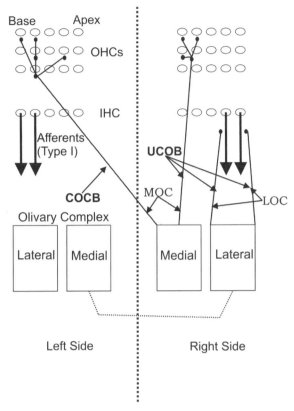

FIGURE 8.13 A simplified schematic diagram showing the olivocochlear bundle (OCB) connections to the inner ear. The crossed (COCB) medial olivary complex (MOC) fibers (26% of the OCB fibers in the cat) synapse directly on the outer hair cells (OCH$_s$) toward the base of the contralateral cochlea, the uncrossed (UCOB) lateral olivary complex (LOC) fibers (48% of the fibers in the cat) fibers synapse on the Type I afferents coming from the ipsilateral inner hair cells (IHCs) located more apically, the uncrossed MOC (11%) and crossed LOC (15%) fibers make up a much smaller proportion of the fibers in the OCB. Based on data from Warr (1992).

1. Afferent fibers
   a. Radial, or Type I, fibers from inner hair cells.
   b. Outer spiral, or Type II, fibers from outer hair cells.
2. Efferent fibers
   a. Lateral olivary complex fibers coming from the lateral areas of the olivary complex that are either uncrossed olivocochlear bundle fibers coming from the same lateral olivary

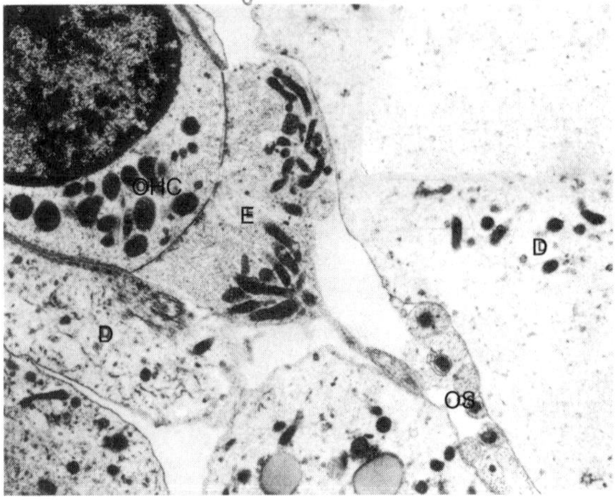

FIGURE 8.14 Transmission electron micrograph showing an efferent nerve ending (E) at the base of an outer hair cell (OHC). Fibers of the outer spiral bundle (OS) are also seen. D = Deiters cells. Chinchilla photograph courtesy of Dr. Ivan Hunter-Duvar, Hospital for Sick Children, Toronto.

complex or crossed olivocochlear bundle fibers that come from the opposite lateral olivary complex.
   b. Medial olivary complex fibers coming from the medial areas of the olivary complex that are either uncrossed olivocochlear bundle fibers coming from the same medial olivary complex or crossed olivocochlear bundle fibers that come from the opposite medial olivary complex.

Both the efferent and afferent fibers are devoid of their insulating myelin sheaths between the organ of Corti and the habenula perforate (see Appendix E). The nerve fibers leave the cochlea through the habenula perforata in an ordered manner and are gathered in a twisted bundle within the modiolus. The nerve fibers that innervate hair cells at the apex are in the middle of the nerve bundle. Fibers from cochlear turns toward the base make up the outside fibers of the nerve bundle. Figure 8.15 shows a cross section of the cochlea with the apex at the top; the middle of the cross section is the modiolus. The fibers from the apex run down the middle of the modiolus, and those from

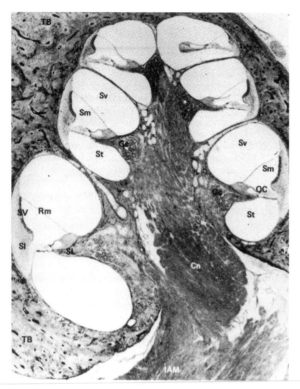

FIGURE 8.15 Light micrograph of a mid-modiolar section of a cat cochlea. The cochlear nerve (Cn) is seen in the modiolus. Fibers from the apical turns form the center of the cochlear nerve, while the basal turn fibers join with the nerve at its outer edges. The nerve leaves the cochlea via the internal auditory meatus (IAM). Photograph courtesy of Dr. Ivan Hunter-Duvar, Hospital for Sick Children, Toronto.

the other turns of the cochlea form the outside of the nerve bundle. Thus, fibers carrying low-frequency information (from the apex) are in the middle of the auditory nerve bundle, whereas high-frequency fibers (toward the base) are on the outside of the bundle. The auditory nerve bundle is joined by nerves from the vestibular system to form the entire VIIIth nerve tract. After the auditory nerve leaves the cochlea, its next junction is the cochlear nucleus in the brainstem. The structure of the nervous system central to the cochlea is discussed in Chapter 15.

There is, therefore, an orderly connection between the inner hair cells and auditory nerve fibers, with the

auditory nerve fibers organized from the center to the outside within the nerve bundle. On an anatomical basis, therefore, we might expect that the discharge patterns of the auditory nerve fibers will reflect the frequency, intensity, and timing encoding performed by the mechanics of the inner ear.

SUMMARY

The electric potentials (CM, SP, AP, and single units) of the inner ear are created as a result of the biomechanical disturbances. Resting potentials are also present regardless of stimulation (especially EP). The likely sources of these potentials are the hair cells for the CM, the stria vascularis for the EP, and simultaneous discharges of auditory nerve single units for the AP. There are numerous possible sources of the SP. The stereocilia of the hair cells are sheared by the differential motions of the basilar and tectorial membranes. This shearing causes neural discharges in the hair cells, probably initiated in the region of the stereocilia at the top of the inner hair cells by means of the tip links between stereocilia. The outer hair cells are motile and change their length as a result of stimulation. The inner hair cells are the auditory biological transducers. Acoustic echoes and cochlear emissions are possible indications of active processes within the inner ear. There are two types of afferent fibers: radial, or Type I, fibers and outer spiral, or Type II, fibers. The radial fibers make up 85% to 95% of all afferents. Each radial fiber innervates only one or two inner hair cells, and each inner hair cell synapses with many radial fibers. The outer spiral fibers comprise the other 5% to 15% of the afferent fibers. Each innervates about 10 outer hair cells in an orderly fashion. The efferent fibers are the olivocochlear bundle, which arises from the medial (MOC) or the lateral (LOC) regions of the olive on the ipsilateral (UCOCB) and the contralateral (COCB) side of the head relative to the inner ear to which the OCB projects. Type I fibers innervating the inner hair cells provide the major sensory transduction mechanism for hearing. The outer hair cells serve to increase the sensitivity and frequency selectivity of the transduction process, most likely as a result of outer hair cell motility. The afferent nerve fibers leave the organ of Corti in an orderly fashion, such that fibers from the base are on the outside of the auditory nerve bundle and fibers from the apex of the cochlea are on the inside.

SUPPLEMENT

There is a vast literature on the function of the cochlea and hair cells. The material covered in this chapter can be found in textbooks by Pickles (1988) and in the first two volumes of the series produced by Webster et al. (1992), Fay and Popper (1992), Dallos, Popper, and Fay (1996), Geisler (1998), Jahn and Santos-Sacchi (2001), and Moller (2003). The work by Hudspeth (2005) should also be consulted.

The study of the cochlea and its potentials has an interesting history. The CM was discovered accidentally by Wever and Bray in 1930 when they were recording from the auditory nerve. They considered the CM to be a neural potential, but this misconception was soon clarified by Adrian (1931) and Saul and Davis (1932). The early work of Tasaki (1954) and Tasaki et al. (1954) suggested that the origin of the CM was the cilia-bearing end of the outer hair cells. Experiments originally performed by Hudspeth (1983) in which recordings were made directly from hair cells have significantly improved our understanding of the CM and its origin.

In the 1970s, minor surgical and nonsurgical techniques were developed to allow for the recording of the AP and, to a lesser extent, the CM and SP from humans. This technique is called *electrocochleography*. The recording electrodes are usually placed somewhere between the earlobe and the cochlea, and the results are similar to those of the round window electrode experiments reported on animals. The most sensitive recording location is the *promontory*, which is the bony protruding wall between the oval and round windows. To make a recording, the tympanic membrane must be penetrated with a fine-needle electrode, the point of which rests on the promontory. This approach to recording cochlear potentials is often called the *transtympanic approach*. In a less severe but less sensitive recording procedure, the recording electrode is placed in the external canal *(extratympanic approach)*. An external canal electrode may rest against the wall of the canal or the tympanic membrane, or it may penetrate slightly the wall of the canal or the annular ligament of the tympanic membrane. Each approach, transtympanic or extratympanic, has its advantages and disadvantages. Measuring cochlear potentials, especially the CM and AP, often occur as part of obtaining *auditory brainstem responses* (ABRs). The ABR is a type of EEG (electroencephalograph) recording made from the scalp; this is discussed in more detail in Chapter 15.

The direction of stereocilia movement (shearing movement toward or away from the outer hair cells) that triggers the hair cell to discharge neurally appears to depend on the level of stimulation and where along the organ of Corti the hair cells are located. It is also possible that the motility of the outer hair cells may alter the excitatory direction of stereocilia movement (see Konishi and Nielsen, 1973; Zwislocki and Sokolich, 1973; and Pickles et al., 1984). The ability to perform in vitro experiments and to record intercellularly from hair cells has enabled hearing scientists to explore in fine detail the function of the hair cells and their stereocilia.

The motility of the outer hair cells was first reported by Brownell et al. (1985). The exact function of the slow and fast types of motility and the possible role of efferent control of motility are much researched topics. Almost all of the work on outer hair cell motility uses in vitro measures of excised other hair cells. No complete in vitro study has been done to fully explain how outer hair cell motility operates in the normal living cochlea (however, see work by Nutall and Dolan, 1993). The theoretical issues surrounding outer hair cell motility, feedback, and the cochlear amplifier are hotly debated. It does seem clear that there is no longer a need to postulate some form of a *second-filter* mechanism to explain differences between the sensitivity and frequency selectivity measured along the basilar membrane and that measured in the auditory nerve (at least for most mammals). These measures are now very similar, and differences obtained in the past were probably due to damaged cochleas in which outer hair cell function is greatly compromised. The idea that the hair cells themselves are tuned adds a new dimension to the role of outer hair cell motility (see Hudspeth, 2005). The discovery of the protein prestin (see Zheng et al., 2000, and Liberman et al., 2002) provides a clue as to the way in which motility may exist at very high rates of sound stimulation. We have talked about tuning mainly in biomechanical terms for the motion of the traveling wave. Fettiplace and Crawford (1980) showed that for many species the hair cells themselves are tuned due to bioelectrical properties of the hair cell and stereocilia. Thus, additional tuning of the cochlea to the frequency of sound may be provided by the electrical tuning of the hair cells (at least in some animals).

Cochlear emissions and acoustic echoes represent a new class of phenomena that may also help us to understand the cochlea. First reported by Kemp (1978), the phenomena have been the subject of a number of subsequent studies. Because the healthy cochlea produces evoked emissions and the damaged cochlea usually does not, cochlear emissions are being tested as a possible means of evaluating hearing in clinical situations, especially in newborns and infants (see Lonsbury-Martin and Martin, 1990, and Culpepper, 2002). The book by Hall (2000) provides a review of the basics of otoacoustic emissions. In addition, these phenomena suggest that the emissions may play a role in understanding *tinnitus*, a disorder in which a person suffers from a ringing or other sound in the ear for which no obvious physical source can be found. However, current research suggests that in only 5% of people who suffer from tinnitus can the tinnitus be traced to cochlear emissions (Bilger et al., 1990). SFOAE have been measured less frequently than DPOAEs and TEOAEs (see Shera et al., 2002).

Spoendlin's work (1970, 1973, 1974) led to the realization that 90% to 95% of the afferent fibers innervate the inner hair cells. Liberman's investigations (1978, 1980, 1982) have also contributed significantly to our understanding of the afferent auditory nerve. When he recorded discharges from several fibers in the auditory nerve, he was then able to trace them to their terminations in the cochlea. All neurons were found to be radial fibers innervating inner hair cells. These data support the notion that essentially none of the single-unit discharge data reported so far has come from fibers that terminate on outer hair cells. These data are consistent with the earlier work by Spoendlin (1978, 1979), which indicated that the outer spiral fibers remain unmyelinated even after they pass through the habenula perforata on their course centrally. The lack of a myelin sheath and their small diameter (less than 0.5 mm) would make it nearly impossible to record from them by traditional techniques. In contrast, radial fibers acquire a myelin sheath as they pass centrally through the habenula perforata and have diameters between 3 and 5 mm.

A number of terms are used interchangeably in describing a neural cell: cell, unit, fiber (in connection with the central nervous system), neuron, and nerve. All of these terms are used in this book to expose the student to the multiple uses found in the literature.

The peripheral efferent fibers have proven difficult to investigate. The first investigator was Rasmussen (1943), who demonstrated the existence of the efferents. Later work of Warr, Guinan, and White (1986) and Liberman and Brown (1986) disproved some earlier ideas about the OCB pathways and have contributed significantly to our understanding of the synapses of the efferent system in the inner ear (see also Geisler, 1998).

9

The Neural Response and the Auditory Code

[handwritten margin note: "Neural spikes are proportional to the velocity of the Basilar Membrane"]

In this chapter we study the function of the afferent and efferent auditory nerves within the VIIIth nerve bundle. We learn how the frequency, level, and temporal properties of sounds change the neural output of the afferent fibers that innervate the inner hair cells and the way in which the efferent fibers might modify this output. The chapter ends with a description of the code for sound provided by the auditory periphery to the auditory brainstem and cortex.

FUNCTION OF THE AFFERENT AUDITORY NERVE

Hair cells initiate the neural part of the auditory process. The mechanical deformation of the stereocilia of hair cells produces graded electrical potentials (that is, potentials whose magnitude is proportional to the amount of stimulation), which are called *receptor potentials* (e.g., CM and SP). The inner hair cell then liberates a chemical transmitter (probably *glutamate-* or *gylcine*-like), which initiates a graded electrical potential in auditory nerve fibers that innervate the base of the hair cell. This graded neural potential is propagated along the nerve fiber to the habenula perforata, where the myelinated portion of the fiber is

reached. At that point neural *spikes*, or *discharges* or *action potentials*, are produced that travel along the auditory nerve to the cochlear nucleus, the first nucleus in the auditory brainstem. Because the graded neural response of the unmyelinated portion of the nerve fiber generates the neural spike, it is called a *generator potential*. Neural spike rate is proportional to the velocity of basilar membrane motion.

The electrophysiologist studies the spike discharge patterns of single neurons by amplifying these minute biochemical potential changes with amplifiers. The discharge pattern of a neural spike initially exhibits a relatively large potential shift (see Appendix E). It then remains in an exhausted condition for a short period (known as the *absolute refractory period*) during which no stimulus, however strong, can be effective in generating a spike. After the absolute refractory period comes a period of *relative refractoriness*, during which the nerve's ability to respond depends on the level of succeeding stimuli. This total refractory period lasts approximately 1 msec and therefore limits the number of discharges a given nerve may be capable of emitting per second. At this point we must be careful to make the distinction between the action potential of an individual neuron and the whole nerve action potential, the AP. The

[handwritten annotation at top: "individual neurons have all-or-none characteristic. An Action-Potential is the sum of many auditory nerves discharges"]

individual neuron's action potential (spike) has an *all-or-none* characteristic. This means the amplitude of the neural discharge does not vary with the level of the stimulus, as the AP does. The AP is a summed combination of the discharges of many auditory nerves. See Appendix E for more details concerning neural physiology.

Spontaneous Activity and Neural Thresholds

Electrophysiologists who record the discharges of a single neuron, or *single-unit* response, as it is often called, employ several methods for dealing with the data. They investigate the characteristics of the neurons by these different methods in an attempt to understand how the relevant aspects (frequency, intensity, and timing) of the acoustic signal are encoded. One method of studying such discharge patterns consists of establishing what the neuron's discharges rate is without a stimulus and then using that as a baseline against which to compare various stimulus-evoked discharge rates. *Spontaneous activity* is the neural activity that occurs without a stimulus. For single units of the auditory nerve, this would be the neural activity occurring without sound. Because establishing a sound-free environment is virtually impossible, there is always the possibility that the neural activity observed without a controlled sound stimulus may be caused by ambient acoustic stimulation. Thus, specifying the exact nature and cause of spontaneous activity is difficult. For our discussion, however, the neural activity without sound introduced by an experimenter will suffice as our definition of spontaneous activity. The discharge rate of spontaneous activity in single units of the auditory nerve may range from no spikes, or discharges, to more than 100 discharges per second.

One of the most useful indicators of neural activity is the discharge rate of the single neuron (single unit). The discharge rate is simply the number of times a unit discharges a neural spike, or "fires," in a given period. The neuron has a 1-msec period after it has

discharged before it can discharge again (the refractory period). Thus, the theoretical maximum discharge rate of a single unit is 1000 spikes/sec, although most auditory nerve fibers have a maximum firing rate of less than 500 spikes/sec.

Once the spontaneous discharge rate of a neuron has been determined, the *single-neuron threshold* to a particular stimulus can be calculated. The threshold of a single neuron may be defined as the <u>minimum</u> stimulus level that will cause an <u>increase</u> in the discharge rate above the spontaneous discharge rate. For instance, consider a neural threshold of a neuron with a spontaneous discharge rate of 14 spikes/sec to a 1-kHz sinusoid. If the system is presented an increase in the level of the 1-kHz sinusoid until the discharge rate is just detectably greater than 14 spikes/sec (e.g., 20 spikes/sec), then that level (20 spikes/sec) will be the threshold. At a lower level the discharge rate will remain at the spontaneous rate, and a more intense signal may significantly increase the rate of discharge above 14 spikes/sec. However, because the spontaneous activity for any given neuron varies randomly, some statistical change in average firing rate is usually used to determine neural thresholds

Figure 9.1 shows the distribution of the single-neuron thresholds for different frequencies of stimulation recorded from the cat. The different areas on the graph refer to the range of spontaneous rates that neurons exhibit. That is, for each neuron recorded, its spontaneous rate was determined without stimulation. Then a tone was presented at different frequencies, and at each frequency the level of the tone that just caused the neuron to fire above its spontaneous rate was determined. This level of the tone was the neural threshold for that frequency. The frequency for which this neural threshold was the lowest was used to determine the best (characteristic or center) frequency (CF) of the neuron as shown on the *x*-axis in Figure 9.1. As can be seen, neurons with high spontaneous activity (rates above 18 spikes/sec) have the lowest thresholds; medium-spontaneous-rate neurons (between 0.5 and 18 spikes/sec) had the next highest thresholds, and neurons with low rates of spontaneous activity (less than 0.5 spikes/sec) had the highest thresholds. Also

"Max spike rate of single-neuron is 1000/sec. However, most auditory nerves have a max discharge rate of 500/sec".

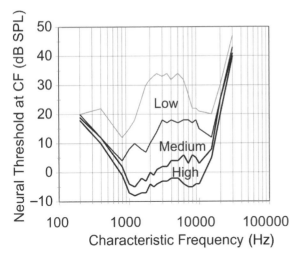

FIGURE 9.1 The neural thresholds (expressed in dB sound pressure level (SPL)) of auditory nerve fibers of the cat plotted for three different ranges of spontaneous activity (low: <0.5 spikes/sec; medium: 0.5–18 spikes/sec; high: >18 spikes/sec). The x-axis represents the frequency at which the neural threshold for that unit was lowest (i.e., the unit's characteristic frequency; see text related to Figures 9.3 and 9.5 for further explanation). Adapted from Liberman (1978), used with permission.

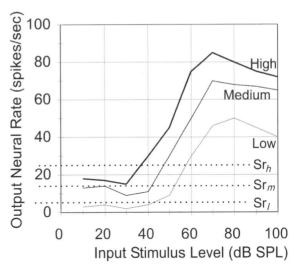

FIGURE 9.2 Intensity, or rate-level, functions for three neurons: high-, medium-, and low-spontaneous-rate fibers. The output of the neurons is plotted in spikes per second as a function of the input level in dB sound pressure level (SPL). Sr_h, Sr_m, Sr_l: spontaneous rate of firings for the high- (h), medium- (m), and low-(l) -spontaneous-rate fibers.

notice that the neuronal thresholds are lowest in the frequency region between 1000 and 10,000 Hz, which for the cat is the frequency region in which it hears best (see Chapter 10 for a discussion of thresholds of hearing).

RATE-LEVEL FUNCTIONS

Increasing the level of the acoustic stimulus and measuring changes in the discharge rate of the single neuron above the spontaneous rate is called calculating an *input–output*, or *rate-level*, *function*. Several such rate-level functions are shown in Figure 9.2. The different curves represent discharge rates from different neurons, each with a different spontaneous rate. Notice that for each neuron the response shows the typical increase in discharge rate for an increase in stimulus level up to 30 to 40 dB above the neuron's threshold, and then the discharge rate remains constant

or declines slightly. Essentially all auditory nerve response rates increase over a range of 20 to 50 dB (called the *neuronal dynamic range*) above their thresholds, after which the discharge rate remains constant or decreases slightly if stimulus level is increased further. The input–output functions for fibers with different amounts of spontaneous activity differ in their intercepts (e.g., in the stimulus level that first causes the fiber to discharge above spontaneous activity). Auditory nerve rate-level functions are somewhat compressive, such as the input–output functions for the basilar membrane (see Chapter 6).

RESPONSE AREAS AND TUNING CURVES

Figure 9.3 shows a family of rate-level functions for one single neuron presented with tones of different frequencies. Any single nerve will respond (that is, increase its discharge rate above the spontaneous rate) to many frequencies of acoustic stimulation. As can be

Threshold = Min stimulus increase
Spontaneous discharge rate

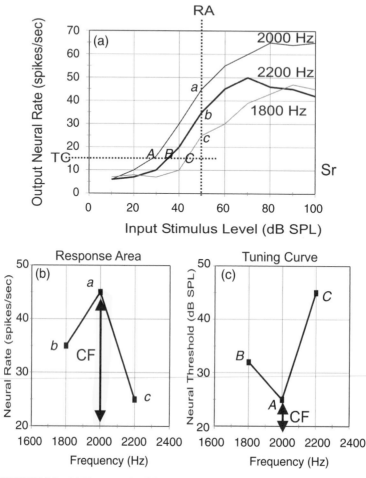

FIGURE 9.3 (a) Three rate-level functions for a single neuron presented with tones with three different frequencies (spontaneous rate, "Sr," is 10 spikes/sec). (b) A response area (RA) plotting discharge rate versus tonal frequency (Hz) obtained from graph (a) by determining at a level of 50 dB the discharge rate for each frequency (in graph (a) the vertical dashed line, "RA," passes through the points *a*, *b*, *c*, which are in turn plotted in graph (b). (c) A tuning curve plotting neural threshold (in dB SPL) as a function of tonal frequency, where the neural threshold is defined as that level required for the neuron to discharge with 15 spikes/sec. The tuning curve (TC) is obtained from graph (a) (the horizontal dashed line, "TC," runs through the points *A*, *B*, *C*, which in turn are plotted in graph (c). CF = characteristic frequency.

seen in Figure 9.3a, the neuron does not discharge equally to all frequencies. We can replot the data in Figure 9.3a in one of two ways to better display how the neuron responds as a function of frequency. We can plot an *isolevel*, or *isointensity*, *curve* (sometimes called a *response area*) by plotting, for each frequency, the neuron's response rate for a fixed level of stimulation (e.g., the discharge rate for a 50-dB SPL signal level). The data are replotted in Figure 9.3b as a response area. Notice that this neuron fires most at

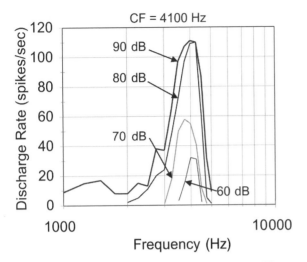

FIGURE 9.4 Response curves for a single unit at four different intensities. The discharge rate is plotted as a function of the frequency of the tone stimulation. Each curve is generated by holding the level of the stimulus constant and recording the discharge rate for each frequency. The unit has a characteristic frequency (CF) of 4100 Hz. Adapted from Rose, Hind, Anderson, and Brugge (1971), with permission.

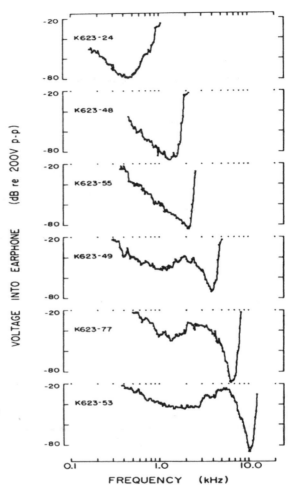

FIGURE 9.5 Tuning curves for six single units with different characteristic frequencies. The stimulus level in dB sound pressure level (SPL) calibrated at the headphones needed to reach each unit's threshold is plotted as a function of stimulus frequency. Note the steep slope on the high-frequency side of the tuning curve and the shallow slope on the low-frequency side. The three units at the bottom have higher characteristic frequencies and show low-frequency "tails" that indicate they are responsive to a wide range of frequencies of stimulation. Adapted from Kiang and Moxon (1972), with permission.

2000 Hz; this frequency is often called the *characteristic frequency* (CF) of the neuron (this was the *x*-axis in Figure 9.1). Figure 9.4 shows a family of response areas for a single neuron. Each curve represents a different level at which the tone was presented.

Suppose this neuron has a spontaneous rate of 10 spikes/sec and, as a result, 15 spikes per second was used as the definition of this neuron's threshold. That is, if the neuron discharges with 15 spikes/sec, then the experimenter is willing to state that the neuron is no longer firing spontaneously and is discharging in response to the stimulus. We can then plot the level of the tone required for the neuron to discharge at this threshold amount of firing (i.e., 15 spikes/sec) as a function of the frequency of stimulation. Such a plot is called an *isorate curve* or a *tuning curve*. Figure 9.3c shows a tuning curve for the data plotted in Figure 9.3a. Notice that the neuron has its lowest threshold at 2000 Hz (the frequency of a neuron's lowest threshold is called its *characteristic frequency,*

or CF). Figure 9.5 shows a series of tuning curves for different neurons. Notice that each neuron has a different tuning curve with a different CF (also note that the data plotted along the *x*-axis in Figure 9.1 are the CFs of each fiber). Tuning curves and response areas are mirrors of each other, as explained in Figure 9.3.

Tuning curves are usually drawn with frequency plotted on a logarithmic scale. The higher-frequency side of the tuning curve appears very steep. The lower-frequency side of the tuning curve is less steep, and for higher CF units, such as the bottom three in Figure 9.5, a long low-frequency "tail" is obvious. Also notice that the difference in threshold level between the tip of the tuning curve at the CF and the low-frequency tail of the tuning curve is approximately 40 to 50 dB for all three units. This *tip-to-tail difference* tends to be 40 to 50 dB for all auditory neurons with relatively high CFs. This means that nerves respond best to their CF, are unlikely to respond to many frequencies higher than the CF, and will usually respond to frequencies lower than the CF if the stimulation is approximately 40 to 50 dB above the threshold of the CF. The *width of the tuning curve* is often calculated as the frequency range at 10 dB above the level of the CF (i.e., one calculates the width of the tuning curve at 10 dB above the lowest point on the tuning curve).

The width of the tuning curve (i.e., the width of tuning) increases as the CF increases. This means that frequency is coded in a roughly logarithmic manner along the basilar membrane, such that in humans each 3.5 mm of basilar membrane equals approximately one octave of frequency (CF). It is also the case that the width of tuning increases with overall level, as can be seen in Figure 9.4 (i.e., the width of the response area is greater for the 80-dB tone than it is for the 60-dB tone).

The data in Figures 9.4 and 9.5 show that auditory nerve fibers are very selective to frequency, with each neuron firing best to a limited range of frequencies, and this range is different (the CF is different) for each neuron. These Type I nerve fibers synapse with one or two inner hair cells along the cochlear partition (see Chapter 8). It is therefore not surprising that the pattern of discharge rate reflects the same type of frequency selectivity obtained at one point along the basilar membrane. That is, <u>the auditory nerve preserves very faithfully the frequency selectivity found along the basilar membrane due to the motion of the traveling wave.</u> Recall that fibers on the outside of the auditory nerve bundle innervate basal hair cells, and these fibers have been shown to have high-frequency CFs, whereas those fibers toward the middle of the nerve bundle that innervate the apex of the cochlea have low-frequency CFs (see Chapter 8). This is a further demonstration of the correspondence between the frequency selectivity found in the cochlea and that measured in the auditory nerve.

This frequency selectivity of auditory nerve fibers is often described in terms of bandpass filtering. That is, a single nerve responds best to a limited range of frequencies (near the CF) and less to frequencies lower or higher than this range. This is similar to the way in which a bandpass filter passes sinusoids with frequencies in its pass band with no change in level and attenuates the amplitudes of sinusoids with frequencies higher and lower than the pass band. Such bandpass filters that simulate the tuning of auditory nerve fibers have very steep roll-offs and are very narrow. The width of the filters increases with the center frequency of the filter and increases in proportion to the level of the sound input.

HISTOGRAMS

The rate at which an auditory nerve fiber discharges depends on the level and frequency of the sound input. What about the temporal properties of sound? How are they processed by the auditory nerve? Single nerves with CFs below 4 or 5 kHz tend to discharge about once per cycle for low-frequency periodic stimulation (below 1 kHz). Figure 9.6 shows the type of discharge pattern we might expect in this situation. This type of response is called a *time-* or *phase-locked response*, or a *following response*, because the single-unit response appears locked to, or follows, the amplitude peaks in the stimulus. Because of the absolute refractory period of the neuron, the unit cannot discharge to every cycle (peak) of a sinusoid with a frequency near or above 1 kHz, although the fiber could discharge to every other or every third (and so on) cycle of the stimulus. Note also that the fiber only fires to positive-going ampli-

Function of the Afferent Auditory Nerve

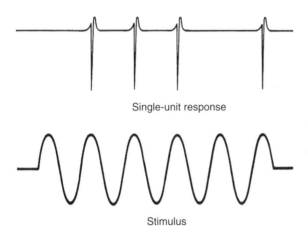

Single-unit response

Stimulus

FIGURE 9.6 Single-neuron discharges to a low-frequency stimulus. Top trace: discharge pattern of the single unit. Bottom trace: the low-frequency stimulus. Note that the neuron responds with a discharge to almost every (but not every) cycle of the stimulus.

tude peaks in the depiction shown in Figure 9.6. That is, the neuron only discharges when the stereocilia are sheared in one direction (see Chapter 8). The fact that the nerve only discharges to one direction of sound movement is called *half-wave rectification*. Finally, the firing of auditory nerve fibers to sound (actually to the vibrations of the cochlea caused by sound) is stochastic, meaning there is a probability that the neuron will fire. Thus, as shown in Figure 9.6, the neuron does not always fire when there is an amplitude peak in the waveform, due to the statistics of neuronal function.

To observe the temporal course of neural firings in the auditory nerve we use a method of data analysis known as *histograms*. Histograms are graphic displays of a single neuron's response to repeated presentations of a given stimulus. The vertical axis of a histogram is usually some measure of the number of responses. It might represent "frequency of responses," "percentage of response," or just "number of neural discharges." The horizontal axis is always time, but it may represent time after stimulus onset or the time interval between successive neural discharges.

Poststimulus time histograms (PST histograms) display the total number of responses at each given moment in time to a repeated stimulus (Figure 9.7). The beginning point in time is usually some point just before the stimulus onset, such as 5 msec. The data shown in Figure 9.7 illustrate two typical PST histograms to tone bursts of different frequency. The greatest number of discharges occurs at the onset of the tone burst ("on" effect). The number of discharges decreases (*adapts*) rapidly over the first few milliseconds of stimulation. Then the *adaptation* (decrease in firing rate) is much slower over the course of the rest of the stimulation. Immediately after the offset of the tone burst the number of discharges in this neuron is zero or near zero (i.e., less than the spontaneous rate). After a short period the number of discharges returns to the normal spontaneous rate. The PST histograms in Figure 9.7 show the number of discharges at each point in time over 1 sec for 1200 presentations of the 500-msec tone burst stimulus (note that the tone is presented for 500 msec, but the spike count continues for another 500 msec after the stimulus is turned off). It should be clear from comparing Figures 9.6 and 9.7 that the PST histogram can reveal response patterns that would never be seen by simply recording discharge rate or studying the response of a unit to each individual stimulus presentation.

Interval histograms, or *interspike interval histograms (ISI histograms)*, provide a method for studying the time interval between each successive pair of neural discharges. The horizontal axis of the interval histogram represents the time interval between successive neural discharges, or the *interspike interval*. The vertical axis shows the number of interspike intervals that occurred. Thus, if an interval histogram had its largest peak at 1 msec, then the time between successive discharges was most often 1 msec. Such an interval histogram is shown in Figure 9.8d, in which the stimulus was a 1000-Hz sinusoid of 1-sec duration repeated 10 times. Because of the 1-msec absolute refractory period of the single neuron, we would not expect an interspike interval of less than 1 msec. Although Figure 9.8d shows that a 1-msec interspike interval occurred more than any other specific inter-

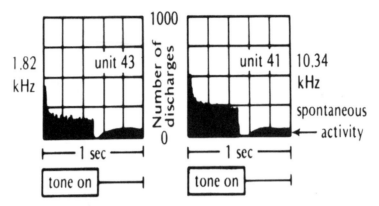

FIGURE 9.7   Typical poststimulus time (PST) histograms to tone bursts. For each histogram, the tone burst is presented 1200 times. The histogram is started 5 msec before the onset of each tone burst. Each time the unit discharges, the histogram increases vertically at the point in time (on the abscissa) the discharge occurred. On average, more responses occur at the beginning of the tone burst than at the end. After the tone burst there is a decrease in spontaneous activity. The PST on the left is for a 1.82-kHz tone, on the right for a 10.34-kHz tone. Adapted from Kiang, Watanabe, Thomas, and Clark (1965), with permission.

val, neural discharges occurred at integral multiples of 1 msec (2, 3, up to 10 msec). That is, there are a lot of times when the time between spikes is 2 msec, 3 msec, etc. When the interval between successive spikes is 2 msec, the neuron fires to one peak of the 1000-Hz waveform, misses the next peak, but fires to the third peak, etc. Although the neuron is not firing all the time to every peak in the waveform, it is mostly firing only at peaks. Thus, the period of the waveform is equal to the time between the major peaks in the interspike histogram (e.g., in Figure 9.8a the time between the ISI peaks is about 2.4 msec, which is the period of the 412-Hz stimulating tone). This phenomenon is also true of other frequencies of stimulation, as illustrated by the interval histograms to other pure tone stimuli shown in Figure 9.8. The relationship between the period of the stimulus (and integer multiples of that period) and the interval between discharges is shown clearly in Figure 9.8. This supports the idea that single neural discharges are locked to the cycles of the stimulus at low frequencies, as shown in Figures 9.6 and 9.8. Some locking of the responses to the cycles of stimulating frequency occurs up to about 5 kHz.

Phase-locked PST histograms (sometimes called *period histograms*) provide additional information about timing in the nerve discharge pattern. The time- or phase-locked PST histogram is generated by obtaining a PST histogram while making sure that the counting of the neural discharges begins at the same phase of the stimulating waveform each time the stimulus is presented. Quite often the histogram shows the neural counts over one period of the stimulating signal. Examples of this type of histogram to the sum of two pure tones of different frequencies are shown in Figure 9.9. As can be seen, the neural discharges occur most frequently during only one phase of the tonal waveform (to positive-going displacements, as depicted in the figure). This is consistent with the example shown in Figure 9.6.

A measure of *neural synchrony* (*coefficient of synchrony*) can be derived from the phase-locked PST histogram that indicates how well the neural pattern conforms to the stimulus waveform period. To calculate the coefficient of synchrony, we measure over one period of the stimulating waveform. If, over one period of stimulation, the discharge pattern in the

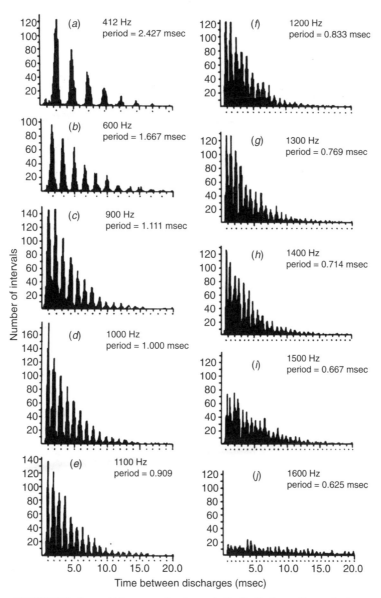

FIGURE 9.8 Interval histograms showing periodic distributions of interspike intervals to pure tones of different frequencies. The stimulus frequency and period are indicated in each graph. The level of all stimuli is 80 dB sound pressure level (SPL), and the tone duration is 1 sec. The responses to 10 stimuli constitute the sample on which each histogram is based. Time in milliseconds between successive neural discharges is plotted on the abscissa. Dots below the time axes indicate integer values of the period of each frequency employed. From Rose, Brugge, Anderson, and Hind (1967), with permission.

Unit 67-135-7

Tone 1: 798 cps
Tone 2: 1064 cps
R = 3:4

Tone 1: 60 dB SPL   Tone 1: 70 dB SPL   Tone 1: 80 dB SPL

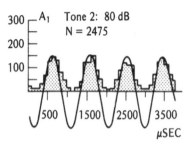
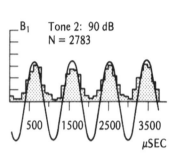
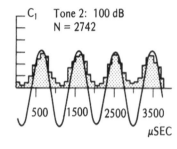

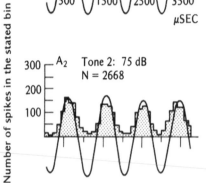
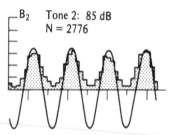
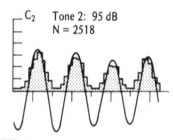

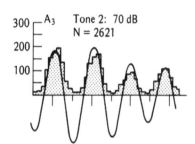
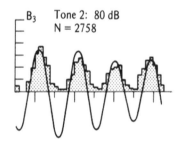
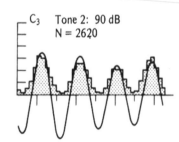

Number of spikes in the stated bin

FIGURE 9.9   Time-locked poststimulus time (PST) histograms to the sum of two pure tones. In the top row, Tone 2 is 20 dB more intense than Tone 1. In the middle row there is a 15-dB difference between the two tones, and in the bottom row the difference is 10 dB. For all cases the time-domain waveform of the summed sinusoids is superimposed on top of the PST histogram. The nerve discharges only during one phase of the waveform (the positive-going sections of the waveform, showing half-wave rectification). The PST histogram displays the ability of the nerve to discharge in synchrony with the period of the input stimulus. Based on a figure from Hind, Anderson, Brugge, and Rose (1967), with permission.

period histogram changes in a sinusoidal fashion (i.e., as if it is following the top half of a sine wave or the half-wave rectified sine wave) then the measure of neural synchrony (or coefficient of synchrony) is nearly 1.0 (the coefficient of synchrony is near 1 for the stimuli shown in Figure 9.9). If the neural pattern of the phase-locked PST histogram shows neural discharges evenly distributed throughout the period of stimulation (i.e., flat), indicating no ability of the neuron to follow the temporal pattern of the sound input, then the coefficient of synchrony is near zero. One can determine the coefficient of synchrony as a function of stimulus level, the function is called the *synchrony-level function*, to differentiate it from the rate-level function described earlier. Typically the coefficient of synchrony is zero for low stimulus levels that result only in spontaneous activity and then increase toward 1 (although the coefficient rarely reaches 1) as stimulus level increases. Recall from Figures 9.2 and 9.3 that rate-level functions do not increase beyond a 30- to 50-dB change in input level. Synchrony-level functions show an increase in synchrony over a much larger range of stimulus levels.

The response of an auditory nerve fiber to a click stimulus reveals several important points concerning neural transduction. Figures 9.10a and b show period histograms to a rarefaction and a condensation click (see Chapter 4). The fact that there are periodic peaks in the period histograms is an indication that the clicks undergo processing by the biomechanics of the inner ear that is like the processing produced by a bandpass filter. In Figures 9.10c and 9.10d, the time-domain waveforms of a rarefaction and condensation click are shown before and after the click has passed through a bandpass filter. The multiple oscillations in the click waveforms at the output of the filter reflect the bandpass filtering, such that the period of oscillations in the filtered click is equal to the reciprocal of the center frequency of the filter (e.g., if the filter's center frequency were 2000 Hz, the period of oscillation would be 0.5 msec). If the nerve discharges to the peaks of the cochlearly filtered click (see Figure 9.9), then the period between the major peaks in the period histogram should be equal to the reciprocal of the CF of

the fiber being measured (see Figures 9.10a and 9.10b). This is further evidence that the biomechanics of the inner ear act as if sound is being bandpass-filtered. Note also that the time-domain waveforms of the condensation and rarefaction clicks are phase reversed (as they should be because the input clicks are phase reversed). If the nerve discharges when the stereocilia move in only one direction, then the peaks in the period histogram of the condensation click should occur one-half period later than those occurring for the rarefaction clicks, as they do, as shown in Figures 9.10a and 9.10b.

TWO-TONE SUPPRESSION AND OTHER NONLINEAR NEURAL RESPONSES

The discussion of afferent activity has centered on tonal, or simple, stimuli. The neural activity to complex stimuli can often be predicted based on what is known about the activity measured for simple stimuli. However, additional phenomena occur when two or more sinusoids are added. One of the more important events arises from presenting two tones together. The presentation of one tone will usually cause a neuron to discharge at a rate well above its spontaneous rate, especially if the tone's frequency is near the fiber's CF. Adding a second tone at a particular frequency and level may cause a decrease in the discharge rate of the fiber to the first tone. This is shown in the top panel of Figure 9.11. When Tone A is on alone, the neuron discharges at a high rate. When Tone B is added to Tone A, the discharge rate of the fiber is greatly reduced. It is as if Tone B inhibited or suppressed the neural activity associated with Tone A. This phenomenon is therefore called *two-tone suppression*. Figure 9.11b indicates the frequencies and intensities of the inhibiting tone (Tone B), which causes a decrease in the firing rate to the exciting tone (Tone A). The darker line shows the tuning curve for Tone A, and the lighter lines indicate the frequencies and intensities of Tone B, which reduced the firing rate of the nerve fiber to stimulation caused by Tone A. Thus, there are inhibitory regions above and below the

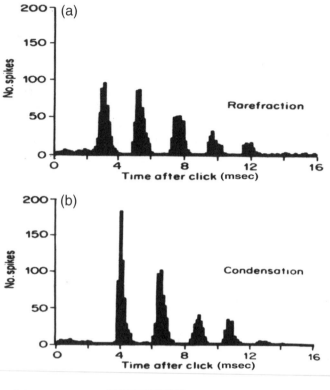

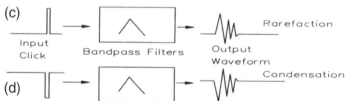

FIGURE 9.10 (a) The period histograms to a rarefaction click. (b) The period histogram to a condensation click. The auditory nerve fiber's characteristic frequency (CF) was 450 Hz. (c) A rarefaction click before and after bandpass filtering. From Kiang, Watanabe, Thomas, and Clark (1965), with permission. (d) A condensation click before and after bandpass filtering. The oscillation, or ringing, of the click in response to the filter occurs with a periodicity equal to the reciprocal of the bandpass filter's center frequency. The multiple peaks in the period histogram that repeat at an interval equal to the reciprocal of the fiber's CF (2.22 msec = 1/450 Hz) and indicate that the fiber reflects a process that is like bandpass filtering.

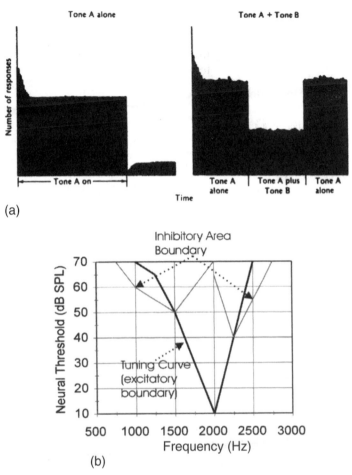

FIGURE 9.11 Schematic diagram showing two-tone suppression. **(a)** The poststimulus time (PST) histogram to Tone A presented alone is shown on the left. If a second tone of the correct frequency and intensity (Tone B) is added to the first tone (Tone A), the discharge rate of the nerve fiber can be reduced during the time Tone B is added to Tone A. **(b)** The typical two-tone suppression result in terms of a tuning curve diagram. The dark borders indicate boundary for the frequencies and intensities of Tone A that excite the nerve (i.e., the tuning curve; see Figures 9.3 and 9.5). The light borders indicate the boundary for the frequencies and intensities of Tone B, which, when added to Tone A, decrease (suppress) the discharge rate of the nerve responding to Tone A.

best frequency of the fiber's tuning curve. The data shown in Figure 9.11 are based on measuring a decrease in the rate of neural discharge due to the interaction of two tones. A decrease in measures of neural synchrony, such as the coefficient of synchrony, also occurs for the proper combination of two tones. Thus, two-tone suppression can be measured neurally as *rate suppression* or as *synchrony suppression*.

Two-tone suppression is a form of a nonlinear response of the cochlea to sound stimulation. The other forms of nonlinearities, discussed elsewhere in this book (e.g., Chapters 5, 7, and 13), can also be found in the neural discharge patterns of auditory nerve fibers. That is, at high sound levels, harmonic and difference-tone distortion, especially that associated with the cubic-difference tone (the difference tone existing at $2f_1 - f_2$, when the primaries are f_1 and f_2) can be measured in the neural response of auditory nerve fibers. Although two-tone suppression and the other nonlinear phenomena are easily measured for neural discharges, they can also be measured for biomechanical motion and for the cochlear microphonic (that is, adding two tones can reduce the magnitude of the CM relative to what occurred when only one tone was presented, as discussed in Chapter 8). Thus, the origin of these forms of nonlinearities is probably not entirely neural. Other excitatory and inhibitory interactions can occur when two or more tones are presented either simultaneously or in temporal sequence. Care must be taken in predicting the neural processing of a complex stimulus based only on what is known about the processing of simple stimuli.

FUNCTION OF THE EFFERENT SYSTEM

The exact function of the efferent system is not well understood, but electrophysiological evidence indicates that the system is inhibitory in nature. By electrical or sound stimulation of the crossed olivocochlear bundle (COCB) and simultaneous measurement of the cochlear potentials and afferent neural activity, investigators have found several effects measurable in the discharges of single auditory nerve fibers, in the action potential (AP), and in the cochlear microphonic (CM). Most neural studies of the OCB are done by monitoring neural function in the ipsilateral ear (ear to which the stimulus is delivered) and either presenting sounds to the contralateral ear (ear opposite to the one stimulated) or directly stimulating the COCB electrically with brief electric shocks at a contralateral neural site (usually at the floor of the *fourth ventricle*, located in the brainstem).

Figure 9.12a shows a PST histogram measured in response to a 4.37-kHz tone presented to the ipsilateral ear along with a brief contralateral noise presented in the temporal middle of the ipsilateral tone. When both the contralateral noise and ipsilateral tone were presented together, the response rate to the ipsilateral tone was suppressed. Thus, it appears as if contralateral noise stimulates the COCB fibers, which in turn causes an inhibition of the neural firing to the ipsilateral tone. Figure 9.12b shows how the rate-level function for ipsilateral stimulation is shifted when the ipsilateral sound is simultaneously presented with a contralateral sound (note that for any input stimulus level the neural rate is lower when both tones are present [light curve] than when only the ipsilateral tone alone was presented [dark curve]). Similar results are obtained when electrical stimulation of the COCB is used rather than acoustic stimulation.

These inhibitory effects may help decrease the neural activity in intense noise situations for protecting the nervous system against noise-induced damage (see Chapter 16). The efferents may also help reduce the effect of background sounds on our ability to detect wanted signals (see Chapter 11, on masking).

ENCODING OF FREQUENCY, INTENSITY, AND TIME

From the information covered in the two preceding chapters we can describe, in a variety of ways, how the auditory system can encode (determine) the frequency, intensity, and temporal/phase characteristics of an acoustic waveform. We have seen that the traveling wave of the basilar membrane vibrates with maximum amplitude at a place along the cochlea that is dependent on the frequency of stimulation, so hair cells have their cilia sheared maximally depending on the frequency of the stimulus. The afferent auditory nerve fibers innervate these hair cells in a systematic fashion, and each auditory nerve fiber is most sensitive to a particular frequency. The individual fibers within the auditory nerve are also organized according to the frequency at which they are most sensitive

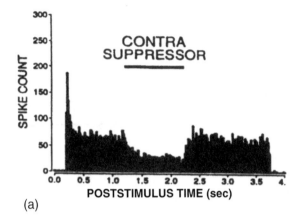

(a)

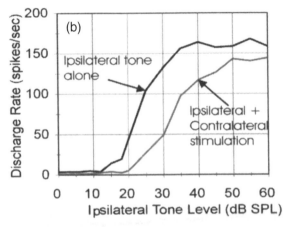

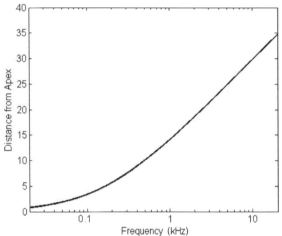

FIGURE 9.13   A cochlear map indicating the place of maximal excitation along the basilar membrane (distance from apex, in mm) as a function of the stimulating frequency (in Hz). This function is based on the work of Greenwood (1990).

FIGURE 9.12   (a) A poststimulus time (PST) histogram for a combined ipsilateral 4.37-kHz, 3.5-sec tone, and a contralateral broadband noise (1 sec long presented midway through the presentation of the ipsilateral tone). The decrease in the discharge rate at 1.5 sec is a result of the contralateral tone's exciting the crossed olivocochlear bundle (COCB) fibers, which in turn inhibit the firing of the ipsilateral auditory nerve fiber. (b) A rate-level function measured from an auditory nerve fiber (characteristic frequency = 1.22 kHz, Spontaneous rate = 1.6 spikes/sec) when it is excited with a 1.22-kHz ipsilateral tone (solid curve) and then with a combination of the 1.22-kHz ipsilateral tone and a 1.0-kHz contralateral tone (dashed curve). As can be seen, the addition of the contralateral tone excites the COCB, which in turn causes the neuron to discharge less to the ipsilateral tone at all levels (i.e., moves the rate-level function to the right). Adapted from Warren and Liberman (1989), with permission.

and the location along the cochlea at which they innervate hair cells; each place or location within the nerve is responding "best" to a particular frequency. The nerve is organized *topographically* (see Chapter 15 for a discussion of *tonotopic* organization) according to the tonal frequency that simulates the auditory system. Thus, the frequency of the input can be determined by noting which nerve fiber (place) within the auditory nerve discharges with the greatest relative discharge rate. This way of determining frequency is called the *place theory*. Figure 9.13 indicates an estimate of the *cochlear map*, which indicates the place of best frequency along the cochlear partition, that is, the tonotopic location along the basilar membrane indicating the tonal frequency that produces maximal displacement and, thus, maximal auditory nerve response.

It is also apparent from the data shown in Figure 9.6 and from the interval and period histograms that auditory nerve fibers also discharge at rates proportional to the period of the input stimulus when the input frequency is less than approximately 5000 Hz. It is possible that information is available to the nervous system about stimulus frequency from an analysis of the periodicity of neural discharge rate. That is, the periodicity of the nerve discharges could be used to determine the frequency of an input stimulus. Using discharge periodicity as the basis for frequency processing is called a *temporal theory* of frequency coding. Thus, for frequencies of less than 5000 Hz, both the place of maximal discharge and the periodicity of the discharge pattern can aid the nervous system in determining the frequency of stimulation.

Intensity is assumed to be encoded by an increase in the discharge rate within the auditory system. This would involve an increase in the discharge rate of single auditory nerve fibers. Notice, however, in Figure 9.2 that a single neuron's discharge rate will increase only for a relatively small range of level changes (usually less than 35 dB). Thus, a single neuron's response rate cannot account for the full 140-dB dynamic range of level to which we are sensitive (see Chapter 10). This would imply that intensity might be determined by the increase in discharge rate of a number of fibers rather than just one. For instance, notice that if we combine the outputs of all three fibers shown in Figure 9.3 that we could cover a larger range of intensities than that covered by anyone fiber. Thus, combining information from low-, medium-, and high-threshold fibers may serve as part of the code for sound level. The inclusion of discharges from many fibers whose CFs are other than those of the stimulus (see, for instance, the low-frequency tails of the tuning curves shown in Figure 9.5) may also help to account for the wide dynamic range of hearing. The processing that takes place in the auditory brainstem (see Chapter 15) may also aid in determining a code for stimulus level that encompasses the entire 140-dB range of level to which many animals are sensitive.

Clearly the fact that nerves discharge in synchrony to the phase of the stimulating sound provides a basis for encoding the phase and dynamic timing aspects of sound. However, such phase and timing information would be limited to periodicities that are less than 0.2 msec, because 5000 Hz appears to be the approximate upper frequency limit to which auditory nerve fibers can discharge in synchrony with a sound

(i.e., 0.2 msec is the reciprocal of 5000 Hz). That is, the fine-structure information in sound as well as envelope fluctuations can only be neurally coded when the rate of fluctuation is less than about 5000 Hz.

Figure 9.14a shows the average rate response of a large number of auditory nerve fibers of a cat to a synthesized speech vowel (the vowel \e\ as pronounced in the word "bet"). This is a *population response* of the

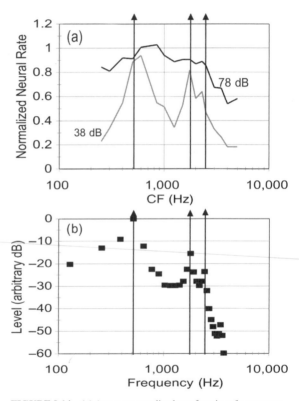

FIGURE 9.14 (a) Average normalized rate functions from a population of auditory nerve fibers to the speech vowel /ɛ/. Normalized rate is the unit's neuronal discharge rate divided by the maximum rate measured. Normalized rate is plotted as a function of the characteristic frequency (CF) of the fibers. The arrows point to the formant frequencies of the vowel, whose spectrum is shown in panel (b). Two different presentation levels of the vowel are shown. Notice how the spectrum of the vowel is well described by the neural data at the low, but not at the high, stimulus level. (b) The amplitude spectrum of the vowel /ɛ/ used in the nerve population studies. The arrows point to the formant peaks. The spectrum was determined near the eardrum of the cat. Adapted from Young and Sachs (1979), with permission.

auditory nerve to a complex sound with an amplitude spectrum that covers a broad range of frequencies. The data are shown for two levels of stimulation. Each data point used to generate the average curve represents the average firing rate of a fiber whose CF is plotted along the horizontal axis (hundreds of auditory nerve fibers were measured in determining the data of Figure 9.14a). The amplitude spectrum of the vowel is shown in Figure 9.14b. The major peaks in the spectrum, called *formant peaks*, result from the way in which the mouth, tongue, throat, etc. filter (resonate to) the sound produced by the vocal cords (see Chapter 14). Formant peaks are a key aspect of speech that account for speech recognition. Thus, it is crucial that these formant peaks be well represented in the neural output of the auditory periphery. The data shown in Figure 9.14a indicate that the spectrum of the sound is well represented at low stimulus levels but that a great deal of information is lost when the level is high (e.g., the neural output is not capturing the formant peaks of the vowel). At high sound levels most of the fibers in the bundle of auditory nerves are firing near their maximal rates due to the limited sound-level range over which they fire and the fact that the width of tuning increases with increased sound level. That is, the neural rate output from many neurons represents, or codes for, the levels and frequencies of a complex sound at low, but not at high, stimulus levels. Because the ability to recognize speech does not change much, if at all, when its level is changed, the information about the spectrum should be preserved at high and low stimulus levels.

Recall that measures of neural synchrony continue to change over a larger range of sound level then do measures of neural rate. Figure 9.15 indicates what happens to a neural measure of the population response if rate information is combined with a measure of synchrony (ALSR, *average localized synchronized rate*, is a measure that combines the rate at which the nerve discharges and its synchrony). Because nerves continue to respond in synchrony to a sound's periodicities at high stimulus levels where the rate has saturated (see Figures 8.4, 9.2, and 9.3), using synchrony information along with rate information

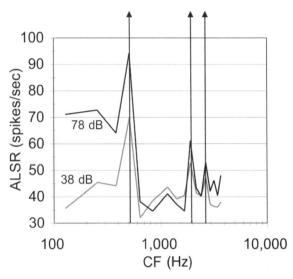

FIGURE 9.15 The average localized synchronized rate (ALSR) functions based on a population of nerve fibers is shown as a function of the fiber's characteristic frequency (CF). The stimulus is the speech vowel, /ɛ/ (its spectrum is shown in Figure 9.14b). The ALSR calculation takes into account both the synchronization of the units to the period of stimulation and the rate at which the unit discharges. The arrows point to the frequencies of the formants in the vowel. Two different levels of stimulation are shown. Compare the ability of the ALSR measure to preserve the spectral information of the vowel (see Figure 9.14b) to that provided by just the rate measure (Figure 9.14a), especially at the high presentation level. Adapted from Young and Sachs (1979), with permission.

preserves the neural code for the speech sound's spectrum at relatively high stimulus levels. These population responses indicate that the auditory periphery at the level of the auditory nerve provides a pretty faithful code of the physical attributes of sound, especially at low stimulus levels. Additional sharpening of this information may also take place in the neural circuits of the auditory brainstem.

MODELING THE AUDITORY PERIPHERY

Enough is known about the function of the inner ear and the auditory nerve that computer models have been developed to simulate the function of the auditory periphery. Such models have three main stages: a stage that simulates the function of the outer and middle ears, a stage that simulates the frequency selectivity of the basilar membrane traveling wave, and a stage for inner hair cell transduction of the vibratory output of the second stage into a neural discharge pattern. Figure 9.16 displays the output of one such computer model to the /e/ vowel sound (shown in Figure 9.14b). Each line is a simulation of the first 50 msec of the PST histogram from an auditory nerve fiber. The fibers are organized vertically, so fibers with low CFs are at the bottom of the display and those with high CFs are at the top of the display. The vertical axis can also represent distance along the cochlea. Note that CF is roughly logarithmically related to cochlear distance.

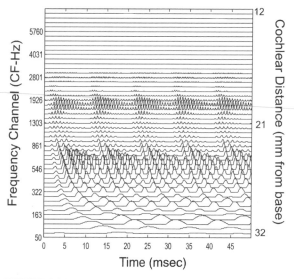

FIGURE 9.16 The output of a computational model of the auditory periphery. The model has two stages, one that represents the traveling wave activity of the cochlea and one that represents the transduction of basilar membrane vibration into neural discharges. The stimulus was the vowel /e/, as shown in Figure 9.14b. Each line is a simulation of a poststimulus time (PST) histogram of a tuned auditory nerve fiber, with low characteristic frequency (CF) fibers on the bottom and high-CF fibers at the top. The right-hand y-axis represents the distance in millimeters from the stapes. The display is a simulation of the pattern of neural activity that is likely to flow up the auditory nerve bundle to the brainstem when the vowel /e/ is spoken. Model from Patterson et al. (1995).

The time delays shown for the low-frequency channels in the model (toward the bottom of the display) correspond to the time it takes the traveling wave to reach the apex (low-frequency end of the cochlea). The higher PST activity in certain channels (e.g., around 550 Hz and around 1900 Hz) represent the fact that the /e/ sound has spectral peaks at 550 and 1900 Hz (e.g., the first and second formants; see Figure 9.14b). The periodic nature of the discharge pattern over time (note that the PST pattern repeats about every 10 msec, or at 100 Hz) represents the periodic nature of the time-domain waveform associated with this /e/ vowel sound (see Chapter 14 for a discussion of speech production). It is also the case that the simulated neural activity is greater at the beginning of the stimulus representing neural adaptation. Thus, the display is a simulation of the neural activity that might flow up the auditory nerve to the cochlear nucleus when the vowel /e/ is spoken. Such computational models do a good job of accounting for a great deal of the data obtained from auditory nerve fibers. These models are useful for studying how the information in complex sounds might be coded in the entire auditory nerve bundle, because it is difficult to perform physiological experiments in which a wide range of nerve fibers are sampled, especially at the same time.

SUMMARY

The responses of the single neurons of the auditory nerve demonstrate that they have a wide range of spontaneous activity, with low-spontaneous-rate fibers having high thresholds and high-spontaneous-rate fibers having low thresholds. The unit's discharge rate increases with an increase in stimulus level for a 20- to 50-dB range above threshold as revealed in rate-level functions. Single nerves respond to a wide range of frequencies but are most sensitive to one frequency, which is called the characteristic frequency (CF) of a unit, as revealed by response area and tuning curve measures. Neurons with high CFs respond to a wider range of frequencies than do units with low CFs.

Interval and period histograms reveal that fibers with CFs below 5 kHz respond to the periodicity of low-frequency stimulation. Two-tone suppression indicates one type of nonlinear interaction that occurs for complex stimuli. Stimulation of the COCB efferent fibers results in changes in a variety of cochlear measures, especially a decrease in single-unit discharge rate. Place and temporal theories are used to account for the neural system's ability to encode frequency. Intensity is encoded by the number of neural discharges, and the phase and dynamic timing information for rates up to 5.0 kHz may be preserved in the synchrony with which auditory nerve fibers discharge to the phase of sound stimulation. Computer models can simulate the neural output of the auditory periphery.

SUPPLEMENT

The material in this chapter may be found in the books by Pickles (1998), Webster et al. (1992), Fay and Popper (1992), Dallos, Popper, and Fay (1996), Geisler (1998), Jahn and Santos-Sacchi (2001), and Moller (2003). The data reported in this chapter are based largely on extracellular recordings, where the recording electrode is near but not actually inside the nerve (see Appendixes E and F). In 1974, Mulroy et al. and Weiss et al. reported the first recordings of intracellular potentials from the hair cells of the organ of Corti of the alligator lizard. Then, in 1977 (a, b), Russell and Sellick were able to record intracellular receptor potentials directly from the inner hair cells of the mammalian cochlea. In 1980, Sellick and Russell compared the intracellular receptor potentials measured from inner hair cells of the guinea pig with the CM recorded from the scala tympani. They concluded that inner hair cells respond to the basilar membrane velocity for frequencies below 100 to 200 Hz. Above that frequency, basilar membrane displacement is the effective stimulus for inner hair cell response. They also noted the presence of two-tone suppression at the receptor potential level. Data on intracellular recordings from outer hair cells have also been measured

(see Dallos and Santos-Sacchi, 1982, and Tanaka et al., 1980). It is now fairly well established that the dc properties of the outer hair cell function contribute to the discharge rate of auditory nerve fibers and that the ac properties determine the synchronous aspects of neural discharges.

Historically, the term CF was defined from the period histograms to click stimuli, where CF equaled the reciprocal of the time between the major peaks in the click-evoked period histogram (see Figure 9.10). *Best Frequency* (BF) was used to define the tip of the tuning curve. Over the years BF and CF have been used almost interchangeably, and CF is used in this book because it appears to be the term most often used to describe the frequency to which a neuron is most sensitive. A number of terms are used almost interchangeably in describing the responses of a nerve: discharges, firings, spikes (e.g., spike rate), and responses. All of these will be used in this book to acquaint the student with their multiple uses in the literature.

Tuning curves for low-frequency CF fibers are about 200 Hz wide (in terms of bandwidth measured at 10 dB up from the tip of the tuning curves) and increase approximately linearly as CF increases, when both bandwidth and CF are plotted on a log axis, such that at a CF of 20,000 Hz fibers have bandwidths that are 2000 Hz wide (the result is that Q_{10dB} [see Chapter 5] values increase from 1 to 10 as CF increases). Narayan et al. (1998) showed that the tuning measured directly in the cochlea is almost identical to that measured in the auditory nerve, indicating that the tuning of the auditory nerve faithfully represents that measured in the cochlea.

The advent of computer processing of the responses of single auditory nerve fibers brought a mass of new information about the auditory system and a new surge of interest. The responses of single neurons in the auditory nerve can be more complex than we have shown in this chapter. We have presented only the single-neuron response data that are consistent with the cochlear mechanics discussed in the previous chapter, but many exceptions exist in which the neuronal discharges do not reflect basilar membrane motion in a simple fashion.

The functional role of the efferent system has not been fully established (see May, Budelis, and Niparko, 2004). The OCB clearly has an inhibitory influence on the neural output of the cochlea, and it may play some role in altering the biomechanics of the inner ear, as is discussed in Chapter 8. Because most neural studies of the auditory system have been conducted with the animals under anesthesia and anesthesia eliminates the normal function of the efferent system, its role may not be fully appreciated. Little data exist that describes how the auditory periphery functions when the efferent system is fully operational. Work by Winslow and Sachs (1988), using electrical shocks of the COCB, and by Liberman (1991), using contralateral sound stimulation, indicates that under the appropriate stimulus conditions, OCB stimulation can act to enhance the neural response to signals in quiet or in a background of noise. These results provide additional data for the possibility that efferent stimulation makes the signal-to-noise ratio larger than it would normally be based on the stimulus, enhancing the auditory system's ability to detect signals in noisy backgrounds. Behavioral studies of the significance of the efferent system are few, and their results are generally inconclusive.

The careful reader of Figures 9.11a and 9.12a will notice that the inhibitory change in the PST histograms due to the simultaneous presentation of two tones is similar in both figures. In Figure 9.11a both stimuli were presented to the same ear, whereas for Figure 9.12a the stimuli were presented to the opposite ears. However, with contralateral stimulation the

experimenter must be careful to rule out the possibility that the contralateral stimulus somehow "leaked" across the head and caused direct ipsilateral stimulation. If such a leak occurred, then the measured suppression may be more a result of two-tone suppression than COCB activity.

The model's output shown in Figure 9.16 is based on the auditory image model (AIM) of Patterson et al. (1995), in which the first stage is a bandpass filter matching the threshold of hearing function (see Chapter 10); the second stage is a bank of bandpass filters (a gammatone filter bank; see Chapter 11); and the third stage is based on the Meddis hair cell (Meddis, 1986). The key elements in such models of the auditory periphery include a representation of the middle ear transfer function (usually with a bandpass filter); the bandpass filtering action of the basilar membrane that indicates the travel time from base to apex and may represent an increase in bandwidth with increase in level (e.g., gammatone filer or chirp-gammatone filter; see Irino and Patterson, 1997); and the transduction of the output of the cochlea into neural responses with appropriate half-wave rectification, nonlinear rate-level characteristics, adaptation, neural refractory properties, and the fact that the hair cell–neural process acts as a low-pass filter (e.g., Meddis hair cell, Meddis, 1986). Greenwood (1990) has documented the relationship between frequency coding and cochlear distance for several species. Greenwood's *cochlear map* equation, relating cochlear frequency (F in Hz) to cochlear place (x in mm) in humans is: $F = A(10^{ax} - 1)$, where $A = 165.4$ and $a = 0.06$.

III

Auditory Sensation

10

Auditory Sensitivity

Chapters 2–5 described sound, the stimulus for hearing, and Chapters 6–9 reviewed some of the key properties of the peripheral auditory system's structure and function. These chapters have established that sound has three basic physical properties—frequency, level, and time—and that the auditory periphery provides a neural code for each. The next few chapters describe some of what is known about how these physical attributes of sound affect our sensations and perceptions related to sound, i.e., hearing.

A great deal of the study of auditory perception is based on measuring the detection of sound, the ability of subjects to discriminate between sounds that differ in frequency, and/or level, and/or time, and the subjective perception of frequency, level, and temporal variation. We also cover the fact that the location of a sound source can be determined based on the interaction of the sound from the source with either the body and head or other objects in the path of the sound.

THRESHOLDS OF AUDIBILITY

A first step in understanding auditory perception is to understand the auditory system's sensitivity to frequency, amplitude, and starting phase. When one understands the sensitivity of the auditory system to these variables for sinusoidal stimuli, the results might form a complete picture of the absolute sensitivity of the auditory system to any stimulus, because all acoustic stimuli can be defined in terms of sinusoids. That is, if the sinusoid is the basic building block of all sounds (see Chapters 2–5), then understanding the detection and discrimination of sinusoidal sounds might form the basic building blocks for understanding the detection and discrimination of all sounds. However, as we will see in this and the following chapters, the solutions are not that simple.

When one pure tone is presented to one ear, the auditory system is actually insensitive to its starting phase. This does not mean, as Helmholtz suggested more than 140 years ago, that the auditory system is phase insensitive. For instance, if two sinusoids of different frequencies are added, the perceived quality of the sound may vary as the relative starting phases of the sinusoids are varied. Also, as mentioned in Chapter 2, if a sinusoid is presented to both ears and there is a change in the interaural (between-ears) phase difference, then observers report a change in the perceived location of the tone (see Chapter 12).

A measure of auditory sensitivity to frequency and level can be made by determining the level required

below 100   above 20,000 Hearing
insensitive

for a listener to detect the presence of a sinusoid at each of many frequencies. There will be very low and very high frequencies to which, no matter how intense the sound, the auditory system is insensitive. These frequency limits define the bounds of the auditory system's sensitivity to frequency. The thresholds relating the smallest level required for detection to the frequency of the tone are called *thresholds of audibility*.

Thresholds of audibility are obtained in the laboratory in the following manner. For each frequency tested, a psychometric function is obtained either directly or indirectly using a psychophysical procedure (see Appendix D). Figure 10.1 demonstrates the results from this part of the experiment. The psychometric functions indicate the percent correct performance for a listener asked to detect tones of different frequencies when presented at different levels. That is, for each frequency the level of the tone is varied, from a level that is so low that the tone is difficult to detect to higher levels when the tone is more easily detected. The listener is asked to detect the presence or absence of the

tone at each sound level. Different psychophysical procedures (see Appendix D) are used to determine how well the listener performs in detecting the presence and absence of the tone and each tonal level. A threshold is determined for each frequency by choosing a performance level on each psychometric function, such as 75%, for $P(C)$, and determining the level (in decibels) of the tone required for $P(C)$ to equal 75%. Percent correct [$P(C)$] is a measure of the percentage of times the listener correctly detected the presence of the tone combined with the percentage of times the listener correctly indicated that a tone was not presented (see Appendix D). The thresholds of audibility are then plotted as the threshold in decibels versus frequency. A listener who has a low *threshold* can also be described as being very *sensitive*. Thus "high sensitivity" and "low threshold" mean the same thing. A great deal of what is known about auditory perception has been gleaned from experiments designed to estimate detection and discrimination thresholds in a manner similar to the one depicted in Figure 10.1.

*Minimum audible field (*MAF) thresholds are sound pressure levels for pure tones at absolute threshold, measured in a free field. The subject listens in a room to tonal sounds over loudspeakers. In the absence of the listener, a microphone is placed where the listeners head was to calibrate the threshold sound pressures, which are then converted to decibels. MAF thresholds are usually determined for listeners facing the source, listening with both ears (binaurally), at one meter from the sound source.

*Minimal audible pressure (*MAP) thresholds describe thresholds in terms of the sound pressure level at the observer's tympanic membrane. The subjects listen to sounds presented over earphones and various procedures are used to determine the sound pressure that occurs at the tympanic membrane. Most earphones are not calibrated in terms of the eardrum pressure they produce. To estimate the actual pressure at the tympanic membrane in a standardized manner, the sound pressure level is estimated from the sound level in a test *coupler* (rather than at the pinna or outer ear) attached to the earphone during calibration. Such couplers are designed to approximate the average acoustic

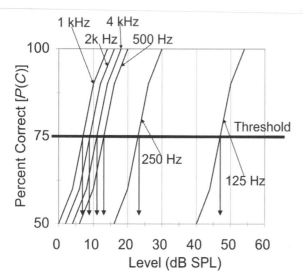

FIGURE 10.1 Psychometric functions obtained for six tones. The thresholds, in decibels of sound pressure level (dB SPL) are obtained for these forced-choice psychophysical data at a $P(C)$ of 75% (indicated by the downward-headed arrows). Adapted from Watson, Franks, and Hood (1972), used with permission.

properties of the outer ear of a listener with normal hearing and contain a microphone for estimating the sound pressure level that would exist at the tympanic membrane. Because there are different types of earphones and couplers, the threshold sound pressure levels vary for each earphone–coupler combination. For a particular earphone–coupler combination, the threshold sound pressure levels measured in the coupler are called the *reference equivalent threshold sound pressure levels* (RETSPLs), and these RETSPLs have been standardized for a variety of earphone–coupler combinations. Each earphone–coupler combination generates a different set of values for RETSPL. That is, the standardized RETSPL measurements indicate the level in decibels (SPL) required for threshold detection of tones of different frequencies presented via different earphones and calibrated with the appropriate coupler.

Three classes of earphones, each with its own coupler type, are typically used for most hearing tests. *Supra-aural* phones fit over the pinna and are calibrated using a *"6-cc" coupler* (6 cc represents the average volume of the adult outer ear canal that lies between the earphone and the tympanic membrane). *Circumaural* phones fit completely over and around the pinna and are calibrated using an *artificial ear*. *Insert earphones* fit directly into the outer ear canal and are often calibrated in an *occluded-ear simulator*, sometimes called a *Zwislocki coupler* after its founder, Joseph Zwislocki, or in a *2-cc coupler* (since 2 cc is the volume between the tip of the insert earphone lying within the outer ear and the tympanic membrane). Figure 10.2 and Table 10.1 show the RETSPLs for examples of a few earphone–coupler combinations.

As can be seen by comparing the MAF with the supra-aural or circumaural earphone MAP thresholds, they do not agree. MAF thresholds are always lower than MAP thresholds. Because the sound impinging on the tympanic membrane should be the same for a threshold response and great care is given to calibrating the actual sound pressure levels for each procedure, all thresholds should be essentially the same. Thus, one might conclude from examining the difference between the MAF and MAP thresholds that a "missing 6 dB" (the average difference between MAF

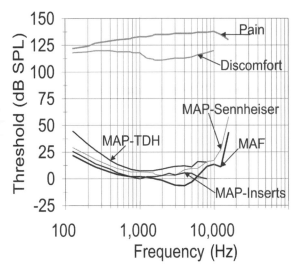

FIGURE 10.2 The thresholds of hearing in decibels of sound pressure level (dB SPL) are shown as a function of frequency for six conditions: reference equivalent threshold sound pressure level (RETSPL) minimal audible field (MAF) thresholds, RETSPL-MAP thresholds for a supra-aural phone and 6-cc coupler, RETSPL-MAP thresholds for an circumaural phone and an artificial ear, RETSPL-(MAP) minimal audible pressure thresholds for an insert phone and a Zwislocki coupler, thresholds for pain, and thresholds for discomfort. The RESTPL measures are from American National Standards Institute (ANSI) 3.6-2004. The thresholds for pain and discomfort represent estimates of the upper limit of the level that humans can tolerate.

and MAP measures in the mid-frequency range) existed between sound field (MAF) and earphone (MAP) thresholds. Experimental difficulties lead to that erroneous conclusion. When estimates of MAP and MAF data are corrected for head diffraction, outer-ear resonances, and the type of calibration procedure used, the greatest difference between the two types of measurements is maximally 2.5 dB, indicating that the different reference sound pressure levels required for calibrating different sound sources reflect differences in the calibration procedure, that the head acts to diffract sound in the MAF procedure, and that the outer ear has a resonant frequency (see Chapter 6). Therefore, there is no "missing 6 dB."

The shapes of the MAP and MAF absolute threshold functions are approximately the same, showing a

TABLE 10.1 Thresholds of Audibility for a Number of Testing Conditions (from American National Standard ANSI 3.6–2004 Specifications for Audiometers)

Frequency (Hz)	MAF[a]	Thresholds—RETSPL (dB SPL)		
		Supra-aural[b]	Circumaural[c]	Insert[d]
125	22	45	30.5	26
200	14.5	32.5	—	18
250	11	27	18	14
400	6	17	12	9
500	4	13.5	11	5.5
750	2	9	6	2
800	2	8.5	—	1.5
1000	2	7.5	5.5	0
1250	1.5	7.5	—	2
1500	0.5	7.5	5.5	2
1600	0	8	—	2
2000	−1.5	9	4.5	3
2500	−4	10.5	—	5
3000	−6	11.5	2.5	3.5
4000	−6.5	12	9.5	5.5
5000	−3	11	14	5
6000	2.5	16	17	2
8000	11.5	15.5	17.5	0
10,000	13.5	—	22	—
12,500	11	—	28	—
16,000	43.5	—	56	—

[a] Binaural listening, free-field, 0° incidence.
[b] TDH type.
[c] Sennheiser HDA2000, IEC 60318-2 with type 1 adaptor.
[d] HA-2 with rigid tube.

loss of sensitivity below approximately 1000 Hz and above approximately 4000 Hz. The loss of sensitivity declines at approximately 6 dB/octave at low frequencies below 1000 Hz and at approximately 24 dB/octave above 4000 Hz (the ability to estimate the slope of the high-frequency side of the thresholds of hearing function is much more difficult than at the low-frequency side due to the difficulty in measuring thresholds above 8000 Hz). Several factors governing the acoustic transfer function of the outer and middle ears (Chapter 6) have been suggested as explanations for the shape of the thresholds of hearing functions. For instance, the loss in middle ear pressure gain at low frequencies (see Figure 6.8) helps explain the loss of sensitivity for low tonal frequencies. The fact that the middle and inner ear structures have mass and inertia and therefore act as low-pass filters helps explain some of the loss of sensitivity to tones of high frequencies. In some general sense, the threshold of hearing curve is an overall functional description of the transfer function of the auditory system to tonal sounds.

The fact that tones over a range of frequencies from 20 Hz to 20,000 Hz can be detected requires a very good loudspeaker or earphone system. Zero dB SPL corresponds to 20 μPa, which is an extremely small pressure. At this pressure and at a signal frequency of 1000 Hz, the tympanic membrane is vibrating through a total distance approximately equal to the diameter of a hydrogen atom. The horizontal axis in Figure 10.2 was constructed so that the intensity is in decibels of sound pressure level, or dB SPL; that is, 0 dB SPL equals 20 μPa of pressure (see Chapter 3). Therefore, a number such as 50 dB SPL means the threshold is 50 dB above a pressure of 20 μPa (or the 50-dB SPL threshold is at a pressure of 6325 μPa; i.e., $20[10^{(50 db/20)}] = 6325$; see Appendix B).

The curves in Figure 10.2 represent the thresholds in dB SPL from the ANSI standard on thresholds (ANSI S3.6-2004). These values have been standardized as the recognized thresholds and are the set of threshold values agreed on when instruments are built and hearing tested. If hearing is tested using such a standard, the thresholds may be expressed in decibels relative to these standardized values. In this case, the thresholds are expressed in dB HL (decibels of *hearing level*). For instance, a person with a 30-dB HL threshold at 1000 Hz measured with a supra-aural earphone has a threshold 30 dB above that shown in Figure 10.2 and Table 10.1, or the threshold is 37.5 dB SPL (i.e., 30 dB HL plus 7.5 dB SPL). When the detection of tones of different frequencies is plotted in dB HL rather than dB SPL, the function is often referred to as an *audiogram*. The audiogram is the common measure of hearing when one is testing for possible hearing impairment. A person who had no hearing loss at all would have an audiogram that was flat as a function of frequency at a level of 0 dB HL. Any hearing loss is indicated as a positive decibel level in dB HL. That is, an audiogram indicating a threshold of 45 dB

A person w/ good hearing will have an ~~flat line~~ audiogram that was flat.

HL at 4000 Hz would mean a 45-dB hearing loss for detecting a 4000-Hz tone.

On average, thresholds of hearing are slightly different for males and females, with females having slightly lower thresholds (usually less than about 3 dB) than males. For many listeners, thresholds of hearing measured at the two ears for the exact same conditions are not always equal. On average the thresholds of hearing increase with age above about 18 years old, more so at high than at low frequencies (the increase in the thresholds of hearing with age is referred as *presbycusis*). On average significant increases in the thresholds of hearing above 4000 Hz occur after the age of 50 years old. And, as is obvious, the thresholds of hearing vary greatly depending on any hearing abnormalities that a subject has (see Chapter 16).

The thresholds of audibility define the smallest amount of pressure to which the auditory system is sensitive. What about an upper limit in terms of the most pressure the auditory system can tolerate? The upper curves in Figures 10.2 show an estimate of this upper limit. The listener can be asked to say when the sound is "felt," when pain is experienced, or when a tickling sensation is felt (these levels form *thresholds of pain* or *feeling*). The listener can also be asked when the sound level has become uncomfortable (*thresholds of discomfort*). These experiences indicate that the sound pressure is reaching a maximum. This maximum limit is approximately 120 to 140 dB SPL, and it remains relatively unchanged as a function of the frequency content of the stimulus. Thus, the *dynamic range* (difference between the threshold in dB SPL and the maximum limit in dB SPL) of the auditory system changes as a function of frequency; e.g., it is approximately 125 to 135 dB at 1000 Hz but 80 to 90 dB at 100 Hz. The upper limit of audibility appears to be less susceptible to factors such as gender, age, and hearing impairment as the thresholds of hearing.

DURATION

One variable that was not specified in the procedures used to obtain tonal thresholds is the duration of the sinusoid. From several points of view one might expect that the longer a sound lasts, the easier it is to hear. For the thresholds of audibility shown in Figure 10.2, the tone's duration was more than 400 msec.

When time (T) is involved in the measurement of intensity, one must be careful in noting whether the intensity is expressed in terms of units of power (P) or energy (E). Remember from Chapter 3 that

$$P = E/T \quad \text{and} \quad E = PT. \tag{10.1}$$

To describe the auditory system's sensitivity to duration, the experimenter can keep the signal level constant in terms of units of either power or energy, but not both, while changing its duration.

Figure 10.3 shows the thresholds for different frequencies as a function of the duration of the signals. In this figure, level is expressed in terms of units of power. Thus, for each tonal duration, a psychometric function was obtained in which the performance of the observer was related to the power of the tonal signal. Then, for each duration, the threshold in units of power was determined from the psychometric functions and plotted in Figure 10.3.

Notice that at durations greater than approximately 250 to 500 msec, the threshold in units of power for various tones does not change much; for durations greater than about 250 to 500 msec, the tone does not become easier to detect. However, as the tone's duration is made shorter than 250 msec, the power of the tone must be increased for the observer to detect the tone (i.e., the tone is more difficult to detect at short durations). This increase is approximately equal to 8 to 10 dB of power increase for each 10-fold decrease in the duration of the tone, although this effect is slightly dependent on frequency. A 10 dB increase in power for each 10-fold decrease in duration means that the signal energy is remaining constant for a constant level of the listener's performance. That is, equation (10.1) states that energy will remain constant if, as duration decreases, power increases. In other words, if $P = E/T$, then $\log P = \log(E/T)$, or $10\log P = 10\log E - 10\log T$. (see Appendix B, rule 2). Therefore, $10\log E = 10\log P + 10\log T$ (if T is less than 1 sec). Thus, for a 10-fold change in duration,

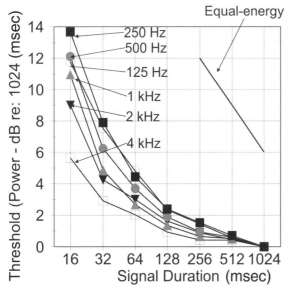

FIGURE 10.3 Thresholds in units of power for six tonal frequencies (ranging from 125 to 4000 Hz) displayed as a function of tonal duration. The thresholds are calculated and plotted in relation to the thresholds obtained at 1024 msec. For instance, the threshold for a 32-msec tone burst with a frequency of 250 Hz (the circles) is approximately 8 dB higher than that of a 1024-msec (1-sec) tone. The straight line with a slope of 3 dB for a doubling of duration indicates performance for equal energy detection. Adapted from Watson and Gengel (1969), with permission.

power must also change 10-fold to keep energy constant (or for a doubling of duration signal power must change by 3 dB). For the data shown in Figure 10.3, it is important to realize that duration is expressed in relation to 1 second. Therefore, a change from 1 second to 1/10 of a second (100 msec) is a change of 1/10, or, in decibels, (10 log 1/10), or −10 dB. So, as duration becomes shorter (less than 1 second), the power must become greater if energy is to remain constant. For example, if a 500-msec tone has a power of 80 dB, then the energy of this 500-msec tone is 77 dB; that is,

$$10 \log E = 10 \log P + 10 \log T,$$
$$E \text{ in dB} = P \text{ in dB} + 10 \log T$$
$$= 80 \text{ dB} + 10 \log 500 \text{ msec}/$$
$$1000 \text{ msec} (1 \sec = 1000 \text{ msec})$$
$$= 80 \text{ dB} + 10 \log 0.5 = 80 \text{ dB} - 3 \text{ dB} = 77 \text{ dB}.$$

If the duration of this tone is changed from 500 msec to 50 msec and energy is to remain at 77 dB, then

$$77 \text{ dB} = P \text{ in dB} + 10 \log 50 \text{ msec}/500 \text{ msec}$$
$$= P \text{ in dB} + 10 \log 0.10 = P \text{ in dB} - 10 \text{ dB}$$

or

$$P \text{ in dB} = 87 \text{ dB}(77 \text{ dB} + 10 \text{ dB}).$$

Thus, the power of the 50-msec tone must be 10 dB higher than that of the 500-msec tone if energy is to remain constant.

Between approximately 10 msec and 300 to 500 msec, the energy of the signal appears to remain approximately constant for constant-detection performance by the listener. Note, however, that the constant-energy property of the auditory system is only approximately true and depends on frequency. A complete understanding of auditory processing requires an explanation of the interaction among frequency, duration, and signal detection.

Once the duration of a sinusoidal signal decreases below about 10 msec, then much more power is required for detection than is needed to keep energy constant. It appears that the auditory system is not a constant-energy detector below 10 msec. In Chapter 4 we showed that a tone turned on and off spreads its energy over a large frequency region. As the duration of the tone becomes shorter and shorter, this frequency region over which the energy is spread becomes larger and larger. Thus, for very short-duration tones (less than 10 msec) the frequency region over which the energy of the tone is spread becomes so large that not all of the energy is contributing to its detectability. Because there is some energy at frequencies to which the ear is insensitive, there will be less energy in the region where the ear is sensitive. This in turn means that the total power or energy of the tone must be increased so that enough energy is in the auditory system's frequency region of sensitivity for the tone to be detected.

In other cases (for example, for a very low-frequency tone, such as a 125-Hz tone) the spread of energy associated with the short duration of the tone might produce energy in a frequency region (higher in frequency, e.g., at 1000 Hz) where the auditory system is more sensitive (see Figure 10.2, and note that at 125 Hz, 22 to 45 dB SPL is required for detection, whereas at 1000 Hz only 0 to 7.5 dB SPL is required). The listener might detect the short-duration tone because the energy available at a frequency other than the tone's frequency is more detectable.

Therefore, the duration of the signal used to establish tonal threshold is important. If it is longer than approximately 300 msec, the thresholds represent intensity in units of power; if the signal is between 10 and 300 msec, the thresholds reflect approximately constant energy; for signals of duration less than 10 msec, the spread of energy makes the determination of thresholds dependent on frequency and is more difficult to determine.

TEMPORAL INTEGRATION

Notice in Figure 10.3 that further increases in duration beyond 300 msec do not change the detectability of a tone. It is as if the auditory system requires about 300 msec for maximal performance. If the signal is shorter than 300 msec, then its level, expressed in units of power, must be increased for maximal performance; but for durations greater than 300 msec, no additional changes in sound power are required for threshold detection. This property of the detection of signals of different durations is often called *temporal integration*. Figure 10.4 diagrams the basic idea of temporal integration. A signal must have some critical amount of energy (in Figure 10.4 energy is the area of the rectangle, i.e., $P \times T$) to be detected (the hashed area is the energy required for detection), and once the signal contains that amount of energy (that area), it is detectable. In addition, the process of summing the power (integration) to generate the required energy is completed by 300 msec (the *integration time*). This means that if the duration is less than 300 msec (the estimate of the integration time from Figure 10.4), then the power of the signal must be increased for the signal to be detected (the height of the rectangle must be increased to achieve the required area as shown in

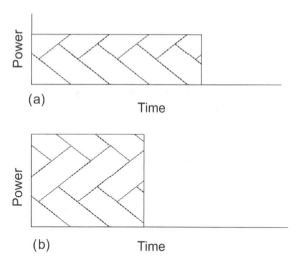

(a)   Time

(b)   Time

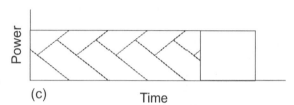

(c)   Time

FIGURE 10.4 Schematic diagram depicting the concept of temporal integration. The hashed area (**a**), represents the energy of a signal required to detect the presence of a tone. In (**b**) the signal is shorter than that in (**a**), so the power of this shorter signal must be increased over that shown in (**a**) to yield a just barely detectable signal. In (**c**) the signal duration is longer than the time required to achieve the necessary energy for detection; thus there is no need to change the power of the signal in order for the signal to remain just detectable.

Figure 10.4b). For durations greater than 300 msec, the threshold expressed in units of power remains constant for a constant level of performance, since the required integration time has been met or exceeded (Figure 10.4c).

The estimate of the integration time for auditory processing can vary a great deal from stimulus condition to stimulus condition. For instance, the detection of a tone requires an integration time of about 300 msec; however, the detection of a click (impulse) stimulus requires an integration time of only a few milliseconds.

Thus, the integration time of auditory processing depends on the type of signal being processed. Estimates range from 1 to 2 msec to more than 500 msec.

DIFFERENTIAL SENSITIVITY

Although the thresholds of audibility define the frequency and intensity range of the auditory system, they do not describe our sensitivity to <u>changes</u> in intensity and frequency. In the early 1800s, Weber observed that it was easy to distinguish between a 1- and a 2-pound weight but not so easy to differentiate a 100-pound weight from a 101-pound weight, although both pairs of weights differ by 1 pound. It was found that the difference between two weights that could just be detected was proportional to the value of the smaller weight. That is, if the *just-noticeable difference (jnd)* for a 1-pound weight as 0.1 pound, then the jnd for the 100-pound weight was 10 pounds (0.1/1 is the same proportion as 10/100). Weber and Fechner stated this relation in equation form: $\Delta S/S =$ constant, where ΔS is the just-noticeable physical difference in some stimulus value and S is the smaller of the two values being discriminated. The ratio $\Delta S/S$ is called the *Weber fraction.* Psychoacousticians have attempted to determine whether the Weber fraction for the level, frequency, and duration of sinusoids is a constant and, if so, over what range of levels, frequencies, and durations.

Extreme care must be taken in studying differential sensitivity, in that the spectrum of a sound changes when any parameter of the sound suddenly changes. As mentioned previously, not all of the energy of a tone is at the tonal frequency if the tone is very short or if it is turned on and off abruptly. This spread of energy also arises if the frequency or level or phase of an ongoing tone is suddenly changed. Thus, one cannot simply study differential sensitivity by changing the level or frequency of an ongoing tone and asking a listener if a change is detected. The listener will probably hear the change because of detecting a click resulting from the spread of energy to other frequencies rather than an intensity, frequency, or dura-

tion change per se. In most studies, two tones are presented in succession: One tone is the standard tone and the second is called the comparison tone, which is presented with a slightly different intensity, frequency, or, in some cases, duration (although as we will discuss later there are other methods for measuring duration discrimination) than the standard tone.

FREQUENCY DISCRIMINATION

Figure 10.5 shows the value of threshold Δf (frequency difference) required to just discriminate a difference in frequency from a given frequency, f. The data are plotted as threshold Δf versus f, with the various curves representing different levels. These data represent the values of the difference threshold (Δf) for frequency. That is, psychometric functions in which the listener's performance was related to various frequency differences could be obtained for many different base frequencies, and then the difference threshold for each base frequency is calculated from the psychometric functions.

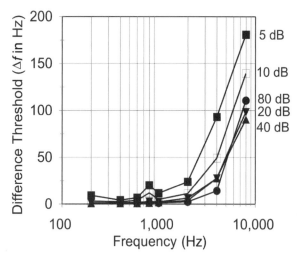

FIGURE 10.5 The value of threshold Δf (Hz) required to just discriminate between two different frequencies is shown as a function of the base frequency for five stimulus levels, expressed in decibels of sound in sensation level (dB SL). Adapted from Weir, Jesteadt, and Green (1977), with permission.

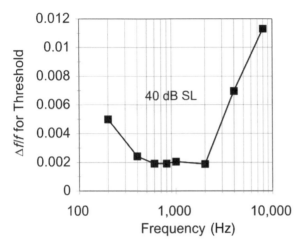

FIGURE 10.6 The value of Δf/f (the Weber fraction for frequency) is shown as a function of frequency for the 40 decibels of sound in sensation level (dB SL) data plotted in Figure 10.5. The results show that over an intermediate range of frequencies the Weber fraction is approximately constant.

As can be seen, the value of threshold Δf increases as f increases above 1000 Hz. In the mid-frequency region, this increase is enough to maintain the Weber fraction for frequency, Δf/f, approximately constant. This can be seen in Figure 10.6, in which the Weber fraction (Δf/f) is plotted as a function of f. Notice that over an intermediate range of frequencies this fraction is nearly constant at approximately Δf/f = 0.002 (or 0.2%). This means that at low frequencies, threshold Δf can be as small as 1 Hz. (For instance, if f is 500 Hz and Δf/500 = 0.002, then Δf = 500 × 0.002 = 1 Hz.)

LEVEL/INTENSITY DISCRIMINATION

Figure 10.7 demonstrates the value of threshold Δf in dB required for the observers to detect a difference in level from the initial value I. The value of threshold Δf in dB is plotted as a function of I, and the different curves represent the results using different tonal frequencies and a wide-band noise. Threshold Δf in dB is the difference threshold for level.

Notice that the auditory system is sensitive to approximately a 0.5- to 1.0-dB change in level across

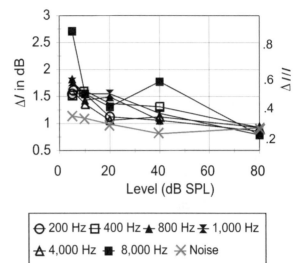

FIGURE 10.7 The value of threshold ΔI in decibels (the difference in decibels between the more and the less intense tones) required for threshold discrimination is shown as a function of overall tonal level in decibels in sound pressure level (dB SL). Data for six tonal frequencies and a wide-band noise are shown. On the right-hand axis is ΔI/I, not in decibels. Adapted from Jesteadt, Weir, and Green (1977) and Viemeister (1974), with permission.

a broad range of frequencies and levels. The fact that threshold ΔI in dB is nearly a constant as a function of I implies that ΔI/I (not in decibels) for pressure, energy, or power (or the Weber fraction) is nearly a constant. This results from the fact that the logarithm (decibels) of a ratio (such as the Weber fraction) is equal to a difference between the logarithm of the divisor and that of the dividend (see Appendix B).

Let ΔI/I = c, a constant (when ΔI and I are not expressed in decibels). This is the Weber fraction. By slightly changing this equation (i.e., adding 1.0 to each side of the equation), one obtains: (ΔI/I) + 1 = c + 1 = K, another constant. This can be written as: (ΔI/I) + 1 = (ΔI + I)/I = K, which is another form of the Weber fraction. Expressing this ratio in decibels, we get 10 log[(ΔI + I)/I] = 10 log(ΔI + I) − 10 log(I) = 10 log K = C, another constant. This last equation is the same as the decibel difference between the more intense stimulus, I + ΔI, and the less intense stimulus, I. This is the same as ΔI in dB or ΔI "in decibels." Thus, if ΔI in dB is a constant, then $\Delta I/I$, not in dB, is also a constant. ΔI "in decibels" is plotted along the left-hand axis in Figure 10.7. From the relations just shown, ΔI in decibels is a simple transform of $(\Delta I + I)/I$, or $\Delta I/I$, as shown on the right-hand axis of Figure 10.7. These relationships also show the various forms that the Weber fraction can take when intensity discrimination is studied.

Intensity discrimination data for a variety of tones of different frequencies and a wide-band noise are shown in Figure 10.7. Notice that the thresholds for threshold ΔI in dB remain very near to 0.5 to 1 dB for a wide range of levels for the wide-band noise, but that the threshold ΔI in dB decreases slightly, but steadily, as the level of the tones increases. The fact that the thresholds for tones are not constant when plotted in terms of ΔI in dB means that they do not strictly follow the Weber fraction. This fact is often referred to as the *near miss to the Weber fraction*. The "near miss" applies to tonal but not to wide-band noise stimuli.

TEMPORAL DISCRIMINATION

If listeners are asked to detect the difference between a 50-msec sinusoid and a 60-msec sinusoid, additional variables besides the tone's duration would be present that might aid the listener in detecting a difference in these two sounds. Recall from Figure 10.3 that because tones of different durations sometimes have different thresholds, the 50- and 60-msec tones might appear different in dectability. Also, the spectrum of pulsed tones depends on the duration of the tone (Chapter 4), thus the two tones differ in spectra. These two additional variables (spectra and detectability) make the study of temporal discrimination difficult.

To measure sensitivity to duration, some investigators have attempted to avoid these confounding problems (see Chapter 1 regarding confounding variables) by presenting the listener with acoustic markers. To measure duration discrimination, the stimuli may consist of the following: a standard stimulus in which a tone of 170-msec duration is followed 10 msec later

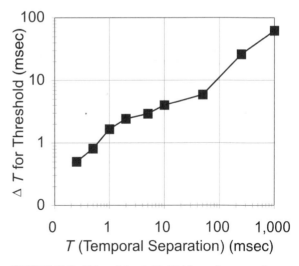

FIGURE 10.8 Value of threshold ΔT (change in temporal separation between two tonal markers in msec) is shown as a function of T (standard separation between the two tonal markers in msec). Adapted from Abel (1971), with permission.

by an identical 170-msec tone; and the comparison stimulus in which the two 170-msec tones are separated by 20 msec instead of by 10 msec. The listener's task is to decide whether these two stimuli are different in the time separation between the two 170-msec tonal markers. If the durations are correctly judged to be different, then one assumes that the auditory system can detect this 10-msec difference in duration between the markers.

The data in Figure 10.8 show the results from such an experiment. At various standard separations of T msec between the two tonal markers, the value of the additional amount of time (ΔT) required to detect the increase in duration is shown for the condition when the markers were 1000 Hz and 85 dB SPL. Thus, as the temporal separation (duration) increases, a greater and greater change in the temporal separation is required to make a temporal discrimination. Although threshold ΔT increases as a function of T, it does not increase at a rate such that $\Delta T/T$ (Weber fraction) equals a constant. Notice that at T equal to approximately 1 msec, threshold ΔT is approximately 2 msec, so the Weber fraction is 2.0. At 300 msec of T, the value of threshold ΔT is 30 msec, so the Weber fraction is 0.1.

Although these results, plus those of other investigations, show that the difference in time required for temporal/duration discrimination increases as the standard time increases, the exact nature of the temporal relationships depends on many different stimulus conditions. For instance, if the frequencies of the two acoustic markers are different, especially if they differ on each trial of the experiment, the listener's threshold for detecting a difference in temporal separation between the acoustic markers is usually elevated well above that when the two acoustic markers are acoustically the same.

TEMPORAL MODULATION TRANSFER FUNCTIONS

The conditions used to obtain the data of Figure 10.8 are based on a single change in the temporal property of sound. Most real-world sounds have fluctuating temporal changes. Detection of sinusoidally amplitude-modulated (SAM) wide-band noise can be used to measure auditory sensitivity to fluctuating changes. Recall from Chapter 4 (see Figure 4.17 and equation 4.6) that sinusoidal amplitude modulation for a noise can be written as $[1 + m\sin(2\pi F_m)]n(t)$, where m is modulation depth, F_m is modulation rate, and $n(t)$ is the noise carrier stimulus.

The basic task for the listener, as shown in Figure 10.9, is to detect which wide-band noise stimulus (10.9a or 10.9b) is sinusoidally amplitude modulated, i.e., which noise sample appears to fluctuate in level (loudness). A psychometric function is obtained for each rate of amplitude modulation (F_m) relating performance, such as $P(C)$, to depth of modulation (m). As the depth of modulation (m) decreases, the modulated noise has a lower depth of modulation and appears to have less level fluctuation and is more like the unmodulated noise. Threshold modulation depth is determined from these psychometric functions and is plotted as a function of modulation rate, such as shown in Figure 10.10. The value of threshold m (threshold

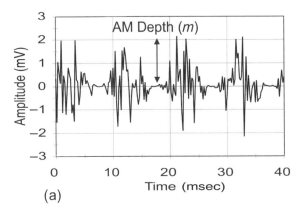

(a)

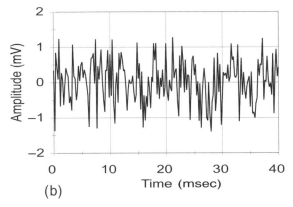

(b)

FIGURE 10.9   An unmodulated (**b**) and a sinusoidally amplitude-modulated noise (**a**) used to determine a temporal modulation transfer function. The listener is to determine which sound is amplitude modulated, and the depth of modulation (where AM depth = m) is adjusted to determine threshold.

modulation depth, where m ranges from 0 to 1) is often expressed in decibel units as $20\log m$, where 0 dB means 100% modulation ($m = 1$), and the more negative threshold depth becomes in decibels, the smaller the depth (for $m = 0.5$, $20\log m = -6$ dB; and if $m = 0$, the noise is unmodulated and $20\log m = -\infty$).

As can be seen, the depth of modulation required to detect sinusoidally amplitude-modulated noise remains fairly constant up to modulation rates of approximately 50 Hz, and as modulation rate increases beyond 50 Hz the thresholds decline, indicating that

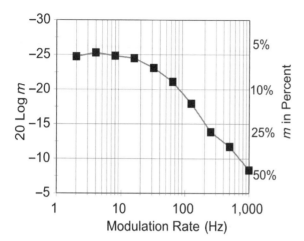

FIGURE 10.10 The temporal modulation transfer function (TMTF) for a wide-band noise stimulus showing threshold depth of amplitude modulation (expressed in decibels as $20 \log m$, where m is the threshold depth of modulation) as a function of the rate of sinusoidal modulation. On the right-hand axis is shown modulation depth (m) in percent. Adapted from Bacon and Viemeister (1985), with permission.

the fluctuations in the amplitude of the noise are more difficult to detect. That is, as modulation rate increases (the time between amplitude peaks in the modulated noise becomes shorter), the depth of modulation must be increased in order for the listener to detect the presence of modulation, i.e., a change in level over time.

The shape of the data curve in Figure 10.10 is like that of a low-pass filter (see Chapter 5 and Figure 5.2). Thus, imagine that the auditory system acts like a low-pass filter, attenuating the depth of modulation for modulation rates above its cutoff frequency (which according to Figure 10.10 would be approximately 50 Hz), making it difficult to detect amplitude modulation for high modulation rates. High rates of amplitude modulation are not processed by the auditory system, at least not as well as low rates of modulation. Such a low-pass filter describes the way in which amplitude-modulated stimuli might be transformed by the auditory system. These data showing the threshold depth of modulation as a function of modulation rate are often described as determining the *temporal mod-*

ulation transfer function (TMTF) of the auditory system.

SUMMARY

The threshold of audibility describes the auditory system's sensitivity to level and frequency. The thresholds are measured in either an MAF or a MAP paradigm, both of which involve a calibration procedure. The duration of the tone used to determine absolute threshold is crucial. If the duration is between about 10 and 300 msec, its energy must remain approximately constant for a constant level of detection by the observer. For durations 300 msec or longer the power must be held constant, whereas for durations shorter than 10 msec much more energy is required for tonal detection because short-duration tones are affected by spread of energy. Temporal integration is often used to describe these duration effects. The data from listeners detecting differences in frequency obey, to a first approximation, the Weber–Fechner law, with $\Delta f/f$ equaling approximately 0.002. The Weber fraction also applies approximately to discriminations of differences in tonal level. In this case only a 0.5- to 1.0-dB difference is necessary for reliable discrimination performance. Temporal discrimination is difficult to study due to dectability and spectral changes associated with changing duration. The temporal modulation transfer function (TMTF) is used to describe detection of amplitude modulation for different rates of modulation.

SUPPLEMENT

Measures of auditory thresholds have existed since the early part of the 20th century, and Sivan and White (1933) conducted the first thorough study of them. Parts of Chapters 1, 2, 3, and 4 in the textbook by Moore (1997) cover topics related to auditory sensitivity. Chapter 2 by Green in the book by Yost, Popper, and Fay (1993) also contains information relevant to this chapter. Laming (1988) provides an interesting discussion of differential sensitivity in audition and vision that pertains to some observations made in this chapter.

Because thresholds of hearing are used to define hearing loss for the hearing impaired, they have been standardized both in the United States and internationally. The ANSI standards establish the thresholds for young adults with normal hearing, as outlined in Table 10.1. In this textbook, the closing section of the References following the appendixes lists ANSI and International Standards (ISO and IEC standards) that are relevant to understanding the fundamentals of hearing.

Sometimes an individual may have a slightly different threshold in the frequency region near 4000 Hz. Because this is the frequency region near the resonant frequency of the outer ear canal, it is usually assumed that alterations in normal thresholds in this frequency region are due to some consequences of these resonances.

The difference between the MAF and the MAP thresholds has been of concern to auditory scientists for years. The differences are almost entirely explained if the impedance properties of the middle and inner ears, along with the resonances of the outer ear, are carefully measured and properly combined. Killion (1978) and Yost and Killion (1997) describe these calculations.

The ability to measure thresholds at very high frequencies (above 8 kHz) is difficult because of the resonance and standing-wave acoustics of the outer ear. There are large differences in the acoustics at or near the tympanic membrane, depending on the type of sound source (external speaker, supra-aural, or insert) used to present the sound. A major difference between measuring thresholds with a supra-aural and an insert earphone is the effect of internal noise due to the *occlusion effect*. When the outer ear is closed with a supra-aural earphone cushion, the effects of internal noise such as that caused by breathing and the pulsing of blood through the arteries near the ear canal interfere with the ability to detect sounds, because the ear is occluded by the earphone. Deeply seated insert

phones produce less of an occlusion effect and, therefore, produce lower thresholds than supra-aural phones at low frequencies (see Yost and Killion, 1997). See ISO-7029 2005, Acoustics—Statistical Distribution of Hearing Thresholds as a Function of Age, for a summary of data on hearing thresholds as a function of age and gender.

As mentioned in Chapters 6 and 7, the inner ear can be vibrated directly via bone conduction. A common hearing test is to vibrate the mastoid (bone of the skull behind the ear) or the forehead with a bone vibrator. One can then measure the bone vibration force required to produce a just-detectable sound for a variety of frequencies in much the same manner as the air-conducted thresholds of Figures 10.1 and 10.2 were obtained. The difference between the air-conducted (through earphones) and bone-conducted thresholds may be used to estimate the site (in the middle ear versus in the inner ear or nervous system) of a hearing abnormality. The values given in Table 10.2 show the force (relative to 1 dyne) required for normal, bone-vibrated thresholds when a vibrator,

TABLE 10.2   RETFLs for Audiometric Bone Vibrators, from ANSI 3.6-2004 (see also Table 10.1)

Frequency (Hz)	Mastoid locations (decibels) relative to 1 dyne	Forehead location (decibels) relative to 1 dyne
250	67	79
400	61	74.5
500	58	72
750	48.5	61.5
800	47	59
1000	42.5	51
1250	39	49
1500	36.5	47.5
1600	35.5	46
2000	31	42.5
2500	29.5	41.4
3000	30	42
4000	35.5	43.5
5000	40	51
6000	40	51
8000	40	50

meeting the specifications of the standard, is applied to the mastoid (column 1) and the forehead (column 2). These values (referent equivalent threshold force levels, RETFLs) can then be used to determine whether a person has a bone-conducted hearing loss in the same way the values in Table 10.1 are used to determine whether someone has an air-conducted hearing loss.

The concepts of temporal integration may be expressed in the following formula: $T(I - I_\infty) = C$, where T is the tonal duration, I is the tonal level at threshold, and I_∞ is the threshold level for a very long (greater than 1 sec) tone, and C is a constant. Thus, in order to maintain the value of C constant, I must decrease as T increases, as is consistent with the data shown in Figure 10.3. Recent discussion of temporal integration and alternative methods for accounting for changes in auditory perception as a function of temporal variables can be found in Viemeister and Plack (1993). Formby et al. (1998) have investigated the ability to determine temporal separations between acoustic markers when the markers differ acoustically (e.g., in frequency).

To be consistent with the definitions given in Chapters 2 and 3, intensity discrimination should be referred to as level discrimination. However, since the term intensity discrimination is used so widely, it has been applied to describe sensitivity to a change in sound level. Riesz (1928) made the first accurate estimates of intensity discrimination thresholds by using a beating stimulus. Riesz reasoned that the ability to hear a slowly beating sinusoid must relate to the ability to detect the change in level that is occurring over time. As Jesteadt, Weir, and Green (1977) argue, this method produces somewhat lower intensity discrimination thresholds than the method they used (see Figure 10.7). The beating has some additional spectral information that aids the listener in discrimination. Thus, a more accurate estimate of intensity discrimination per se is probably obtained in a forced-choice procedure, using two tones of slightly different levels rather than a beating stimulus.

The section of the book on Terms, Measurements, Equations, and Conversions (following the appendixes) provides equations for various ways of measuring the Weber fraction for intensity based on the work of Grantham and Yost (1982). As Grantham and Yost showed, there are a variety of methods used to calculate the intensity discrimination thresholds. The more intense tone may be generated by adding two tones, s (the signal) and m (the masker). The less intense tone is m and the more intense tone is $m + s$ (see Chapter 11 for a discussion of signals and maskers). When adding two tones, the phase relationship (α) between the tones (see Appendix A) must be used to compute the summed level. The work of Viemeister (1974) and Viemeister and Plack (1993) should be consulted with regard to the near-miss to Weber's law, the differences between tonal and noise intensity discrimination, and issues pertaining to coding of level by the auditory system (see also Green, 1993).

Shower and Biddulph (1931) used a frequency modulation (see Chapter 4) technique to measure frequency discrimination thresholds, for approximately the same reason that Riesz used beats to measure intensity discrimination thresholds. The results of Weir, Jesteadt, and Green (1977), as displayed in Figures 10.5 and 10.6, are in fair agreement with these earlier data. Jesteadt and Bilger (1974) discuss problems in measuring frequency discrimination thresholds.

The potential power of the TMTF is based on treating the obtained TMTF as a low-pass filter transfer function for predicting auditory sensitivity to other forms of amplitude modulation that might be imparted to a sound. The TMTF predicts how a listener loses sensitivity to modulation as the rate of modulation increases. One such form of modulation is square-wave (see Chapter 4) modulation, in which the noise is turned on and off abruptly in a repeating fashion, which happens if the noise is multiplied by a square wave rather than by a sine wave. The TMTF does a good job of describing a listener's ability to detect square-wave modulation. One version of square-wave modulation is a noise with a temporal gap in the middle. A sound with a temporal gap is also similar to stimuli like those discussed for Figure 10.9, in which two identical sounds mark a temporal interval. A great deal of work has been done on listeners' ability to detect temporal gaps of different widths for assessing temporal auditory sensitivity (see Viemeister and Plack, 1993).

One can also measure modulation detection for sinusoidal carriers (see Dau et al. 1997). However, recall that sinusoidally amplitude modulating a sinusoidal carrier produces a stimulus with sideband components (see Chapter 4) that are separated from the carrier frequency by a frequency difference equal to the modulation frequency. Thus, at fast rates of modulation (high modulation frequencies) these sideband components are at frequencies that differ significantly from the carrier frequency. As a result, listeners might detect these sideband components as their cue for discriminating an unmodulated tonal carrier from a modulated one. Such sideband detection would confound the ability to measure modulation processing per se.

The measure of the temporal processing abilities of the auditory system is sometimes referred to as *temporal acuity*. Green (1971) and Viemeister and Plack (1993) provide excellent reviews of some of these concepts and experiments. Viemeister and Plack (1993) describe the procedures used to estimate temporal processing time from TMTF experiments. Such TMTF estimates of temporal processing time are usually much shorter than most estimates of temporal integration times. Viemeister and Plack (1993) suggest a possible way to reconcile the different estimates of temporal processing time. Dau and colleagues (1997) have suggested that the auditory system's sensitivity to modulation might be modeled by assuming that a bank of bandpass "modulation" filters exists in the upper brainstem or cortex. This modulation filter bank consists of bandpass filters "tuned" to different rates of modulation, in a way that is analogous to a frequency-tuned filter that is tuned to different sound frequencies. The modulation filter bank is discussed again in Chapter 14.

11

Masking

Sounds in our environment rarely occur in isolation; often many stimuli occur either simultaneously or close together in time. The study of masking is concerned with the interaction of sounds. The experimenter is interested in the amount of interference one stimulus can cause in the perception of another stimulus. A change in stimulus threshold is a typical measure of the amount of interference produced. Tonal masking, for instance, deals with the change in tonal threshold of one tone associated with the interference, or masking, produced by another tone.

TONAL MASKING

It is logical to assume there is a great deal of interaction, or masking, between two stimuli with frequencies that do not differ by much. To investigate this interaction, the listener is asked to detect the presence of a weak-intensity sinusoid (perhaps 5 dB SL) at one frequency (perhaps 1000 Hz)—*the signal tone*. Another tone (the *masking tone*), usually with a frequency different from that of the signal, is presented simultaneously with the signal. The level of the masker that leads to threshold detection of the signal is used as the indicator of the amount of masking the

masker has provided for the signal. If the masker is very intense and the listener can still detect the signal, the masker is not very effective in interfering with detection of the signal. On the other hand, if a weak-intensity masker causes the signal to be undetected, then the masker is effective in interfering with signal processing. Figure 11.1 shows the results from just such an experiment. In this experiment, the listener was presented with either the signal-plus-masker tones followed by the masker tone or the masker followed by the signal-plus-masker. In this two-alternative, forced-choice procedure, the listener had to decide whether the signal appeared the first time (first observation interval) or the second time (second observation interval). At masker frequencies either lower or higher than the signal frequency, the masker level required for threshold detection was higher than when the masker frequency was near the signal frequency. This indicates that frequencies different from the signal frequency are not as effective at masking as those near the signal frequency. Figure 11.1 shows a family of masking curves obtained with different signal frequencies. In general, their shapes are similar.

Both your intuition and your knowledge about the neural activity of the auditory periphery should enable you to understand the shape of the curves in

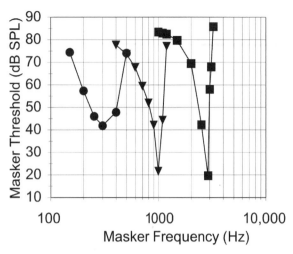

FIGURE 11.1 Three psychophysical tuning curves for simultaneous masking are shown. The different curves are for conditions in which the signal frequency was 300, 1000, and 3000 Hz. Based on data from Wightman, McGee, and Kramer (1977), with permission.

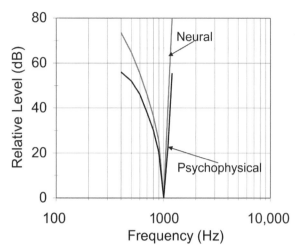

FIGURE 11.2 A comparison of an auditory nerve tuning curve (from Figure 9.5) and a psychophysical, simultaneous tuning curve (from Figure 11.1). The auditory nerve tuning curve is narrower than the psychophysical tuning curve.

Figure 11.1. Consider the "tuning curves" for auditory nerve fibers described in Chapter 8. These curves show that a particular neuron is most sensitive to one frequency of stimulation and that as the frequency of stimulation differs from the nerve's best frequency, a higher level of stimulation is required to drive the neuron at its threshold value. The similarity between the procedure used to obtain the neural tuning curves and that described earlier to obtain the masking data shown in Figure 11.1 has led to the name *psychophysical tuning curves* for these masking functions. The procedures are similar, and so are the derived functions. Both the psychophysical and neural tuning curves have a sharp tip at the best or test frequency, and the high-frequency sides of the curves are steeper than the low-frequency sides. However, the psychophysical tuning curves are not as narrow as the neural tuning curves. These comparisons are shown in Figure 11.2.

A variety of interactions can take place when two tones are presented together. These interactions are important, both for a greater understanding of how the auditory system functions and in terms of recognizing

the precautions that must be taken when measuring masking. In Chapter 4 the phenomenon of beats was described. When two tones are close together in frequency, the time-domain waveform has a modulated pattern that is called *beating*, and we often experience a waxing and waning in loudness, or *beats*. In this situation (that is, when two tones are close together in frequency, one with frequency f_1 and the other with frequency f_2), we hear a tone with a pitch equal to the average of the two frequencies $(f_1 + f_2)/2$ wax and wane in loudness at a rate equal to the difference between the two frequencies $(f_1 - f_2)$. The "best beating" sensation for a continuously presented sound is usually heard at a rate of 3 to 5 HZ (the difference between f_1 and f_2 equals 3 to 5 Hz). The beats are strongest when the amplitudes of the two tones are equal. Thus, it is possible in masking experiments that when the tonal masker frequency is close to the tonal signal frequency, the listener will hear beats. This is especially true because under these conditions the signal and masker are likely to be close together in level (see Figure 11.1). One way to avoid, or at least reduce, the extra sensation of beats during a masking experiment is to present a very short-duration signal. Because the best beats occur with a rate of 3 to 5 Hz, the signal must be 200 to 333 msec long for just one period of the beat to occur (that is, the period of 3 to 5 Hz is 333 to 200 msec). Thus, if the signal is 30 msec long, as it was for the data shown in Figure 11.1, such a short portion of the beat period is presented that the listener usually does not hear any loudness change, or beating.

Another independent property of the auditory system that could influence the detection of the signal in a masking experiment is the nonlinearity of the peripheral auditory system (see Chapter 5). This non-linearity can produce audible tones (aural harmonics and combination tones; (see Chapter 13) in addition to the signal and masker, especially at high stimulus levels. Although aural harmonics and combination tones can occur in a masking experiment, they are usually not detected in a psychophysical tuning experiment because of the low signal level and the short signal duration.

To indicate how beats, aural harmonics, and combination tones can influence results from a study of masking, consider the following experiment conducted by Wegel and Lane in 1924. They asked listeners to detect the presence of signals of different frequencies while an 80-dB SL, 1200-Hz tone served as the masker. For the fixed 1200-Hz masker, the level of the signal was adjusted until the subject could just barely discriminate a difference between the masker and the signal plus masker. The data are shown in Figure 11.3 as the threshold of the signal (expressed in dB SL) versus the frequency of the signal. These data indicate that there is an *upward spread of masking*, in that a masker of a given frequency masks higher-frequency signals more than lower-frequency signals. Because signal frequency was varied in this experiment, the masking data are sometimes referred to as *masking patterns*, to differentiate this pattern from the psychophysical tuning curve patterns shown in Figures 11.1 and 11.2, where the signal frequency was kept constant.

The shaded areas above the data curve (e.g., at the signal frequency of 1200 Hz) in Figure 11.3 indicate

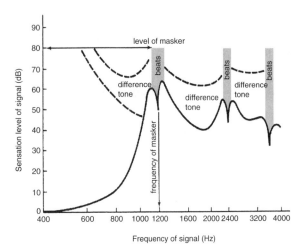

FIGURE 11.3 Masked threshold of signal in dB SL as a function of signal frequency in Hz with a 1200-Hz, 80-dB SL masker. The figure indicates that in addition to detecting the masker and the signal, the observer can also detect beats and nonlinear difference tones. Adapted from Wegel and Lane (1924), used with permission.

that when the signal was close in frequency to the masker, the observer heard beats that indicated the presence of the signal. Notice that beats were also reported at harmonics (2400 Hz and 3600 Hz) of the 1200-Hz masker. If a nonlinear system is excited with a single frequency, higher harmonics of the input frequency can be detected. When a pure tone of one frequency is presented to the auditory system at a high level, listeners report hearing tones at that frequency and tones at frequencies equal to harmonics (usually the first two or three harmonics) of the frequency presented. These audible higher harmonics are called *aural harmonics*, and their presence indicates that the auditory system is nonlinear. Figure 11.3 shows that at a signal frequency of 2400 Hz (the second aural harmonic of the masker frequency, 1200 Hz) and at 3600 Hz (the third aural harmonic of the masker), the signal frequency is beating with the masker harmonics. In other words, the intense 80-dB SPL, 1200-Hz masker has produced aural harmonics at 2400 and 3600 Hz (see Chapter 13). When the signal frequency is close to those of these aural harmonics (e.g.,

2403 Hz or 3603 Hz), the beating occurs between the signal frequency and that frequency produced by the nonlinear properties of the auditory system (e.g., a 3-Hz beat is generated by a 2403-Hz signal and the 2400-Hz second aural harmonic produced by the 1200-Hz masker).

In addition to the aural harmonics produced by the nonlinearity of the auditory system, combination tones are present when the signal and masker are presented simultaneously. The two types of combination tones (produced by the signal and the masker) heard in this experiment were the *primary and secondary difference tones*. The frequency of the primary difference tone is equal to the difference in frequency between the masker and the signal. The frequency of the secondary difference tone (also called the *cubic difference tone*; see also Chapters 8, 9, and 13) is produced by the difference between twice the masker frequency minus the signal frequency or twice the signal frequency minus the masker frequency (see Appendix A). Wegel and Lane's pure tone masking experiment shows that listeners do detect these difference tones. Although both beats and combination tones can be heard when two tones are presented together, the two phenomena (beats and combination tones) represent very different aspects of hearing.

NOISE MASKING

Because white noise (see Chapter 4) contains a wide range of frequency components, we would expect it to mask tones of many different frequencies. In a noise-masking experiment, a broadband white Gaussian noise, whose spectrum level (N_o; see Chapter 4) was varied, is used to mask a tonal signal with different frequencies. The masked threshold of the signal was measured. The data from this type of experiment are shown in Figure 11.4. With no noise present, the thresholds of hearing show that the threshold for a tone depends to a large extent on the tone's frequency. However, as the noise background level is increased, the masked threshold for the pure tone is less dependent on the frequency of the tone. Another

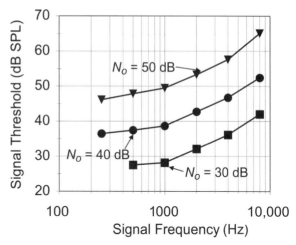

FIGURE 11.4 The signal level (dB SPL) required for noise-masked threshold is shown as a function of signal frequency for three levels (expressed in spectrum level, N_o) of the wideband masking noise. Based on data from Reed and Bilger (1973), used with permission.

important aspect of these data is that above an N_o of approximately 20 dB, an increase in the spectrum level of the noise means that the signal level must be increased by approximately the same amount for the signal to be detected (i.e., for each decibel increase in the level of the masker, the signal must be increased by the same amount to maintain a constant detection threshold). The data indicate that over a wide range of levels and frequencies the signal energy must be 5 to 15 dB more intense than the spectrum level of the noise for the signal to be detected, as shown in Figure 11.5.

In these masking experiments the ratio of the signal energy to the spectrum level of the noise is used to describe the masked threshold. The signal-to-noise ratio (E/N_o) is expressed as the energy of the signal (E) divided by noise power per unit bandwidth (N_o). In decibels, the signal-to-noise ratio equals the signal energy (in dB) minus the spectrum level (in dB). The data in Figure 11.5 from the noise-masking experiments suggest that E/N_o must be approximately 5 to 15 dB for the signal to be detected, with E/N_o being lower for low signal frequencies and increasing as the signal frequency increases.

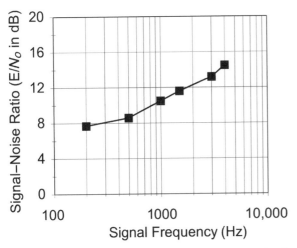

FIGURE 11.5 The signal- (energy) -to-noise (spectrum level) ratios required for detection are shown as a function of signal frequency. Adapted from Reed and Bilger (1973), used with permission.

CRITICAL BAND AND THE INTERNAL FILTER

The data of Figures 11.1–11.3 suggest that those masker frequencies near that of the signal are important in determining masking. Thus, we might expect that when a noise was passed through a narrower and narrower bandpass filter (that is, a narrower and narrower band of noise is providing the masking), the detection of a tone whose frequency was in the center of the noise's pass band would become easier. Conversely, one expects that a signal with a frequency that was not in the pass band of the filter would be very easy to detect because there would be no energy in the masker at the same frequency as the signal frequency.

Fletcher performed a band-narrowing experiment in 1940 and made some assumptions about the frequency region of the noise that would be effective in masking the tone. He assumed that some sort of "internal filter" was centered on the frequency of the signal and that the total noise power coming through that internal filter determined the amount of masking for the signal. That is, the detection of a tonal signal is

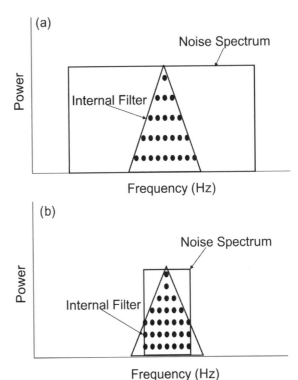

FIGURE 11.6 Schematic diagram of the "internal filter" (the triangle). **(a)** Broadband noise "produces" maximum power (maximum area) at the output of the internal filter. **(b)** The bandwidth of the noise is less than the bandwidth of the internal filter (less area under the filter). There is more masking for a signal whose frequency is at the center of the internal filter for the broadband noise (a) than for the narrowband noise (b).

determined by the amount of total power present in a narrow range of frequencies. This narrow range of frequencies is determined by the internal filter. Figure 11.6 shows this idealized internal filter schematically for two noise spectra. In Figure 11.6a, the noise spectrum is much broader than the pass band of the internal filter, and, hence, the maximum amount of masking occurs because the maximum amount of total power is coming through the filter. In Figure 11.6b, the spectrum of the masking noise is narrower than the pass band of the internal filter, and the signal is easier to detect than that indicated in Figure 11.6a because less than a maximum amount of noise power is

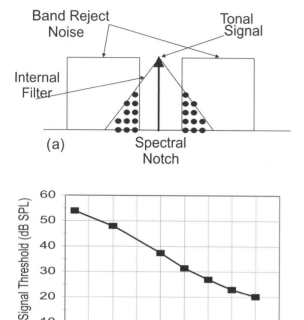

(a)

(b)

FIGURE 11.7 **(a)** A noise band with a spectral notch, or gap, is used to mask a signal whose frequency is in the center of the spectral gap. **(b)** The masked thresholds for detecting a 1000-Hz signal are shown as a function of increasing the spectral notch of the band-reject noise. Adapted from R. D. Patterson and Moore (1989), with permission.

coming through the filter. Fletcher called the internal filter the *critical band*, because the frequencies within the pass band of the internal filter were <u>critical</u> for masking.

A band-reject filtered noise such as that shown in Figure 11.7 offers an excellent masker for estimating the shape of the critical band. Thresholds for detecting a tonal signal whose frequency is centered in the spectral notch of the band-reject noise are determined as a function of the spectral width of the spectral notch, as indicated in Figure 11.7a. The resulting masking data (Figure 11.7b) can be used to estimate the shape of the critical band filter. It is assumed that the total power coming through the filter determines

the amount of masking. As the spectral notch is widened there will be less total power coming through the filter and therefore less masking, as indicated in Figure 11.7b.

The shape of these masking data can be used to estimate the shape of the internal, critical band filter. The bandwidth of the derived critical band filter (called the *equivalent rectangular bandwidth*, ERB) can be obtained for different signal frequencies. Figure 11.8 shows the ERB as a function of frequency, and the results indicate that the width of the critical band (ERB) is proportional to its center frequency (i.e., the signal frequency). Figure 11.8b displays estimates of auditory filters centered at different center frequencies (signal frequency). The estimated shape of the filters does not change much with signal frequency, but bandwidth does. The width of the critical band (or ERB) also increases with increasing signal level, as indicated in Figure 11.9. This increase in critical bandwidth with level may represent nonlinear properties of cochlear transduction, as discussed in Chapters 8 and 16.

RELATIONSHIP BETWEEN EXCITATION PATTERNS AND CRITICAL BANDS

We have used the concept of an internal filter (or critical band) to explain masking data when the masker contains frequencies different from the signal. The data of Figures 11.1 and 11.2, involving the psychophysical tuning curve, and those of Figures 11.7, 11.8, and 11.9, involving noise maskers with a spectral gap, can be used to derive estimates of the shape and bandwidth of the critical band. In these experiments the signal is kept fixed in frequency, and we assume that the listener detects the signal by monitoring the critical band centered on the signal frequency.

For the masking pattern data shown in Figure 11.3, the frequency of the masker was kept constant and the signal frequency changed. Thus, the listener is assumed to monitor a different critical band for each signal frequency (each critical band with a center frequency at the signal frequency). In order to explain the

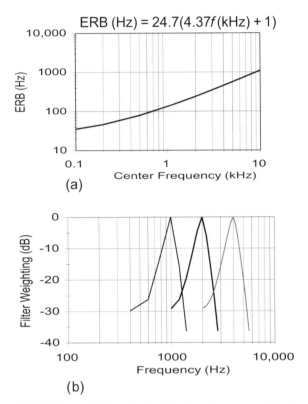

$$\text{ERB (Hz)} = 24.7(4.37f(\text{kHz}) + 1)$$

(a)

(b)

FIGURE 11.8 (a) The width (in Hz) of the estimated critical band (ERB, or equivalent rectangular bandwidth) is shown as a function of signal frequency. Data were obtained from experiments in which noises with spectral gaps masked tonal signals. The equation in the graph (a) shows a fit to the data that can be used to estimate ERB critical bandwidths for critical bands centered at any frequency. In the equation, f is the center frequency of the critical band (i.e., the signal frequency) and is expressed in terms of kHz. Adapted from Moore (1989), used with permission. (b) Estimates of three critical-band, internal filters based on the ERB experiments described in Figure 11.7 are shown. (The filters are based on the rounded exponential filter model, *roex*, from Patterson and Moore, 1989.)

masking pattern data, it is assumed that the masking tone stimulates a number of different neurons, one set of neurons with their best frequencies at the masker's frequency and other neurons with best frequencies removed from that of the masker's frequency. The neuron with its best frequency equal to that of the masker would be stimulated the most, and the other

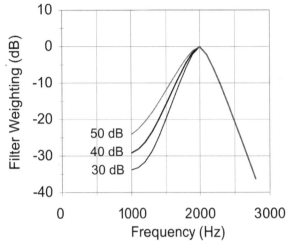

FIGURE 11.9 Estimates of the critical-band internal filters from experiments in which the level of the tonal signal was increased in the notched noise-masking experiment. The width of the filters increase with increasing level. (The filters are based on the rounded exponential filter model, *roex*, from Rosen and Baker, 1994.)

neurons would be stimulated less, depending on how close their best frequencies were to the frequency of the masker and on the overall level of the masker. That is, the masking tone sets up a pattern of excitation in the bundle of auditory nerves. If we imagine that the detection of a signal tone masked by a masking tone is mediated by this *excitation pattern*, we can explain results shown in Figure 11.3. That is, the excitation caused by the masker spreads to critical bands located above and below the masker in frequency. When the listener monitors the critical band centered on the signal frequency, the critical band will contain energy due to the spread of excitation from the masker (assuming that the masker and the signal are not too far apart in frequency and the level of the masker is sufficiently high for the excitation to spread to that critical band), and this energy will mask the signal whose frequency is at the center of the critical band. Figure 11.10 describes how an excitation pattern can be obtained from critical-band, internal filters. Notice the similarity in the shape of the excitation pattern of Figure 11.10b and the masking pattern data of Figure

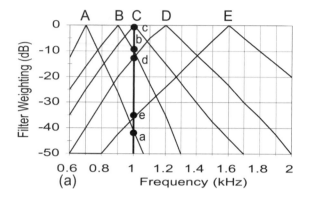

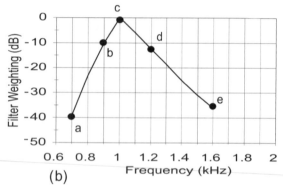

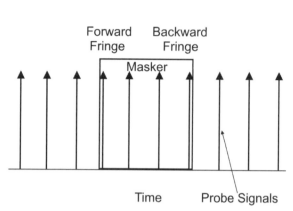

FIGURE 11.11 Schematic diagram of temporal positions of probe signals in relation to a pulsed masker. Signals can occur before the masker (backward masking), during the time of the masker presentation (simultaneous masking), or after the masker (forward masking). Forward and backward fringes also produce masking.

FIGURE 11.10 (a) Five critical-band internal filters are shown. (b) If a masker tone is placed at 1000 Hz (1 kHz), the masking pattern is obtained by assuming that the excitation produced in any critical band by the masker at 1000 Hz is equal to the amount of energy coming through that critical band at 1000 Hz. Thus, for the filter labeled "A", the amount of excitation for this filter at 1000 Hz is "a," or −40 dB. Thus, in the excitation pattern (b) at the frequency equal to the center frequency of filter "A" (500 Hz), the amount of excitation is −40 dB (point a). Similar calculations can be made for filters B, C, D, and E, yielding the other points, b, c, d, and e, on the excitation pattern (b).

11.3, indicating that excitation-masking patterns are directly related to the critical band.

TEMPORAL MASKING

In the masking experiments just described, the masker and the signal occurred simultaneously. There are many acoustic events in which two stimuli follow one another. For instance, in music the notes usually appear sequentially, and in speech words appear in sequence. Psychoacousticians have, therefore, studied the amount of masking provided for a signal that occurs before or after the masker.

Figure 11.11 is a schematic diagram of the stimulus conditions used in studies of *temporal masking*. Signals, or probe tones, can occur at different times relative to the masker (rectangle in Figure 11.11). The signal probes in the middle of the masker represent the *simultaneous masking* conditions we have already studied. When the signal is presented near the beginning or end of the masker, *backward fringe masking* or *forward fringe masking* occurs. When the signal precedes the masker in time, the condition is called *backward masking*; when the signal follows the masker in time, the condition is *forward masking*.

Various stimuli have been used in temporal masking studies (tones, noises, speech, clicks), and the results shown in Figure 11.12 demonstrate the salient data from these experiments. More masking occurs in the fringe conditions than in the simultaneous situation, such that a signal placed in the forward fringe is masked more than one placed in the backward fringe

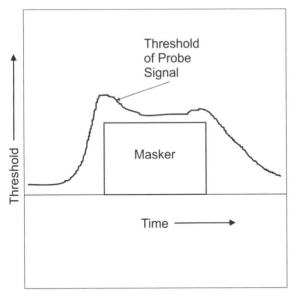

FIGURE 11.12 Schematic diagram of the relative change in signal thresholds as a function of the temporal position of the probe signal in relation to the masker.

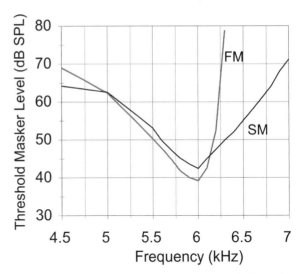

FIGURE 11.13 A comparison of a forward-masked (FM) and a simultaneously masked (SM) psychophysical tuning curve obtained for similar stimulus conditions. The signal was 6000 Hz. Forward-masked tuning curves are very similar to neural tuning curves obtained from the basilar membrane and eighth nerve (see Figures 7.18 and 9.5). Based on data from Moore (1978), used with permission.

(the masking that occurs when the signal is in the forward fringe is sometimes referred to as *overshoot*, as if the extra masking caused by the masker onset has overshot the masking caused by the steady-state portion of the masker). Forward masking of a stimulus can take place when a temporal difference between the two stimuli is as large as 75 to 100 msec, and backward masking occurs up to 50 msec. Thus, the amount of backward masking declines more quickly than does the amount of forward masking as a function of increasing the temporal separation between the signal and the masker.

TONAL-TEMPORAL MASKING

At the beginning of this chapter we described the psychophysical tuning curve. If there is forward masking, then we might expect that the effect of the forward masker would be frequency dependent, as it was for simultaneous masking (see Figure 11.1). The data shown in Figure 11.13 marked as FM were

obtained in the same manner as described for Figure 11.1, except in this case the signal appeared immediately after the masker was turned off (forward masking, FM). These forward-masking results show that the masker does influence signal detection when it does not overlap the signal. The effects are about the same as when the signal and the masker overlap in time (Figure 11.1). Figure 11.13 shows a direct comparison of psychophysical tuning curves obtained in simultaneous masking (SM) and in forward masking (FM). As can be seen, this comparison indicates that the psychophysical tuning curve is sharper in forward masking than in simultaneous masking. The sharper tuning curve means that the auditory system is better able to detect the presence of the signal in forward masking than in simultaneous masking for the same masker frequency.

These tuning curves are based on one pure tone masking another pure tone. We have already studied the use of noise maskers, but what happens for other, complex maskers? Let us consider the case of using a two-tone complex as the masker. In this experiment, the actual masker (M) will be fixed at a particular level (40 dB SPL) and frequency (1000 Hz), and the level of the signal (the signal also has a frequency of 1000 Hz) is varied to determine a threshold. In a test, or baseline, condition, the signal threshold is determined when the masker is equal in frequency to the signal (that is, both are at 1000 Hz). In the test conditions, a second tone is added to the masker, so the masking stimulus consists of two tones, M, the initial masker, and SU, the second masking tone. The level of the second tone (Su) is 20 dB above the level of the masker tone, or M tone; the second tone, SU, is, therefore, 60 dB SPL. The frequency of the second tone (SU) was varied to determine the threshold for detecting the signal for each value of the frequency of SU. Finally, this experiment was performed for both simultaneous masking and forward masking.

Figure 11.14 shows the two stimulus conditions and the results. The vertical axis in each figure is the change in signal threshold from the test condition. Recall that in the test condition only the masking tone (M) was presented and the signal and the masker were equal in frequency (1000 Hz). The solid horizontal line at 0 decibels represents this masking condition. Thus, if the second tone, SU, provides masking in addition to that caused by M presented alone, the signal thresholds should increase above 0 dB. As can be seen, in simultaneous masking most masking (about 20 dB of masking) occurs when the second tone, SU, is equal in frequency to the masking tone, M (SU, M, and the signal are all 1000 Hz). As the second tone (SU) becomes different in frequency from the masking tone (M) and signal tone (S), the amount of threshold change above 0 dB decreases until the difference between the two masking tones is so large that only the original masking tone, M, continues to provide masking (that is, masking is back at the baseline amount of masking, 0 dB). These data are similar to those shown in Figure 11.4.

Let us compare this simultaneous masking effect to what happens in the forward-masking condition. Notice that in forward masking the values of signal threshold are negative when the second masking tone,

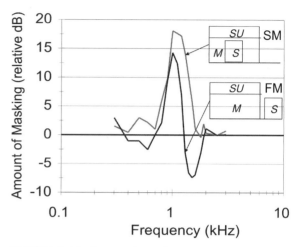

FIGURE 11.14 A comparison of two-tone tonal masking in simultaneous (the SM condition shown with the light curve) and forward masking (the FM condition shown with the dark curve). The frequency of the suppressor tone (SU) is shown on the horizontal axis and the level of the 1000-Hz signal (S) required for threshold detection is shown on the vertical axis. Signal threshold is shown relative to that required to detect the signal when only the masking tone (M) was present. The masking tone is presented at 40 dB SPL and with a frequency of 1000 Hz. The suppressor tone is presented at 60 dB SPL. In the simultaneous masking condition the signal is presented in the temporal middle of the masking stimulus (either M alone or M and SU presented together), while in the forward masking condition the signal is present after the offset of the masking stimulus. Signal thresholds above 0 dB mean that the suppressor tone (SU) increased the amount of masking provided by the masker tone (M), thresholds below 0 dB mean that the suppressor tone (SU) caused less masking than that produced by the masker tone (M) when it was presented alone (e.g., SU suppressed the masking ability of M), and thresholds at 0 dB mean that only the masker tone (M) was providing masking. Adapted from Shannon (1974), used with permission.

SU, is slightly greater in frequency than the masking tone (M). That is, when SU is added to M, signal threshold can be lower than that obtained when just M is presented. In this example, the 1000-Hz signal is easier to detect when the 1000-Hz masker (M) is present along with a second tone (SU) of slightly higher frequency (e.g., 1250 Hz). It is as if the second tone (SU) has made the 1000-Hz masking tone (M) a less effective masker. The second tone (SU) is sometimes referred to as a *suppression tone* because the second tone (*SU*) is suppressing the masking ability of the masking tone (*M*).

Labeling the second tone the *suppression tone* allows us to describe the two-tone masking effect. Care should be used, however, in drawing too many conclusions about the nature of this suppression-like effect. Some investigators refer to the effect as "unmasking," in that the second tone has "unmasked" the effect of the masker (*M*). "Unmasking" is viewed as a more neutral term than suppression because it does not imply that the second tone (*SU*) actually interacts in a direct fashion with *M*. The unmasking, or suppression, phenomenon is another factor that must be considered in attempting to account for the way in which the auditory system operates when two or more stimuli exist in the environment.

MASKING USED TO MEASURE NONLINEAR COMPRESSION

Previously in this chapter, we described some of the nonlinear effects that can be measured with masking, e.g., aural harmonics and difference tones. Chapters 7, 8, and 9 described how the biomechanical and neural output measured at the auditory periphery is a nonlinear compressive function of sound level (i.e., the input–output functions are often compressive). That is, as sound level increases there is a smaller and smaller increase in biomechanical vibration, or neural spike rate. However, this compressive nonlinearity is only present when the sound's frequency is near or at the center frequency (CF) of the nerve fiber whose input–output function is being measured (see Chapters 7 and 8). That is, if the sound's frequency is not near the fiber's CF, changes in sound level result in a fairly linear change in neural spike rate, rather than the compressive change that exists when the signal frequency is near or at the fiber's CF (see Figure 7.19).

We have argued that masking is determined to a significant degree by the properties of the nerves within the bundle of auditory nerves. Thus, one might predict that the compressive nonlinearity of cochlear and auditory nerve function would affect masking and that the

effects
tions
phy
we
a

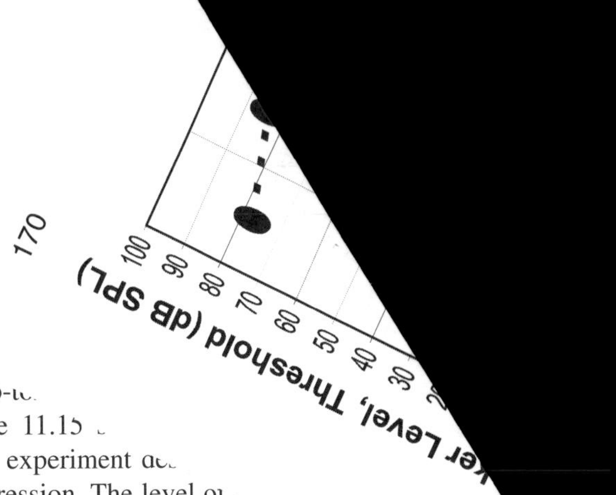

signa
fore, two-t

Figure 11.15
masking experiment a
of compression. The level of
to forward mask a tonal signal whe
tonal signal was varied is plotted in Figur
two conditions: (1) the frequency of the maske
signal were the same (both 6000 Hz), and (2) the frequency of the masker (3000 Hz) and the signal (6000 Hz) were different. As can be seen, there is a linear relationship between masked threshold and signal level when the masker and the signal are equal in frequency but a compressive relationship when the masker and signal differ in frequency, very much like the results shown in Figure 7.19.

The following argument suggests that these results are consistent with the idea that they are a result of compression in the auditory periphery. To explain masking, it is assumed that the listener uses (attends to) those neural fibers with CFs that are equal or nearly equal to the signal frequency. When the signal and the masker are the same in frequency, the change in neural output (e.g., spike rate) for each stimulus would be the same as their level is changed. Thus, one would predict that a 1-dB change in signal level would require about a 1-dB change in masker level to yield a masked threshold, which is what the data of Figure 11.15 indicate. However, when the signal and the masker differ in frequency and the listener is assumed to use fibers with CFs near the frequency of the signal, the neural output to the signal is compressed as its level changes (the signal frequency is at the fiber's CF), but the neural output of the masker is not (the masker

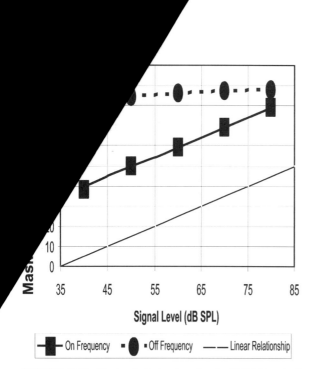

(legend) On Frequency — ■ Off Frequency ■● — Linear Relationship

10
0
35   45   55   65   75   85

Signal Level (dB SPL)

FIGURE 11.15 The level of a tonal masker (in dB SPL) required to forward mask a brief tonal signal (6000 Hz) presented at different sound levels (dB SPL). In the on-frequency condition the masker frequency was the same as the signal frequency (6000 Hz), and in the off-frequency condition the masker frequency (3000 Hz) was different from the signal frequency. The thinner line indicates a linear relationship between masker level at threshold and signal level. The masking relationship is linear in the on-frequency condition and compressively nonlinear in the off-frequency condition, as is consistent with the nonlinearity measured at the auditory periphery. Adapted from Plack and Oxenham (1998), used with permission.

frequency is not at the fiber's CF; see Figure 7.19). As a consequence, the neural output for the signal does not change a lot when its level is increased, and less masker level would be required to mask the signal as its level is increased, as is indicated in Figure 11.15 (note the relationship between the functions of Figures 7.19 and 11.15, and recall that in the physiological experiment the output of one place along the basilar membrane was measured, whereas psychophysically the masking of one tone by another was measured).

A great deal of the results from the masking research described in this chapter appears to be dependent on the biomechanics of cochlear function and the neural processes that occur in the auditory nerve. Thus, one might conclude that masking and the interference that one sound can impart to another sound is determined almost solely by the properties of the auditory periphery. While the peripheral properties of auditory processing play a crucial role in masking, we will learn in Chapter 14 that many interactions that occur between "maskers" and "signals" involve processes that are probably located in neural areas of the brainstem and cortex.

SUMMARY

Masking of a tonal signal by a tonal masker has been used to study the interaction of sounds occurring simultaneously and to probe the frequency selectivity of the auditory system. Psychophysical tuning curves are often used to describe the masking effect of one tone on another tone. The results indicate that low-frequency tones mask high-frequency signals more than high frequencies mask low frequencies. Sometimes, due to the presence of beats and combination tones, the exact relationship between tonal signal threshold and tonal masker frequency is difficult to determine. Beats indicate that the auditory system has a limited frequency-resolving power but that it can follow the amplitude of the input stimulus. Combination tones indicate the extent to which the auditory system is nonlinear. When white Gaussian noise is used as a masker for tonal signals, the ratio of signal energy (E) to masker level of spectrum level (N_o) required for masked threshold is approximately 5 to 15 dB as the spectrum level of the noise or the frequency of the signal is varied over a considerable range. Critical bands and excitation patterns are used to estimate the bandwidth properties of the frequency-resolving capability of the auditory system. Fringe masking and forward and backward masking are used to determine the masking interaction of sounds not occurring simultaneously. Tuning curves obtained in forward masking are sharper than those obtained

in simultaneous masking. **Psychophysical suppression, or unmasking, can occur when the masker consists of two or more frequencies. Temporal masking can also be used to measure the compressive nature of the input–output relationships measured at the auditory periphery.**

SUPPLEMENT

Throughout the discussion of masking, we have stressed the concept of the "internal filter." The psychophysics of hearing suggests that the nervous system operates as if there is a bank of bandpass filters that process sound. We have already learned (in Chapters 7–9) that both the biomechanics and the neural aspects of auditory physiology demonstrate the existence of neural tuning that resembles bandpass filtering. A challenge for auditory scientists is to determine to what extent the neural tuning, observed in the cochlea and auditory nerve, accounts for the psychophysics of masking. Many of these issues and data are reviewed in the book edited by Moore (1989), in Chapter 3 of the textbook by Moore (1997), and by Moore in a chapter in the book edited by Yost, Popper, and Fay (1993).

Another variable that can affect a listener's ability to detect signals in masking experiments is "off-frequency listening." The basic idea behind off-frequency listening is that the listener may be able to perform the detection task by listening in a frequency region different from that in which the signal occurs (that is, off the signal frequency, or off-frequency). In many situations the signal may excite a wide frequency region, and a larger signal-to-masker ratio may exist in a frequency region that is different from that of the signal. Using a noise with a spectral notch (see Figure 11.7) reduces the ability of the listener to "listen off-frequency" to detect the signal in the notch-noise-masking procedure, because this noise energy exists in all frequency regions except the narrow region near the signal. An excellent discussion of off-frequency listening can be found in Moore's (1989) book.

Patterson and Moore (1989; see also Moore and Patterson, 1986) used a particular filter shape called the *rounded exponential* (*roex filter*) to fit masking data like those shown in Figure 11.7. The roex filter function can be written as

$$W(g) = (1 + pg)\exp(-pg),$$

where $W(g)$ is the linear (nondecibel) value of the filter output ($0 \leq W(g) \leq 1$), $g = f - f_o/f$, f_o is the signal frequency (filter's CF), f is a frequency on the filter function, p is determined by the bandwidth and slope of the filter such that the higher the value of p the more sharply tuned the filter, p is obtained by finding the best-fitting function $W(g)$ to the data, and "exp" is the exponential argument. Once p is determined from the data, the ERB, or the equivalent rectangular bandwidth, (see Supplement to Chapter 5) can be obtained from the roex filter as ERB $= 4f_o/p$. The *gammatone filter* (see Patterson et al., 1995, and Rosen and Baker, 1994) is another filter function used to describe the shape of the critical-band filter. The time domain (*the impulse function*) description of the gammatone function is

$$t^{n-1}\exp(-2\pi bt)\cos(2\pi f_o t),$$

where n and b are constants and f_o is the CF of the filter. In the frequency domain the filter function is approximately equal to

$$(1-r)\left[1 + \left\{(f - f_o)^2\right\}/b^2\right]^4,$$

where f_o is the filter's CF, f is a frequency on the filter, b controls the filter's sharpness, and r is proportional to the slope of the filter. In these measurements filter bandwidth is sometimes referred to in terms of the number of ERBs (#ERBs):

$$\#ERBs = 21.4\log(4.37f + 1)$$

or

$$f = \left[10^{(\#ERBs/21.4)} - 1\right]/4.37;$$

f in kHz. So, a frequency of 1000 Hz is 15.6 ERBs ($15.6 = 21.4\log 5.37$); or 1 ERB is 26 Hz ($0.26 = [10^{1/21.4} - 1]/4.37$).

Weber (1983) has suggested that there are at least three explanations for the narrower forward-masked tuning curves (see also Lutfi, 1988). Psychophysical suppression appears to be much more effective for high-frequency suppression tones on a lower-frequency masker tone than for low-frequency suppression tones on a high-frequency masking tone. Suppression by low-frequency suppression tones on the masker tone has been observed, but usually only when the suppression tone is fairly high in level (see Shannon, 1974).

Although comparisons between psychophysical suppression and two-tone neural suppression (see Chapter 7) are tempting, there are some arguments that the two may not be the same (see Moore and Glasberg, 1982).

The two stimuli in the intensity discrimination experiment described in Chapter 10 differ only in that one is more intense than the other. The more intense stimulus could have been produced by adding two tones of the same frequency: tone A, with a level of I in decibels, and tone B, with a level such that when it was added to tone A the summed level in decibels would equal $I + \Delta I$ in decibels (recall that when two stimuli of equal frequency are added, the sum depends on the phase difference between two tones). Thus, data from the intensity experiment could be plotted as the level of tone B required for the subject to determine that it was added to tone A versus the level of tone A. The fact that the level of tone B must be raised above absolute threshold due to the presence of tone A is defined as tone A masking tone B.

Fletcher observed that when the spectrum of the noise was broad (i.e., the internal filter contained the maximum total noise power required for masking; see Figure 11.6), the power of the just-detectable masked signal (the signal at masked threshold) was equal to the total power contained within the critical band that he had measured. Fletcher's observation makes it possible to predict the width of the critical band without performing a band-narrowing or band-reject experiment. According to Fletcher's assumptions, masked signal power (P_s) equals the power of the noise in the critical band (P_{ncb}): $P_s = P_{ncb}$. Since $P_{ncb} = N_o \times CBW$ (see Chapter 4), where N_o is noise spectrum level and CBW is an estimate of the critical bandwidth, CBW = P_s/N_o. Expressed in decibels, 10 log CBW = P_s in dB

$- N_o$ in dB, and 10 log CBW is referred to as the *critical ratio*. Thus, CBW can be estimated directly from a single masking threshold by computing the signal-to-noise ratio (P_s/N_o). However, the signal level (P_s) required for detection depends on how efficient the auditory system is at detecting the signal as well as on the width of the critical band. Thus, if the total power within the critical band does not <u>equal</u> the power of the masked signal at threshold (i.e., P_s does not equal P_{ncb}), then the basic assumption of the critical ratio calculation is violated and the critical ratio will not yield a valid estimate of the width of the critical band. In most experiments performed since those by Fletcher, the power of the signal at masked threshold rarely equals the power within the critical band, so one should probably no longer use the critical ratio as an estimate of critical bandwidth.

Another type of signal has been used in masking experiments to measure the effects of how the phase of sound is altered in the auditory periphery (see Figure 7.16) *Schroeder tones* are harmonic sequences of tones in which the starting phase of each tone (the nth tone) in the harmonic sequence has the value of $\pi n(n - 1)/N$ for positive Schroeder-phase tones and $-\pi n(n - 1)/N$ for negative Schroeder-phase tones, where n is the harmonic number of the tonal component and N is the total number of components. Because the biomechanics of the traveling wave impart a phase shift to sounds of different frequencies, the starting phases of the various harmonics of the Schroeder-phase tones arrive at the auditory nerves with different phase relationships than those provided by the stimulus. The neural phase relationships for positive Schroeder-phase tones are considerably different than those for negative Schroeder-phase tones. These peripheral phase transformations can be measured psychophysically using Schroeder-phase tones (both positive and negative) in forward-masking experiments (see, for instance, Carlyon and Datta, 1997). The book by Bacon, Fay, and Popper (2004) provides a thorough review and explanation of the compression and phase changes measured physiologically and psychophysically in people with normal and impaired hearing.

12

Sound Localization and Binaural Hearing

LOCALIZATION

The source of a sound can be localized in the three spatial dimensions: the *horizontal plane* (*azimuth*), or the left–right dimension; the *vertical plane*, or the up–down dimension; and *distance* (*range*), or the near–far dimension (Figure 12.1). Sound has no spatial dimensions. The ability to perceive the location of a sound source based on sound alone is the result of the auditory system's processing of the interaction of sound with objects (e.g., the head) that the sound encounters as it travels from its source to the outer ear canals. While we can use vision to locate objects, vision does not help locate objects when the objects are out of sight (e.g., behind us or at night). Thus, sound localization is valuable for determining the location of sound sources.

LOCALIZATION IN AZIMUTH

To understand one set of stimulus cues responsible for our localization abilities, picture a person sitting in a room listening to a sound source without moving his or her head. Figure 12.2 illustrates the temporal and level information arriving at the person's ears that can be used to locate stimuli in the azimuth plane. Notice that the sound travels a shorter distance to the right ear than to the left ear. Hence, it will arrive at the right ear earlier than at the left ear; this yields an *interaural time difference* (ITD) in arrival of the sound. Recall that the speed of sound in air is relatively constant, independent of frequency. Thus, the interaural temporal difference for any frequency is theoretically the same for all frequencies for a particular stimulus location and a particular person, whereas the *interaural phase difference* (IPD) will vary according to the frequency of the stimulus. That is, if a tonal sound with a frequency of 1000 Hz (a period of 1 msec) arrives at the right ear 0.5 msec after it has reached the left ear, the tone at the right ear is half a period (or 180°) out of phase with the tone at the left ear. If a 500-Hz sinusoid (a period of 2 msec) arrives at the right ear the same 0.5 msec later than at the left ear, there is only one-quarter of a period (or 90°) phase difference between the two ears. Thus, two different tones (1000 and 500 Hz), both with a 0.5-msec interaural time difference, produce different interaural phase differences.

There is also an *interaural level difference* (ILD) for the condition shown in Figure 12.2 due to two aspects of the physics of sound. First, because the

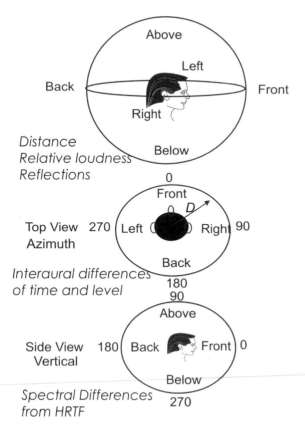

FIGURE 12.1   The three spatial dimensions: azimuth (left–right), vertical (up–down), distance (near–far). HRTF = head-related transfer function.

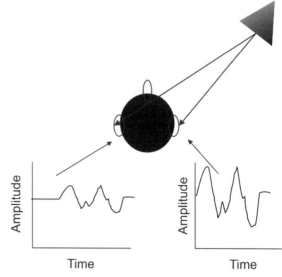

FIGURE 12.2   Schematic diagram of a sound source on an azimuth plane around the head. Distance of the sound from the ears is the range. The sound reaches the right ear first, and thus there is an interaural difference in the arrival time; and the sound at the left ear is less intense than that at the right ear, leading to an interaural level difference.

stimulus arrives at the left ear after it reaches the right ear, it has traveled a greater distance and is therefore less intense at the left ear (inverse square law relationship; see Chapter 3). However, the difference in level caused by the inverse square law produces extremely small interaural level differences. Like any object, the head can produce a sound shadow (see Chapter 3), yielding reduced sound level at the ear opposite the sound source, assuming that the size of the head is close to the sound's wavelength. Because wavelength is directly proportional to frequency, the interaural level difference caused by the head's sound shadow depends on frequency. The higher the frequency, the shorter the wavelength and the greater the sound shadow caused by the head in establishing the

interaural level difference. Thus, large interaural level differences exist at high frequencies and could be used to indicate the location of the source. Figure 12.3 shows the interaural temporal difference measured at the ears for a stimulus located at different azimuth angles. Figure 12.3 also shows the interaural level difference for different azimuth angles and frequencies. Notice that the interaural temporal difference is a smooth function of frequency and varies from 0 to 0.8 msec as the azimuth of the source changes. The interaural level difference varies considerably, especially at high frequencies. The binaural auditory system therefore could determine the location of a sound coming from, say, the right side by noting that the right ear received the sound first and that the stimulus was more intense at the right ear.

Figures 12.4 and 12.5 show how well listeners localize sound sources. Figure 12.4 shows the errors in localizing sinusoids of different frequencies. These data indicate that listeners have more errors localizing

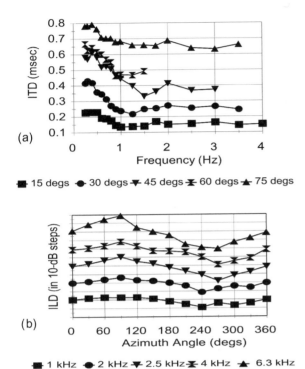

15 degs ● **30 degs** ▼ **45 degs** ✖ **60 degs** ▲ **75 degs**

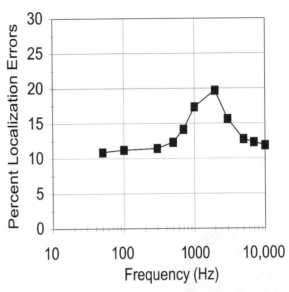

FIGURE 12.3 (a) Values of interaural time difference (ITD in msec) measured at different azimuth angles (see Figure 12.1). (b) Values of interaural level difference (ILD in dB) measured at different azimuth angles and frequencies (each tic mark on the vertical axis represents 10 dB of ILD). Adapted from Kuhn (1987), used with permission.

FIGURE 12.4 Errors (in terms of percentage of judgments made) in judging the location of a sinusoidal sound source shown as a function of frequency. Adapted from Stevens and Newman (1936), used with permission.

sounds with frequencies in the mid-frequency region, around 2000 Hz, than for sounds with lower or higher frequencies. The data in Figure 12.5 indicate how well a listener locates a broadband noise. Perfect localization would be represented by the data following on the diagonal straight line, because the data are plotted as the judged location of the source versus the actual location of the source. As can be seen, this listener is very good at determining the location of broadband noise in the azimuth plane.

Figures 12.6 and 12.7 represent the data from an experiment in which blindfolded listeners were asked to discriminate between the location of two small loudspeakers, each placed approximately 100 cm from

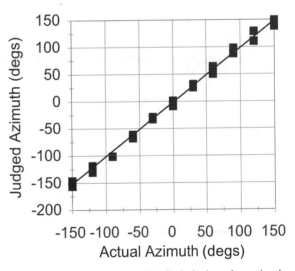

FIGURE 12.5 The judged location in the horizontal, or azimuth, direction of a broadband noise source presented at different locations. The diagonal straight line represents perfect judgments (data from one listener). Adapted from Wightman and Kistler (1989b), used with permission.

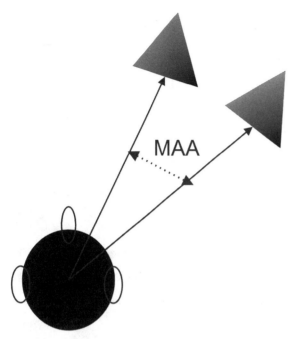

FIGURE 12.6 Schematic diagram of measuring the minimum audible angle (MAA).

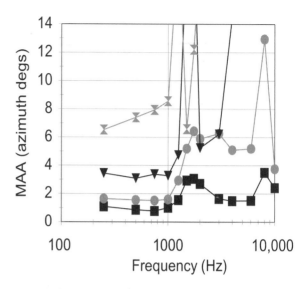

FIGURE 12.7 Values of MAA are plotted as a function of sinusoidal frequency for different azimuths. The MAA increases as the source moved away from in front of the listener and is large in the mid-frequency region, between 2 and 4 kHz. Adapted from Mills (1972), used with permission.

the listener's head. As shown in Figure 12.6, the smallest angular separation between the two loudspeakers that the listener could just detect is called the *minimal audible angle* (MAA). Thus, the MAA in degrees of angular separation was measured as a function of the frequency of the sinusoid. The various curves of Figure 12.7 represent various azimuth positions at which the discriminations were made. That is, the curve labeled 0° means that the loudspeakers were directly in front of the listener, whereas the curve labeled 75° means that the loudspeakers were placed 75° toward one ear (the speakers were to the side of the listener). Notice that the listener required larger and larger angular separation (the MAA increases) between the loudspeakers in order to detect a difference in loudspeaker location as the loudspeakers were moved from directly in front of the listener toward one ear (the listener's head was held stationary). In other words, when the sound is in front of the listener, a change in location can be better discriminated than

when it is toward one side. Of course, in the real world this poses no severe limitation because a person can generally move so that the sound source is in the front.

The MAA results also show, as do the data from Stevens and Newman (see Figure 12.4), that listeners made more mistakes in locating sound sources when their frequency content was in the mid-frequency range than at high or low frequencies. Stevens and Newman, and earlier Lord Rayleigh, believed that the mid-frequency region represented those frequencies for which the interaural temporal and level differences were each relatively too small to be used as accurate cues for localization. They concluded that there were two cues for determining location: the interaural temporal difference, which provides information for low-frequency stimuli, and the interaural level difference, which provides location information at high frequencies. This idea is referred to as the *duplex theory of localization*.

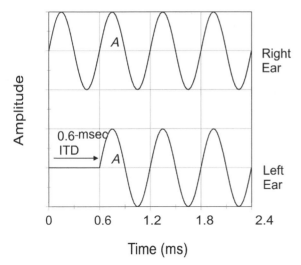

FIGURE 12.8 A 1666-Hz tone presented to the right side of a listener so that it reaches the right ear 0.6 msec before it reaches the left ear. **(top)** Sinusoid at right ear. **(bottom)** Sinusoid at left ear. After the first peak, the waveforms arriving at each ear are in phase, which would indicate that the sound is in front rather than to the right.

The sound shadow effect demonstrates why the physical interaural level difference is small at low frequencies and hence why listeners would have trouble using interaural level as a cue at low frequencies. That is, the interaural level difference caused by the head's sound shadow decreases (see Figure 12.2) as the frequency decreases (wavelength increases), so at low frequencies the interaural level difference may not be large enough to detect.

One explanation of why the interaural temporal difference might provide location information at only low frequencies is diagramed in Figure 12.8. Assume that the low-frequency tone (1666 Hz) shown in the top panel was presented so that it arrived first at the right ear. Thus, the sinusoid arriving at the two ears would appear in time as shown in Figures 12.8. The difference in the timing pattern at the ears could be used by the auditory system to determine that the sound source was toward the right ear. In these panels we assume that the period (time between peaks) of the sinusoid was 0.6 msec (1666 Hz), nearly the maximum

time it takes a sound to travel from one ear to the other (see Figures 12.2). A 1666-Hz sinusoid would appear at the two ears as in Figure 12.8. Notice that although the 1666-Hz sinusoid is on the right side and the first period of the left and right waveforms are displaced, the waveforms are identical thereafter (as at point *A*). Thus, except for the first period, there is no difference between the stimulation at the two ears, so the listener might assign the sound to a location in front since stimuli that are directly in front of the listener produce no interaural differences. In this case, that judgment is incorrect because the stimulus was presented opposite the right ear. For this frequency and this interaural time difference, an ambiguous temporal cue would exist for locating the sound source. This confusion would not exist for frequencies lower than 1666 Hz but would occur for those of 1666 Hz and greater, assuming the time it takes sound to travel from one ear to the other is 0.6 msec. Thus, interaural time produces ambiguous information about spatial location (i.e., the onset interaural time difference suggests one location and the ongoing time difference a different spatial location) when the frequency is too high (too high relative to the width of the head).

LOCALIZATION IN THE FRONT–BACK DIRECTION AND IN THE VERTICAL PLANE

The cues of interaural time and level have been shown to be of great importance in localizing sounds in the horizontal plane. If a listener's head remains steady, then there are a number of locations that would produce the same interaural differences of time and level; for instance, a sound directly in front would produce the same interaural differences as one directly behind a listener as well as one directly overhead and one directly below the listener (see Figure 12.1). Sounds that lie in this plane are in the *mid-sagittal plane*, and this plane forms a *cone of confusion* where all sounds that are located on the cone produce the same interaural differences (for the mid-sagittal plane the interaural differences are zero because the sound source is always midway between the two ears). For each sound source location, there is a cone of confusion that describes the location of other sound sources that produce the same interaural differences. While cones of confusion exist for a stationary head, small head movements would potentially enable a listener to accurately localize sound, because the head would be in a different position and the original cone of confusion would no longer exist. Even when we do not move our heads, we can still localize sounds on cones of confusions, such as in the mid-sagittal plane. That is, we can determine that the sound comes from in front as opposed to behind (we do not often make front–back confusions) or that the sound came from directly overhead as opposed to from directly in front (we do not often make cone-of-confusion errors). However, when sound localization mistakes are made, it is often the case that the mistakes occur along cones of confusion.

Because the sources of sounds that lie on cones of confusion can be localized, cues in addition to the interaural differences must aid us in determining the location of sound sources in the vertical direction. These cues, usually referred to as *spectral cues*, are derived from the head-related transfer functions (HRTFs), as explained in Chapter 6. As explained in Chapter 6 (see Figure 6.5), the many external parts of our head and body, especially the pinna, act as small sound shadows for the path of the sound to the ears. These parts of the body can also delay the sound in reaching the outer ears. These obstacles to sound transmission are most important for high-frequency sounds because the wavelength of high frequencies may be close to the size of these small obstacles (see Chapters 3 and 6).

If the sound is complex, such as a noise, then different frequencies in the sound will be attenuated and delayed by different amounts, depending on the interaction between the size of the objects the sound encounters before it reaches the ear (such as the pinna and various parts of the pinna, the nose, and the torso) and the sound's wavelength. The delay will lead to different phases and, thus, will establish a phase spectrum for the HRTF. Thus, the head and torso provide a spectral HRTF alteration of the sound source. The

amount of attenuation and delay (i.e., the spectral characteristics of the HRTF) provided by any obstacle will also depend on the direction the sound is coming from. For instance, the pinna offers more attenuation from sounds coming from behind than those coming from in front. Thus, the spectral shape of the HRTF for a complex sound arriving at the outer ear will differ depending on the location of the sound source relative to the body. Because the major changes in the HRTF occur for high frequencies due to the interaction between wavelength and obstacle size (as explained earlier), it is not surprising that the major cues for vertical localization occur for the higher frequencies. Figure 12.9 displays the HRTFs obtained at four elevations in the mid-sagittal plane ($0°$, $30°$, $60°$ and $90°$) for the left and right ears of a subject. Because the sound source is located midway between the ears in the mid-sagittal plane, the overall level at both ears for all elevations is about the same. Notice, however, that there are deep spectral valleys in the spectral region near $10,000\,Hz$, especially at $30°$ and $60°$ of elevation. Aspects of the spectral location of these valleys (and sometimes peaks) are the presumed HRTF cues for vertical localization. For instance, in Figure 12.9, the location of the major spectral valley seems to increase in frequency from the vertical positions of $0°$ to $30°$ to $60°$ and then the valley disappears at $90°$. Thus, the spectral shape of the HRTF probably provides information about the location of a sound source, especially vertical location. Such HRTF differences are also presumably used in solving back–front and front–back confusions along the azimuth plane.

Figure 12.10 shows data indicating the ability of a listener to judge the vertical location of a broadband noise source, where the angle is the vertical angle of the source relative to the listener (see Figure 12.1). The fact that the data are scattered about the diagonal line representing perfect vertical localization indicates that the listener is not as good at determining the vertical location of sound as at determining horizontal location (vertical localization is usually poorer than horizontal localization; see Figure 12.5). Thus, cone-of-confusion localization and localization in the vertical direction with a stationary head is the result of the

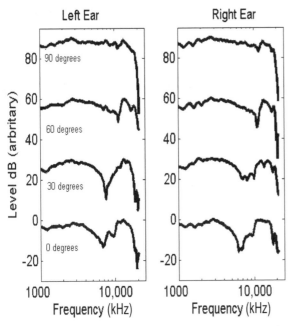

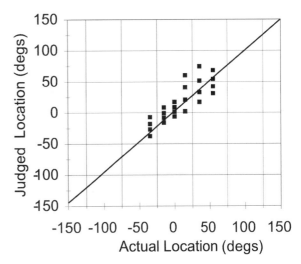

FIGURE 12.9 Two sets of HRTFs are shown, those measured for the left ear on the left and those for the right ear on the right. The HRTF measurements were made in the mid-sagittal plane at 0° (directly in front), 30°, 60°, and 90° (directly overhead) elevations. Note the deep spectral valley and how it changes spectral location with elevation.

FIGURE 12.10 The judged location in the vertical dimension of a broadband noise source. Data are plotted in the same way as for Figure 12.5 and are for the same listener whose data are shown in Figure 12.5. Adapted from Wightman and Kistler (1989b), used with permission.

sound's interaction with the torso, head, and pinna in generating an HRTF.

LOCALIZATION AS A FUNCTION OF DISTANCE

Less is known about the cues used to determine the distance, or *range*, of a sound source. A possible cue for distance is the sound's loudness, or level: Loud sounds appear closer than far sounds. However, soft sounds can be close and loud sounds far away. Thus, relative sound level can logically be a cue for distance only if the listener has other information about the sound source that might suggest what its overall level is likely to be. For instance, if the source is someone speaking, then from experience we know what speech should sound like, and this information could allow one to use the overall loudness of someone's speaking to infer the relative distance of the speaker from the listener.

Early-arriving reflections from a sound source off nearby surfaces also provide important cues for determining the distance (range) of a sound source. That is, the ratio of the level of the direct sound to reach the listener to the level of the reflected sound decreases as the sound source is located at a greater distance from the listener (i.e., near the listener the level of the reflected sound is low relative to the direct sound; at a distance, both the direct and the reflected sound travel a longer distance and will arrive at the listener with levels that maybe somewhat equal). As a result, the ratio of the sound levels of direct versus reflected sound could be a cue for judging the distance of a sound source. Listeners are much poorer at judging the distance of a sound source than they are in judging either azimuthal or vertical location.

INTERACTIONS OF THE SOURCE SOUND AND THE CUES USED FOR SOUND LOCALIZATION

Thus, sound interacts with the head to produce interaural differences of time and level that allow us to determine the azimuthal location of a sound source. The interactions of sound traveling across the body, head, and pinna produce a spectral alteration of the sound (the HRTF) that could provide cues for vertical location and sound localization along cones of confusion (e.g., differentiating sound sources from in front from those from in back). Sound that reflects off of surfaces in our environment (e.g., the ground) could interact with the sound that arrives at our auditory system directly from a sound source. As stated earlier, the ratio of the levels of direct versus reflected sound provides a possible cue for judging the relative distance of a sound source. The location of a sound source can therefore be determined in all three spatial dimensions, and the cues for sound source location differ for each spatial dimension but are the result of sound's interacting with objects in its path as it travels from its source to the auditory system.

PRECEDENCE-LOCALIZATION IN REVERBERANT SPACES

Everyday experience will tell you that even in rooms where there are many reflections from walls, floors, and so on, we are still able to localize acoustic events accurately. The reflections cause a complicated pattern of stimulation at the ears, because the reflections come from many different directions (see Chapter 3). How does the auditory system assimilate these conflicting cues to accurately determine the actual location of a sound source rather than misperceiving the source as the location of one of the reflections? A number of experiments have shown that it is the first wave arriving at the ears that dominates in establishing the location of the actual sound source. That is, in locating sound sources, the auditory system appears to process the first wavefront and suppresses the location information in later wavefronts coming from the reflections. Because the first wave that comes directly from the sound source will almost always arrive at the ears before those coming from any reflections, the first wave contains the information about the sound source. The phenomenon is called the *law of the first wavefront*, or the *precedence effect*. In Figure 12.8, although the later peaks present confusing information, there is no doubt concerning stimulus location if the first peak arriving at each ear is used as the basis of the location judgment. By using only the first positive peak in each sinusoid, one can determine that the stimulus arrived at the right ear before it reached the left ear. However, for sinusoidal stimuli the sounds must come on and go off slowly in order to reduce the spread of energy associated with turning sounds on and off abruptly (see Chapter 4). Thus, these slow onsets and offsets for sinusoidal stimuli eliminate the use of the first wavefront for localization. However, for most stimulus conditions the information arriving first at the ears will contain reliable data about the source of the sound, and work on the precedence effect suggests that this early-arriving information dominates our ability to localize sound sources.

In many precedence experiments and acoustic environments, reflections are not perceived as separate from the sound from the source (*echoes* are not usually perceived in most acoustic environments). This suggests that the sound from the source and that from reflections are perceptually <u>fused</u> into one perceived sound. The location of the sound in most acoustics environments is at or near the actual location of the sound source (the actual sound source <u>dominates</u> the perceived location) rather than at a location of a reflection. And acoustic information about reflections is <u>suppressed</u> relative to information about the sound from the actual source. For instance, the location of echoes is more poorly determined than that of the actual sound source.

LATERALIZATION

In studying localization of actual sound sources, it is impossible to separate the variables of interaural time from interaural level because both differences always coexist in localization experiments. In addition, the HRTF-derived differences in spectra cannot be accurately controlled in a free-field study, and the precedence effect will almost always be present. One simple way to control stimuli more accurately than can be done in the free field is to present them over headphones. The experimenter can directly manipulate interaural temporal difference or an interaural level difference or some particular spectral difference over headphones, thereby controlling the variables. When a tone is presented to a listener by means of headphones, the listener will, under most conditions, perceive an image that lies within his or her head and that has a location that moves as a function of changes in interaural temporal and level differences. To differentiate the perception of the internal (or intracranial) image that usually occurs with headphone-delivered sounds from the external image associated with external sound sources, the term *lateralization* is used to describe the former and *localization* for the latter. The image formed from binaural presentations over headphones is sometimes referred to as a *fused image* because the listener reports hearing one image as if the sound sources arriving at both ears were perceptually fused. A listener will not perceive a fused image if the interaural temporal difference or the interaural frequency difference is too large. If the interaural temporal difference is very large (more than many milliseconds depending on the stimulus), the listener will report hearing two images, one at each ear. Also, if the two ears receive independent sinusoidal signals differing greatly in frequency, the listener perceives two images, one at each ear, and both frequencies can be identified.

It has been shown that a fused image in a lateralization experiment appears toward the ear that receives the stimulus first or receives the more intense stimulus, in about the same manner that an external image is perceived more toward the ear that receives the sound first (and therefore receives the more intense sound). Thus, a lateralization procedure appears appropriate for studying the effects of interaural temporal and level differences on the ability of the auditory system to locate sound sources.

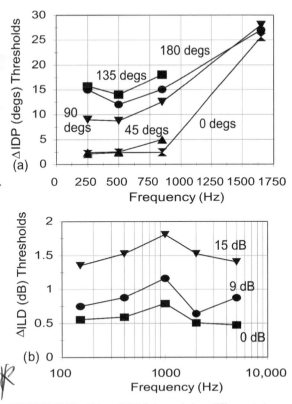

FIGURE 12.11 Value of IPD (interaural phase difference) change threshold (ΔIPD) and ILD (interaural level difference) change threshold (ΔILD) required for a $P(C)$ of 75% discrimination as a function of frequency (Hz). The various curves represent the values of the standard IPD or ILD. (a) ΔIPD as IPD changes from 0° to 180°. (b) ΔILDs are shown as a function of frequency, with each curve representing a different base value of ILD. Adapted from Yost and Dye (1991), used with permission.

Figure 12.11 shows the results from experiments in which tones were presented at different frequencies and the interaural temporal (actually interaural phase) and level difference thresholds were obtained. These and other results show that as the interaural phase difference increased toward 180°, the fused image was located closer toward the ear that received the tone first (leading in time). As the interaural phase difference exceeded 180°, the image was located on the other side of the head (toward the ear lagging in time); and as the interaural time difference approached 360°, the image was located back toward the middle of the head. A tone presented with no interaural difference was perceived toward the middle of the head or at midline. By introducing an interaural level difference, the tone was perceived closer to the ear receiving the louder tone. Thus, an image was placed in different perceptual positions within the head by introducing an interaural phase or level difference. Assuming that the image was at some location, due to a given interaural phase or level difference, the additional amount of interaural phase or level difference the listener required to detect a change in the perceived location of the fused image was determined. The amount of additional phase difference required for threshold detection is called ΔIPD (delta IPD), and the additional interaural level difference is called the ΔILD (delta ILD). The various curves in Figure 12.11 represent the initial interaural phase or level differences introduced such that for phase differences less than 180° the image was located on the left side of the head (Figure 12.11a) and for phase differences greater than 180° the image was on the right side of the head; data for interaural level discrimination are shown in Figure 12.11b.

A number of aspects of these data are important. First, notice that for any initial phase difference, the amount of ΔIPD required for detection remains constant up to frequencies of approximately 900 Hz and then increases. This indicates that at frequencies greater than 900 Hz, interaural (time) phase is a poor cue for processing an interaural time difference (for tonal frequencies above 1500 Hz, investigators have been unable to move the fused image as a function of changing the interaural phase or time difference). This agrees with Stevens and Newman's prediction that interaural time is not a usable cue for localization of high-frequency sinusoids. Thus, the binaural system does not use interaural time at high sinusoidal frequencies in order to localize sound.

The second interesting aspect of these data is that as the image is moved toward one side of the head by introducing phase differences close to 180° or a large interaural level difference, the amount of additional interaural phase or level difference required to discern

a change in perceived location (ΔIPD or ΔILD) also increases. This is consistent with Mills' MAA finding that listeners are less sensitive to changes in sound source location when the source is located toward one ear than when it is directly in front.

The fact that over headphones the interaural level difference is approximately the same for all frequencies (notice that there is a slight increase in ΔILD for frequencies in the 1000-Hz region) does not mean that in localizing a sound in the free field a listener could use interaural level at low frequencies. That is, even though a listener can detect a 2-dB change in interaural level at 200 Hz with headphones, this 2-dB interaural level difference will not occur in the free field at 200 Hz. The physical interaural level difference at 200 Hz is smaller than 2 dB. Thus, at 200 Hz the listener will not be presented a large enough interaural level difference in the free field to use for localization (see Figure 12.3).

The data described in Figures 12.8 and 12.11a imply that the binaural system can process interaural time for only low-frequency stimuli. This is not the case for complex sounds. If a high-frequency complex sound is presented such that there is a low-frequency repetition in the temporal waveform's envelope, then the binaural system appears almost as sensitive to differences in interaural time as for low-frequency sinusoids. Consider the case for a 300-Hz low-frequency tone, a 3600-Hz high-frequency tone, and a 3900-Hz tone amplitude modulated (SAM; see Chapter 4) by a 300-Hz tone. As predicted from Figure 12.11, listeners cannot detect a change in interaural time differences for the 3600-Hz tone and they can for the 300-Hz tone. However, they can also detect an interaural time difference change for the 300-Hz amplitude-modulated 3900-Hz carrier tone almost as well as they could for the 300-Hz tone. Thus, the high-frequency carrier with the slow amplitude modulation (300 Hz) has about the same interaural time difference threshold as the low-frequency tone. In this example, the 300-Hz sinusoidally amplitude-modulated 3900-Hz carrier tone produces a spectrum with components at 3600, 3900, and 4200 Hz (see Chapter 4), all well above the region where interaural time based on the spectrum operates (see Figure 12.10a). Many stimuli that contain only high spectral frequencies but have a low-frequency repetition in the time domain can be discriminated on the basis of interaural time differences. Some examples, in addition to AM stimuli, are beating tones (i.e., adding two high-frequency tones together that differ by a small amount in frequency; see Chapters 4 and 10), narrow bandpassed, filtered noises (i.e., the repetition in the time-domain waveform is proportional to the bandwidth of the noise; see Chapter 4), and a slowly repeating click stimulus that has been high-pass filtered so that only high frequencies are present. The facts of physics along with observations from lateralization experiments lead to the duplex theory for localization being restated as: <u>Interaural level is a cue used for locating high-frequency sounds. Interaural time is the cue used to locate any sound with low frequencies or any high-frequency complex sound with a low-frequency repetition in the time-domain waveform.</u>

The binaural system is remarkably sensitive to changes in interaural time and level. Figure 12.11 shows that the listener could detect a change of 3° of interaural phase. At 1000 Hz, this phase difference corresponds to a 0.01-msec change in interaural time. The data from lateralization experiments have also shown that the auditory system is sensitive to temporal differences equal to 10 one-millionths of a second (0.01 msec, or 10 microseconds).

In Chapters 7 and 8, we showed that the discharges of auditory nerve fibers were phase locked to the periodicity of low-frequency stimuli. The fact that interaural temporal differences are a cue for localization for low frequencies and for complex stimuli with low-frequency repetitions suggests that the phase locking might be crucial for understanding how the nervous system processes interaural temporal information. If the phase-locked activity of the nervous system is responsible for encoding interaural temporal differences, this would also explain why interaural time is a cue only at low sinusoidal or repetition frequencies (see Chapter 15 for the discussion of a possible neural mechanism that might code for interaural time differences).

LOCALIZATION VERSUS LATERALIZATION

We have already commented on the fact that sounds presented over headphones are usually perceived as "inside the head" rather than "out in space," where actual sound sources are usually located. Usually when sounds are presented over headphones they do not have all of the spectral complexity of a real sound source, since the headphone-produced sound does not pass over the torso, head, and pinna of the listener like the sound from an actual sound source would. That is, the headphone-delivered stimuli do not preserve the spectral complexities described by the HRTFs. In a real sense, the head and torso filter the sound (see Chapter 5) before it reaches the tympanic membrane, and the HRTF describes the amplitude and phase spectra of this filter function. If a complex sound is actually filtered by a filter made to reflect the amplitude and phase spectra of the HRTF and then presented over headphones, the sound arriving at the tympanic membrane should have all of the spectral complexities of a real sound that had passed over the head and torso. When sounds are presented through headphones after such HRTF filtering, most listeners report that the sounds appear much more like those occurring in space than when the sounds are not filtered by the HRTF.

Table 12.1 shows a comparison of a listener locating actual sounds versus "locating" sounds presented over headphones when they have been filtered by the appropriate HRTFs. For each listener and for each sound source location, an HRTF was computed for both ears and then used to determine HRTF filters so that over headphones the waveform arriving at the two tympanic membranes for each listener was as close as possible to what occurs naturally. In listening to both the actual sound sources and the "simulated (virtual) headphone sources," the listener indicated where in space he or she thought the sound occurred. In the actual localization experiment, the listener's location judgments are compared to the location of the actual source. For the headphone-delivered sounds, the listener's location judgments are compared to the location of the sound source for the HRTF filter used to

TABLE 12.1 Comparison of Location Judgments for Two Listeners (S1 and S2) Judging the Vertical and Horizontal Locations of Actual Noise Sound Sources and Simulated Sources Using HRTF-Filtered Noises Presented over Headphones

Listener	Actual	Simulated
S1	0.99	0.96
S2	0.97	0.83

The judgments are in terms of correlation coefficients, which means how well the listeners judged the position relative to the actual position. A coefficient of 1.0 means the listener indicated for all locations exactly where the source was, whereas a coefficient of 0.0 means that the listener had no idea where the sounds were coming from (from Wightman, Kistler, and Perkins, 1987).

filter the stimulus for that judgment. As can be seen, there is little difference, in that judgments remain excellent in the two listening conditions (i.e., the correlations between perceived and actual locations are very high), which indicates that reproducing the complex spectrum of real sounds is an important variable in auditory localization.

BINAURAL MASKING

In the preceding section, we described the auditory system's sensitivity to changes in interaural time and level, which are principally used to locate sound sources in the azimuth plane. Many experiments have shown that the threshold for detecting a signal masked by noise is lower when the noise and signal are presented in a particular way to both ears. In these experiments, subjects first determined their masked thresholds when both the noise and tonal signal were presented equally to both ears. In one test experiment, the tonal signal was removed from one ear such that the noise was at both ears and the signal at only one ear. In this case the signal was easy to detect, and therefore the level of the tone had to be reduced to obtain masked thresholds. Subsequently, many investigators have studied the improvement in detection associated with presenting signal and maskers to both

ears. A certain nomenclature has been developed to describe the various types of binaural configurations of signal and masker.

monotic: stimuli presented to only one ear
diotic: identical stimuli presented to both ears or no interaural differences for the signal and the masker presented to each ear
dichotic: different stimuli presented to the two ears

Investigators have found that the masked threshold of a signal is the same when the stimuli are presented in a monotic or diotic condition. If the masker and the signal are arranged in a dichotic situation, however, the signal has a lower threshold than in either the monotic or diotic condition. There are several ways to present the signal (S) and the masker (M) in a dichotic or diotic manner; again, a set of symbols is used to describe these stimulus conditions.

S_o: signal presented binaurally with no interaural differences (diotic)
M_o: masker presented binaurally with no interaural differences (diotic)
S_m: signal presented to only one ear
M_m: masker presented to only one ear
S_π: signal presented to one ear 180° out of phase with the signal presented to the other ear
M_π: masker presented to one ear 180° out of phase with the signal presented to the other ear

For the binaural conditions described previously, the signal or masker is identical in all dimensions except that denoted by a subscript. Thus:

monotic: $M_m S_m$
diotic: $M_o S_o,$ $M_\pi S_\pi$
dichotic: $M_o S_\pi,$ $M_o S_m,$ $M_\pi S_\pi,$ $M_\pi S_o,$ $M_\pi S_m$

To compare detection in one binaural condition with that in another, the data are usually presented as the difference between the signal level required for detection (masked threshold) in a monotic condition and that required in a diotic or dichotic condition. That is, the signal level required for detection in the relevant diotic or dichotic condition is subtracted from the signal level required for detection in the $M_m S_m$ condi-

TABLE 12.2 The Masking-level Difference in dB for a Variety of Stimulus Conditions

Interaural condition compared to M_mS_m	MLD
M_mS_m, M_oS_o, $M_{M\pi}S_\pi$	0 dB
$M_\pi S_m$	6 dB
M_oS_m	9 dB
$M_\pi S_o$	13 dB
M_oS_π	15 dB

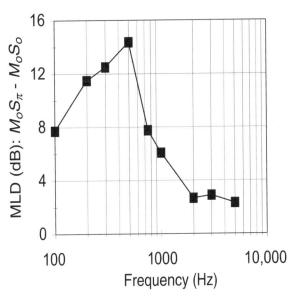

FIGURE 12.12 Difference in masked thresholds (in dB) between M_oS_π and M_oS_o conditions (MLD) plotted as a function of signal frequency. Adapted from Webster (1951), used with permission.

tion (monotic condition). Such a difference when expressed in decibels is called a *masking-level difference* (MLD) or a *binaural masking-level difference* (BMLD).

Table 12.2 shows the type of improvement in detection provided by dichotic presentation of maskers and signals (MLD). These data represent approximately the maximum MLD obtained when the masker is a continuous, broadband white Gaussian noise presented at moderate to intense levels and the signal is a pulsed sinusoid of low frequency (below 1000 Hz) and long duration (greater than 100 msec). Figure 12.12 describes the MLD obtained between the M_oS_o condition and the M_oS_π condition as a function of signal frequency. Notice that as the frequency of the signal increases, the MLD decreases. However, the MLD never goes to zero; the signal is always easier to detect in the dichotic case than in the diotic case.

The fact that the MLD decreases as a function of frequency has suggested to many hearing scientists that the MLD might be related to the interaural differences of time and level. When the stimulus condition is dichotic, there are differences in the interaural temporal and level information between the stimuli arriving at the ears. However, in the diotic condition there are no interaural differences. It is therefore logical to assume that interaural differences associated with dichotic presentations result in the improvement in detection over that obtained in the dichotic condition.

The MLD phenomenon may also be related to another important aspect of spatial hearing. If two or more sound sources are separated in space, it is easier both to locate *and* to attend to the individual sounds.

For instance, recognizing a particular voice in a choir, distinguishing an instrument in an orchestra, or hearing a particular conversation at a noisy party may be made easier because the sound that is of interest is in a different location than other, interfering sounds. This ability to discriminate sounds in complex acoustic environments based on the sources' spatial separation is often called the *cocktail party effect*. The MLD is a result of the signal plus masker having a different interaural configuration than the masker alone. Thus, like in the cocktail party effect, this interaural separation between the masker and the masker plus signal may make it easier to detect the signal. Recall that the main MLD effect is the ability to detect a signal, whereas the cocktail party effect refers to recognition or identification of a signal. Thus, although the two effects (MLD and cocktail party effect) are probably related, they may not be measuring exactly the same aspect of binaural processing. The ability to locate a sound in space is important, therefore, not only as an aid for determining the position of sounds, but also perhaps for attending to a particular sound in an environment with many sound sources.

SUMMARY

For localizing sound sources in the azimuth plane, interaural time is the relevant cue for stimulus location at low frequencies and for complex stimuli with low-frequency repetition, and interaural level is the cue at high frequencies. Spectral differences provide by the head-related transfer function (HRTF) are probably the cues used for vertical localization and on cones of confusion. Loudness and early reflections from reflective surfaces are the probable cues for localization as a function of distance. The precedence effect stresses the importance of the first wave in determining stimulus location. In the lateralization procedure stimuli are presented over headphones, and the location of the fused image is dependent on interaural time for low-frequency tones and on interaural level at all frequencies. By using the spectral differences of the HRTF, sounds presented over headphones may be judged similarly to naturally occurring sound sources. Signals and maskers presented in dichotic stimulus configurations have lower thresholds (MLDs) than signals and maskers presented in either diotic or monotic configurations. The MLD and the cocktail party effect demonstrate how binaural cues can be used to detect and recognize signals in noisy environments.

SUPPLEMENT

A number of books describe in more detail binaural hearing, localization, and lateralization: Blauert (1997), Yost and Gourevitch (1987), Gilkey and Anderson (1997), and Popper and Fay (2005). Chapter 6 in the textbook by Moore (1997) and a similar chapter by Yost and Dye (1991) cover many aspects of binaural hearing. Also see Wightman and Kistler

(1993). The article by Litovsky et al. (1999) provides a review of the precedence effect.

All of the data described in this chapter relate to stationary sound sources and not sensitivity to moving sound sources. Chandler and Grantham (1992) and Saberi and Perrott (1990) have published a number of articles on auditory motion. These studies involve the study of sound sources that actually move and of simulated moving sound sources. If a sound is presented to one loudspeaker at one location at one instant in time and then is presented to a different loudspeaker at another location at the next instant in time, listeners almost always report that the sound appears to move from one location to the other, even though nothing actually moved. By changing the time interval between exciting one loudspeaker and then the other, the velocity of the apparent motion can be varied.

The fact that we can move our heads when localizing sounds was briefly mentioned in this chapter. Head motion (see Mills, 1972, for a brief review) may be an important variable for many aspects of localization, especially when one tries to present sounds over headphones in order to produce the illusion that there are sound sources in actual space. These experiments in which headphone-delivered sounds are judged to be "externalized," are often referred to as experiments in *auditory virtual environments*. That is, it is possible to present sounds over headphones such that listeners report that actual sound sources exist, and as such the headphone-delivered stimuli have produced a "virtual" rather than a "real" acoustic environment.

While the spectral structure of the HRTF is known to be important in vertical localization and along cones of confusion, the exact aspect of the HRTF spectral structure that mediates localization is not known (see Colburn and Kulkarni, 2005; see also Wightman and Kistler, 1989a and 1989b)). Using HRTF-filtered stimuli delivered to headphones allows one to carefully control for the spectral differences that might provide localization cues. For instance, Wightman and Kistler (1997) present data that suggest that vertical localization may not be processed based on the HRTF configuration at only one ear. They presented properly filtered HRTF-processed sounds to only one ear of listeners and asked them to indicate the sounds' location. Their data suggest that vertical localization can't be based on the acoustic information arriving at only one ear, implying that some form of binaural comparison is required to completely account for vertical localization (see also Colburn and Kulkarni, 2005).

Binaural beats are another phenomenon not described in the chapter. Binaural beats occur when two tones of slightly different frequencies are presented, one to each ear. In this case, listeners report hearing a movement of the sound image between the two ears that occurs at a rate equal to the frequency difference. For instance, if a 500-Hz tone is delivered to one ear and a 505-Hz tone to the other ear (5-Hz difference), a movement of an image between the two ears will occur at a rate of five times per second (see McFadden and Passenan, 1975). Henning (1977) studied interaural time discrimination for low rates of amplitude modulation (see also the book by Yost and Gourevitch, 1987).

Cherry (1953) first coined the term *cocktail party effect* when he discussed how we perceive one world with two ears. Another way to explain the MLD (see Green and Yost, 1975) has been provided by Durlach (1972; see also Colburn and Kulkarni, 2005) in his equalization-cancellation (EC) model of binaural hearing. In the EC model, the waveforms at the two ears in an MLD procedure are first assumed to be equalized, and then the neural information at one ear is subtracted from that at the other ear. Consider what would happen in the M_oS_o and M_oS_π conditions if the waveforms at both ears were subtracted. In the M_oS_o condition, there would be a complete cancellation because both ears receive the same waveform.

However, in the M_oS_π condition only the masker would completely cancel because the masker but not the signal is identical at both ears. The signals would actually add (i.e., subtracting one waveform that is $180°$ out of phase with another waveform is the same as adding the two waveforms; see Appendix A). Thus, the cancellation process provides a large signal to detect in the M_oS_π condition and nothing to detect in the M_oS_o condition, predicting a lower signal threshold in the M_oS_π condition. The EC model makes additional assumptions about the equalization and cancellation processes so that exact predictions for MLD data can be obtained.

Another "model" of binaural processing assumes that the sounds at both ears are compared via a process called *cross-correlation* (see Trahiotis et al., 2005). Jeffress (1948; also see Trahiotis et al., 2005 and Colburn and Kulkarni, 2005) suggested that cross-correlation could be implemented by a neural network that measures the coincidence of neural inputs arriving at each ear. Cross-correlation and binaural coincidence models have provided excellent accounts of many data from lateralization, localization, and binaural masking experiments. Neural networks that appear to operate something like a coincidence network have been observed in some species of birds (see Kubke and Carr, 2005).

Although this book is largely about human hearing, a variety of different neural methods appear to enable different animals to localize sound sources (see the books by Yost and Gourevitch, 1987; Fay and Popper, 1998; and Popper and Fay, 2005). Studies of animals that echolocate (e.g., bats and dolphins) present a particularly interesting and well-studied area of sound localization (see the books by Yost and Gourevitch, 1987, and Au, 1993).

means that the contributions of very high and very low frequency components to the dBA measure are small. Thus, only those frequency components to which human listeners are most sensitive (see Chapter 10) contribute most to the dBA measure.

Figure 13.2b is also a plot of loudness versus level, but in this case curve B represents the loudness of a tone that was masked by a 30-dB spectrum level (N_o) wideband noise. Curve A is the same as the one in Figure 13.2a. Notice that the threshold for the masked tone is 40 dB above the unmasked tone's threshold. Because both tones are at threshold (one at absolute threshold, the other at masked threshold), the two tones are of equal loudness when their actual levels are 40 dB apart. When the actual level of both tones is 80 dB SPL, they are both also judged equally loud. This, in turn, means that the loudness of the masked tone (curve B) increased faster (steeper slope) than the unmasked tone. This increase in loudness (or the steep loudness slope) is sometimes called *loudness recruitment*. The loudness of the masked tone changes much more for each 10-dB increase in level than does the loudness of the unmasked tone. Curve B might also represent the data from someone whose threshold of hearing was 40 dB above the normal threshold (i.e., the person had a 40-dB hearing loss) but who judges an 80-dB SPL tone the same in loudness as a subject with normal hearing would. The fact that the individual's loudness function shows loudness recruitment is important in treating certain hearing abnormalities. Note, for instance, that amplifying sound (e.g., by use of a hearing aid) will lead to a more rapid increase in loudness for the person with a hearing loss than for the person with normal hearing.

Most of the results that have been studied using threshold as a psychoacoustic measure can also be investigated using loudness. For instance, the duration of a tone can be varied, and the listener can adjust the tone's power so that it remains equally loud. In so doing, loudness measures are used to determine temporal integration (see Chapter 10). A short sound will not be as loud as a long sound if their powers are equal and their durations are less than approximately 250 msec. The loudness of a sound can also be main-

tained at a constant phon level as the bandwidth of a stimulus is narrowed in order to measure a critical band (see Chapter 11). In this case, narrowing the bandwidth of a stimulus will decrease the loudness once the bandwidth is less than a critical band. In these and other cases the data from threshold experiments are not substantially different from those obtained in loudness studies, but significant differences do exist.

Loudness adaptation (or *perstimulatory fatigue*) occurs during exposure to a long-duration (on the order of seconds or minutes) adapting stimulus. The change in loudness adaptation takes place while the adapting stimulus is being presented. That is, a stimulus appears to become softer if it is kept on for a very long time (seconds or longer). The loudness of the stimulus is typically measured by having the listener match a comparison stimulus (usually presented to one ear) to the adapting stimulus (usually presented to the other ear) in terms of loudness. As the adapting stimulus remains on for longer and longer periods of time, listeners decrease the level of the matching stimulus in order to achieve a loudness match, indicating that the loudness of the adapting stimulus has decreased over time while it is on. Thus, the context in which a sound occurs can affect its perceived loudness.

As we mentioned in Chapter 2, although changes in level are highly correlated with loudness changes, the relationship is not perfect. That is, changes in frequency, duration, intensity, and bandwidth all affect the perceived loudness of a stimulus even though the level of the stimulus remains fixed. Remember that loudness is a subjective evaluation of sound, whereas intensity is an objective measure of vibratory magnitude or sound pressure.

PITCH

The pitch of sound is perceived in many auditory contexts: The melody of a song is determined by pitch changes, a female has a higher-pitched voice than a male, the perceived sound from many sound sources differ in pitch, etc. Just as sound contains no variable called *loudness,* it also does not contain a variable called *pitch.* Loudness and pitch are properties of perception that provide information about sound sources. Different physical attributes of sound yield the perceptions of loudness and pitch (as well as other perceptual attributes), and these perceptual attributes are a result of the auditory systems processing the neural code for these physical variables of sound (e.g., frequency, level, and time).

Experiments on pitch are usually performed with a pitch-matching procedure in which a standard stimulus (sometimes a sinusoid) is used as the basis for pitch matches of comparison stimuli. As in a loudness-matching experiment, the listener adjusts some acoustic aspect of a comparison sound such that it is perceived to have the same pitch as a standard sound. The standard sound is often either a sinusoidal sound or a pulse train of periodically repeating transients (see Chapter 4). The frequency of the standard sinusoid or the repetition frequency of the standard pulse train, expressed in hertz, that is judged equal in pitch to the comparison sound is used as the measure or scale of pitch in pitch-matching experiments. That is, pitch can be expressed either in terms of spectral frequency or in terms of repetition frequency. While spectral and repetition frequency are often directly related (see Chapter 4) in terms of pitch perception, there are cases in which they are not, as we discuss later in this chapter.

Musical scales, such as the seven-tone musical scale (B C D E F G A), are often used to generate a pitch scale. In general, the relationships among musical notes in a musical scale are arranged in an octave manner, with 12 intervals per octave. In the *equal temperament scale,* the octave is divided into 12 equal logarithmic intervals called *semitones* and each interval is divided into 100 equal logarithmic steps called *cents.* Thus, an octave has 1200 cents. A semitone is 100 cents in the equal temperament scale. These relationships are shown in Table 13.1. For this table, assume that the note A is 440 Hz. Other schemes are often used to express the physical relationship among intervals. The *just intonation* and the *Pythagorean schemes* have a slightly different number of cents between intervals (in a semitone) than the equal temperament scale. Different scales are preferred by different musicians. Thus, musical notes or cents or semitones can be used to indicate the pitch of a sound.

Scaling procedures (see Appendix D) have been used in the measurement of pitch, but listeners often respond in a different manner when they are asked to judge pitch than when they are asked to judge loudness. This difference stems from the qualitative aspects of pitch. That is, as the pitch of a stimulus changes, it does not appear to vary along a single dimension of greater to smaller or more to less. One tone can be said to be greater in loudness than another tone, but one pitch may not be greater in magnitude than another pitch. The *mel scale* is a scale derived for pitch in the

TABLE 13.1 Relationship Between Musical Note, Cents, and Frequency (Hz) for the Three Major Scales of Musical Pitch

Musical note	Just Intonation		Equal Temperament		Pythagorean Tuning	
	Cents	Frequency	Cents	Frequency	Cents	Frequency
C	0	264	0	264	0	264
D	204	297	200	296	204	297
E	386	329	400	333	408	334
F	498	352	500	352	498	352
G	702	396	700	395	702	396
A	884	440	900	443	906	445
B	1088	495	1100	498	1100	501
C	1200	528	1200	528	1200	528

same way the sone scale was obtained for loudness, by using direct scaling techniques. However, the mel scale is difficult to obtain, probably due to the qualitative nature of the subjective dimension of pitch.

In discussing the threshold of audibility, we mentioned that listeners might be asked to detect the presence of a tonal-sounding stimulus instead of just detecting any sound. Tonality implies that the observer is detecting the presence of pitch. Von Bekesy found that a tone with a frequency that was less than 1000 Hz must have a duration equal to 3 to 9 periods if the tone was to have a definite pitch. Above 1000 Hz this critical duration for the perception of tonality, or pitch, was 10 msec regardless of the frequency of the tone.

COMPLEX PITCH

There is a strong correlation between the pitch of a stimulus and the spectral location of its frequencies. That is, if a complex sound has a spectral structure that can be *resolved* by the auditory system, then aspects of this spectral structure (e.g., the spectral region with the greatest level) is often highly correlated with the sound's perceived pitch. Recall from Chapters 7–9 and 11 that the auditory system is limited in its ability to resolve spectral differences, in that small frequency differences are resolvable in the low-frequency region of the spectrum but not in the high frequencies. Thus, small spectral differences at high frequencies are unlikely to contribute to pitch perception.

Listeners can perceive a pitch for complex sounds that do not have any spectral components at the perceived pitch. For instance, listeners report a 100-Hz pitch associated with a stimulus consisting of a sum of the frequencies of 700, 800, 900, and 1000 Hz. Although there is absolutely no energy at 100 Hz, listeners judge the sound to have a 100-Hz pitch. These four tones are all harmonics of 100 Hz (in fact, 100 Hz is the highest frequency for which the tones could be harmonically related). The observation that a pitch could be associated with the fundamental of a complex stimulus even when the fundamental was absent in the spectrum of the complex stimulus is called the *case of*

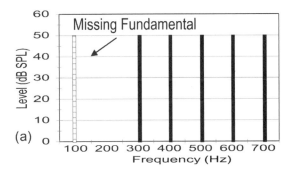

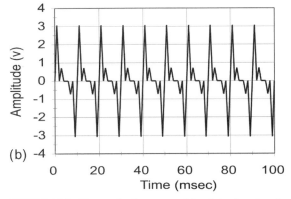

FIGURE 13.3 The amplitude spectrum **(a)** and the time-domain waveform **(b)** of a missing-fundamental pitch stimulus consisting of a complex sound with frequency components of 700, 800, 900, and 1000 Hz. The pitch is 100 Hz, which is the missing fundamental (dotted) component in panel (a). The time domain has an envelope with a 10-msec period, the reciprocal of 1000 Hz.

the missing fundamental or *missing fundamental pitch*.

The amplitude spectrum and the time waveform (assuming all the tones had the same phase) associated with the tonal complex (700, 800, 900, and 1000 Hz) are shown in Figure 13.3. Notice that there is a 10-msec spacing between the major peaks in the complex time waveform. Since the frequency associated with a 10-msec period is 100 Hz, it may be possible that the auditory system perceived the 100-Hz pitch because of the 10-msec periodicity of the time waveform. In fact, most stimuli that have a periodic time waveform will have a perceived pitch equal to

194

the reciprocal of the period, called *periodicity pitch*. For instance, because the time waveform of the square wave shown in Figure 4.8 consists of a periodically occurring square wave whose period is 2 msec, this waveform will have 500-Hz periodicity pitch. In this case, as can be seen from Figure 4.8b, there is also energy at 500 Hz in the amplitude spectrum. Thus, one can perceive a periodicity pitch when the complex stimulus has energy at the frequency of the pitch (the square wave) or when there is not energy at the frequency of the pitch (the missing fundamental tonal complex). It is also possible that the pitch of the missing fundamental stimulus is based on some other spectral analysis performed by the auditory system (e.g., the spectral spacing between the harmonics is equal to the missing fundamental, which equals the perceived pitch). Thus, the missing fundamental pitch clearly indicates that pitches can be perceived even when complex sounds have no spectral components at the perceived pitch. However, the pitch of the missing fundamental could be determined by temporal and/or spectral processing performed by the auditory system.

Although the periodicity concept might account for the data of the missing fundamental pitch, there is a counterexample. The sound with the spectrum and time-domain waveform shown in Figure 13.4 produces a 250-Hz pitch (i.e., listeners indicate that a 250-Hz tone has the same pitch as the stimulus described in Figure 13.4). The spectrum of the sound is continuous and there are noisy spectral peaks at 750, 1000, 1250, 1500, 1750, and 2000 Hz. Thus, the spectral peaks are somewhat like the tonal components for a missing-fundamental pitch stimulus. However, there is neither any energy at the reported pitch (250 Hz) nor any periodicity in the envelope of the noisy waveform. Thus, neither a concentration of energy in a particular frequency region nor the periodic nature of the envelope can be used to determine the sound's 250-Hz pitch. Data involving other complex waveforms indicate that although the envelope-periodicity theory might be correct in some cases, other processing is taking place in addition to envelope-period analysis. The pitches of these complex sounds are referred to in

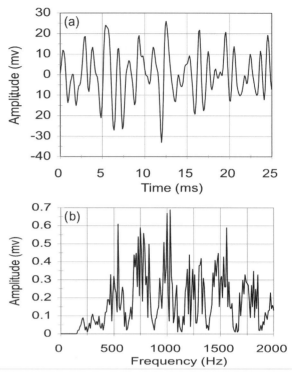

FIGURE 13.4 The amplitude spectrum **(a)** and the time-domain waveform **(b)** of a complex sound that leads to a perceived pitch of 250 Hz. The amplitude spectrum has noisy peaks at integer multiples of 250 Hz but not a spectral peak at 250 Hz. There is no periodicity in the time-domain waveform envelope at 4 msec, the reciprocal of the pitch (1000/250 = 4 msec).

a number of ways: *pitch of the missing fundamental*, *complex pitch*, and *virtual pitch* (as opposed to the *spectral pitch* of a sound, whose pitch is determined entirely by the spectral location with the most energy).

Figure 13.5 indicates one more aspect of complex pitch. In this case the tones of the complex are at 425, 525, 625, 725, 825, and 925 Hz. This sound is generated by shifting the spectrum of a 100-Hz missing-fundamental pitch stimulus consisting of components at 400, 500, 600, 700, 800, and 900 Hz up in frequency by 25 Hz. Notice that although all frequencies are equally spaced at 100-Hz intervals, 100 Hz is not the "missing fundamental"; 25 Hz would be the highest fundamental of this complex sound. Listeners match

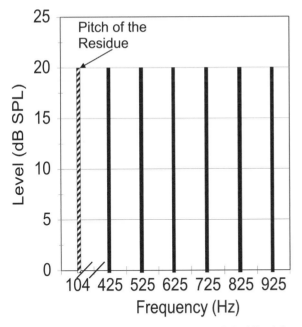

FIGURE 13.5 The amplitude spectrum of a pitch shift of the residue stimulus consisting of a complex sound with frequency components of 425, 525, 625, and 725 Hz. The pitch is 104 Hz, which is neither the missing fundamental (25 Hz is the fundamental) nor the frequency spacing among the frequency components.

the pitch of this complex to that of a sinusoid with a frequency of 104 Hz, indicating that this complex has a perceived complex pitch of 104 Hz, which is neither the frequency of the missing fundamental nor the frequency spacing of the tones. This pitch is referred to as the *pitch shift of the residue*. Again there is no energy in the spectrum at 104 Hz, nor is there a clear periodicity in the time-domain envelope at the reciprocal of 104 Hz.

The pitch of a sound can also vary as a result of several other variables, including bandwidth. If a harmonic series with a low-frequency fundamental (less than approximately 1000 Hz) is high-pass filtered, the complex pitch remains at the missing fundamental, although the pitch will be very weak as the high-pass-filter cutoff is increased. In other cases, a *dichotic pitch* (see Chapter 12) can be produced when a noise is presented to one ear exactly as it is to the other ear,

except in a small spectral region where this is an interaural phase shift. The perceived dichotic pitch is associated with the spectral region containing the interaural phase shift (i.e., if the interaural phase shift is maximal at 500 Hz, the dichotic pitch as determined by pitch matching is 500 Hz) and the strength of the perceived pitch is strongest when the interaural phase shift is 180°. In some cases, the pitch of a broadband sound is closely associated with the high-frequency edge of the sound's spectrum (*edge pitch*).

In many cases, a single sound from a source may contain several pitches. For instances, a missing-fundamental sound consisting of 400-, 600-, 800-, 1000-, 1200-, and 1400-Hz components might be perceived as having the missing fundamental pitch of 200 Hz along with pitches of 400 and perhaps 600 Hz. The ability of the auditory system to resolve spectral differences in the low frequencies may allow one to "hear out" the 400- and 600-Hz components of this complex in addition to the 200-Hz missing fundamental pitch. Another example of the ability of the auditory system to process more than one pitch exists for *inharmonic tonal sequences* in which one component is *mistuned*. A stimulus consisting of 250, 500, 825, 1000, 1250, 1500, and 1750 Hz comprises all multiples of 250 Hz, except 825 Hz, which is a mistuned inharmonic tone in an otherwise harmonic sequence of spectral components. If an inharmonic tone differs by about 8% or more from it harmonic frequency (825 Hz is 10% different than 750 Hz), then listeners are likely to match both a frequency near (but not exactly at) that of the fundamental (250 Hz in the example) and a frequency near that of the mistuned harmonic (825 Hz in the example).

When the pitch of a stimulus can be determined on the basis of periodicity in the time-domain waveform, hearing scientists believe that some aspect of the auditory nerve's ability to be phase locked to the periodicity of low-frequency stimuli accounts for the way in which the auditory system processes these pitches. The area of pitch perception still poses a real challenge for auditory theorists, in that complex pitch perception is determined neither by only the spectral content of the sound nor by only its temporal structure.

NONLINEAR TONES

In Chapter 11, we described the aural harmonics and difference tones produced by the nonlinearity of the auditory system. The first and second *aural harmonics* ($2f_1$ and $3f_1$), *difference tone* ($f_1 - f_2$), and a *cubic-difference tone* ($2f_1 - f_2$) are those nonlinear tones most often perceived (see Chapter 5 and Appendix A for a discussion of nonlinearity). That is, when a complex sound consisting of a number of sinusoids is presented to a listener, especially at loud levels, listeners hear pitches in addition to those corresponding to the frequency of the sinusoids in the stimulus. These additional pitches are associated with the aural harmonics and difference tones produced by the nonlinear properties of the auditory periphery (see Chapters 8 and 9). The cubic-difference tone is of particular interest because in many conditions it is the most perceptible nonlinearly produced tone. For instance, if 1400-Hz and 1680-Hz primary tones are summed, a cubic-difference tone of 1120 Hz is perceived; that is, $2 \times 1400\,\text{Hz} - 1680\,\text{Hz} = 1120\,\text{Hz}$. This cubic-difference tone can be heard when the levels of the 1400-Hz and 1680-Hz primary tones are less than 40 dB SL, whereas the difference tone of 280 Hz ($1680\,\text{Hz} - 1400\,\text{Hz} = 280\,\text{Hz}$) cannot be detected at these low primary tone levels. Remember that the perception of the 1120-Hz or the 280-Hz pitch is not due to the presence of these frequencies in the stimulus. The pitches result from the nonlinear distortion caused by the peripheral auditory system.

In order to completely describe the nonlinear tones, we must specify their levels and phases as well as their frequencies. The *cancellation method* is often used to obtain estimates of the level and phase of nonlinear tones. In the cancellation method one complex stimulus is used to elicit the nonlinear tone, for instance, an 840-Hz and a 1000-Hz primary tone pair that produces a 680-Hz cubic-difference tone; that is, $2 \times 840\,\text{Hz} - 1000\,\text{Hz} = 680\,\text{Hz}$. Another stimulus is presented along with the primaries and is used to cancel the pitch of the nonlinear tone, in this case a 680-Hz *cancellation tone*. That is, a 680-Hz cancellation tone is added to the 840-Hz and 1000-Hz primary tones. Without the addition of the 680-Hz cancellation tone, listeners can detect sound with pitches of 840 and 1000 Hz (the primary tones) and 680 Hz (the nonlinearly produced cubic-difference tone). If the 680-Hz cancellation tone is presented 180° out of phase with that of the nonlinear 680-Hz cubic-difference tone, then the 680-Hz pitch might be canceled, and the listener would detect only the two primary tones. This cancellation should only occur when the two tones (cancellation tone and cubic-difference tone) are at equal levels and 180° out of phase (i.e., the addition of two tones of the same frequency and level but 180° out of phase will lead to complete cancellation). In the cancellation procedure, the listener is presented the 840-Hz and 1000-Hz primary tones (tones used to elicit the 680-Hz cubic-difference tone) and the 680-Hz cancellation tone. The listener is instructed to adjust the level and phase of the 680-Hz cancellation tone until the listener no longer hears a pitch of 680 Hz (the cubic-difference tone). The level of the cancellation tone and 180° minus the phase of the cancellation tone that the listener picked that eliminated the pitch of the cubic-difference tone is used to estimate the level and phase of the cubic-difference tone (or other nonlinear tones).

Figure 13.6 displays the results from a cancellation experiment. The upper curve shows the level of the 680-Hz tone required to cancel the cubic-difference tone as a function of the overall level of the two primary tones (840 and 1000 Hz) used to elicit the cubic-difference tone. The lower curve shows the phase (minus 180°) of the 680-Hz tone required to cancel the cubic-difference tone.

The intensities and phases of the nonlinearities of the auditory system are crucial values to be determined if we are to describe how the system produces these nonlinearities. The cubic-difference tone has been of special interest because it appears at low levels, and the level and phase of the cubic-difference tone change in a complex way as a function of its pitch (that is, as a function of separation in frequency between f_1 and f_2). Because of these relations, most scientists believe that the source of the cubic-difference tone is in the inner ear; the perceived pitch of the cubic-difference tone probably results either from the nonlinear motion of the basilar membrane or from some nonlinearities that exist when the hair cells stimulate auditory nerve fibers.

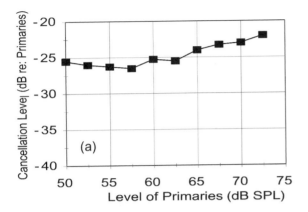

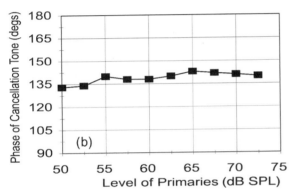

FIGURE 13.6 (a) The level of a cancellation tone (680 Hz, with its level expressed relative to the levels of the primaries) required to cancel a 680-Hz cubic-difference tone produced by 840- and 1000-Hz primaries presented at different levels (dB SPL). The cancellation-tone level is about 25 to 28 dB below that of the primaries for primary levels ranging from 45 to 75 dB SPL. (b) The phase of the cancellation tone required to cancel the 680-Hz cubic-difference tone shown as a function of the level of the primaries. The estimated phase of the cubic-difference tone is 180° minus the values shown in curve (b). Based on data from J. L. Hall (1975), used with permission.

instance, the quality difference between a violin and a cello playing the same musical note at the same loudness and for the same duration would be defined as a difference in timbre between the two instruments. Timbre appears to be related to the bandwidth of the complex stimulus, especially for complex waveforms consisting of harmonically related sinusoids. A stimulus with a larger number of harmonics is usually perceived as having a fuller or richer timbre than more narrowband stimuli, such as a pure tone.

In addition to timbre, musicians often refer to the *consonance* and *dissonance* of complex stimuli, such as notes of music. Consonant pairs are those notes played at intervals that result in a "pleasant" sound. Dissonant pairs are played at intervals that sound "unpleasant" to many musicians. We have already discussed (Chapter 10) the beats associated with mixing two sinusoids whose frequencies differ by a few hertz. The sensation of beats gives way to *flutter* and then to *roughness* as the frequency difference between the two tones is increased.

S. S. Stevens determined that sounds also have attributes of *density* and *volume*. The density of a tone increases as its frequency or intensity increases. Increases in volume are generally associated with decreases in frequency and level. Thus, volume and density are approximate opposites. The fact that different sounds elicit different subjective descriptions is not surprising. Many scientists believe that the labeling of the subjective dimensions of sound may also depend on culture and experience. For instance, many modern composers are writing music with dissonant intervals. Because some of this music is becoming popular, perhaps which musical intervals are labeled as consonant and dissonant might change over time.

OTHER SUBJECTIVE ATTRIBUTES OF SOUND

Complex stimuli have subjective attributes in addition to pitch and loudness, one of which is *timbre*. Timbre is often defined as that subjective attribute of a sound that differentiates two or more sounds that have the same pitch, loudness, and duration. For

SUMMARY

From equal-loudness contours and loudness-scaling experiments, we can construct the phon and sone scales of loudness. These scales enable us to relate the subjective description of loudness to the physical descriptions of frequency and intensity. Pitch is often measured in a pitch-matching task.

The musical scale of pitch contains octaves, intervals, semitones, and cents. The mel scale of pitch is constructed from a pitch-scaling experiment. Scales of pitch are more qualitative in nature than are loudness scales. Pitch and loudness are not perfectly correlated with their physical counterparts: frequency and intensity. The concept of the missing fundamental illustrates that pitch processing is sometimes dependent neither on spectral information at the frequency of the pitch nor on envelope periodicity information associated with the period of the pitch. Edge pitch, dichotic pitch, resolved pitch, and the pitch of mistuned harmonics are all examples of the variety of situations in which complex sounds produce pitch. The levels and phases of nonlinear tones (especially the cubic-difference tone) can be measured by the cancellation technique. Complex stimuli have additional subjective attributes, such as timbre, consonance, dissonance, beats, flutter, roughness, density, and volume.

SUPPLEMENT

Loudness and pitch as subjective attributes of sound have been studied extensively by S. S. Stevens. His book *Psychophysics* (1975) and his article in *Science* (1970), "Neural Events and the Psychophysical Law," provide an insight into his work. Fletcher and Munson (1933) used the loudness-matching technique to obtain the equal-loudness contours. The book by Hartmann (1998) should also be consulted for more details about pitch, loudness, and nonlinearities. The book by B. C. J. Moore (1997) also covers topics on loudness and pitch. Plack et al. (2005) provide a thorough review of pitch.

Loudness is often measured in an alternating binaural loudness balance (ABLB) technique. In this procedure, the standard tone is presented to one ear and the comparison tone to the other ear. The tones are alternated in time, and the listener adjusts the comparison tone until it appears as loud as the standard. Steinberg and Gardner (1937) provided insights about

the relationship between masking and loudness that led to the concept of recruitment. Buus, Florentine, and Poulsen (1999) should also be consulted for a view of loudness and loudness recruitment.

S. S. Stevens devised a method that has become standard for determining loudness of complex, non-tonal sounds (ISO standard 532 (1975)—Method A; see the supplements to Chapter 10 and the section on Standards at the end of the References, following the appendixes). This method involves combining the sone measurements for various frequency bands. Another method, devised by Zwicker (ISO standard 532 (1975)—Method B), has also been used to measure the subjective magnitude of a complex stimulus. In general, critical bandwidths estimated using loudness methods are three to four times wider than those obtained from masking studies (see Chapter 11).

The book by Plack et al. (2005) should be consulted for a history of the study of pitch perception. The student might have noted for the missing fundamental pitch (in Figure 13.3, where the frequencies added together were 700, 800, 900, and 1000 Hz) that a nonlinear difference tone exists at 100 Hz. Thus, the 100-Hz pitch might be due to the nonlinearity of the ear. This, however, does not seem to be the case. Licklider (1954), for instance, showed that the difference tone due to nonlinearity could be masked by a noise with frequencies near 100 Hz. Licklider then showed, however, that the pitch of the missing-fundamental stimulus was unaffected by a masking noise with a frequency of 100 Hz. Since the nonlinear tone at 100 Hz was masked and the pitch was still perceived, nonlinearity did not yield the missing fundamental pitch.

There is considerable evidence that the pitch of a tone changes (usually increases) as its level increases. Although Stevens (1975) studied this effect extensively, the pitch changes are highly variable and usually fairly small. Jesteadt (1980) provides an interesting procedure for determining pitch shifts associated with intensity changes. Moore et al. (1985) and Hartmann et al. (1990) have studied the pitch of mistuned harmonics. Hartmann and Zhang (2003) can be consulted for more about both edge pitch and dichotic pitch (also see Bilsen and Raatgever, 2000, for dichotic pitch). The chapter by de Cheveigne (2005) should be consulted for a review of models and theories of pitch.

A few people, without a reference, can produce an exact pitch or recognize a sound as having an exact pitch. This ability is often referred to as *absolute pitch*. A more common form of pitch performance is *relative pitch*, in which some listeners can identify the musical interval between two musical notes. Relative pitch is found among many musicians. Ross, Gore, and Marks (2003) provide an interesting theory of absolute pitch.

There is evidence that we hear primarily the following aural harmonics and combination tones: $2f$, $3f$, and $4f$, $f_1 - f_2$, $2f_1 - f_2$, $2f_1 - 2f_2$, $3f_1 - 2f_2$. Summation tones have generally not been reported as audible. This is presumably because low-frequency tones mask high-frequency tones very well (upper spread of masking; see Chapter 11). Because summation tones are higher in frequency than the primary tones but also usually close to the frequency of one of the primaries, the summation tones are masked by the primary tones.

The cancellation method is usually used with one additional tone added to the input stimulus. Because the pitch of the nonlinear tone is often difficult to detect, it can be made easier to perceive if a tone is added that is slightly different in frequency than the cancellation tone (thus, the input stimulus consists of the primaries, the cancellation tone, and a tone that is slightly different in frequency, e.g., 3 Hz, from the cancellation tone). This additional tone and the cancellation tone (and the nonlinear tone) will produce a beating sensation. If the cancellation tone is now added out of phase and at the same level as the nonlinear tone so that the nonlinear and cancellation tones are eliminated, then the beating stops and the listener hears the pitches of two primary tones and the tone used to beat with the nonlinear tone. Most listeners find it easier to make the cancellation procedure measurements when they are asked to eliminate the beating rather then to eliminate the pitch of the nonlinear tone.

A review of the cubic-difference tone can be found in Zwicker and Fastl's book (1991). Appendix A shows how one could obtain difference tones and summation tones from a nonlinear equation ($y = x + x^2$). The cubic-difference tone ($2f_1 - f_2$) is obtained if the nonlinear equation is in the form $y = x + x^2 + x^3$. Thus, the name *cubic-difference tone* occurs because the tone is obtained by including the cubic (x^3) term in the nonlinear equation. Also, as mentioned in Chapter 8, the cubic-difference tones is important for measuring cochlear emissions, especially the distortion product otoacoustic emission (DPOAE).

The stimulus shown in Figure 13.6 is a regular interval stimulus (RIS) called *iterated rippled noise* (IRN). It can be generated by delaying a noise and adding the delayed noise back to the undelayed noise. The perceived pitch of IRN stimuli is equal to the reciprocal of the delay (Yost et al., 1996). Thus, in Figure 13.6 the delay was 4 msec, yielding the 250-Hz pitch (4 msec = 1/250 Hz) and 250-Hz spacing between the noisy spectral peaks. Research involving IRN stimuli suggests that the temporal fine structure of complex sounds plays a role in complex-pitch processing (see Yost et al., 1996).

IV

Auditory Perception, the Central Nervous System, and Auditory Disorders

14

Auditory Perception

The preceding chapters have described the physical aspects of the sound field (frequency, level, and time), how those physical attributes are processed by the peripheral auditory nervous system, and the behavioral consequences of this neural processing (e.g., detection and discrimination of frequency, level, and/or time). Such descriptions are often described as the study of *sensation*, i.e., how the basic physical properties of the environment are processed by the initial sensory transducers (e.g., the inner hair cells), how the output of this transduction is relayed to the brainstem and brain, and the consequences of this processing on the sensations that one experiences (e.g., pitch or loudness).

However, the major advantage of many sensory systems, such as hearing, is that they allow one to use these sensations in many ways to better cope with the world. They may allow an animal to determine the source of a sound so as to avoid predators, find prey, mate, navigate, etc.; to communicate using sound (e.g., to perceive speech); to have an appreciation of sound (e.g., music); etc. In order for the sensory information to assist an organism in performing these tasks, the sensory information needs additional processing, and this additional processing is often referred to as *perception*. Thus, perceptual processes operate on the

neural sensory information to allow one to determine sound sources, understand speech, appreciate music, etc.

Let's consider a trivially simple example of a complex sound that might have been generated from two different sound sources. Figure 14.1 shows the output of a model (the same AIM model used for Figure 9.16) used to simulate the coding of sound by the auditory periphery. The sound in this case is a complex consisting of four tonal components. Let's imagine that this complex sound is the sound field generated by two sound sources, where the spectrum of each sound source consists of two tones. Let's further assume that the tonal components that make up each source are intermingled in the complex sound field as indicated in the sound field spectrum shown in Figure 14.1. Recall from Chapter 9 that the display in Figure 14.1 is not unlike the spectral-temporal pattern of neural information the auditory periphery provides to the central nervous system about the complex sound field.

Figure 14.1 captures the major aspects of the frequency, intensity, and timing characteristics of the complex sound field that are coded in the auditory periphery. However, little in this display or code indicates that there are two different sound sources.

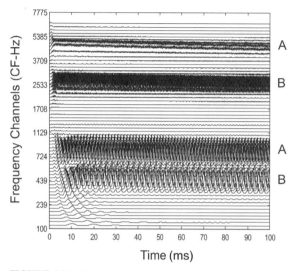

FIGURE 14.1 The outputs of a computational neural model of the auditory periphery (Patterson et al., 1995). The neural output is plotted for 100 msec of a complex sound containing four tonal components. Each line represents the output of one filter channel or one place along the basilar membrane. The filter channel center frequencies begin at 100 Hz, and the highest center frequency is 7114 Hz. This display provides an estimate of the spectral and temporal information available in the auditory periphery concerning this complex sound of four tones. The tones from one source (source A) were 450 and 2500 Hz, while those from the other source (source B) were 725 and 5000 Hz. Thus, the spectral components from the two sources overlap. Although the temporal and spectral information regarding the four tonal components that make up the complex sound are well preserved at the auditory periphery, there is little information displayed in this figure, which indicates that two components are from one source and two from another source.

Somehow the information in the neural codes for the two tones that make up sound source A need to be perceptually *fused* together and then perceptually *segregated* from those associated with sound source B. The physical characteristics of the sound from source A must differ in some way from those from source B if the nervous system is to determine that the complex field consists of two sources. The ultimate ability of the auditory system to use the information that there are two sound sources probably depends on analysis beyond sensory and perceptual processing. The information about the sources probably will have to be stored in memory, and the attention that one might pay to one source or the other might change over time. Thus, auditory memory and auditory attention are probably required for one to function in the real world, and such analyses may also play a role in the perceptual processing that fuses and segregates sounds. This chapter briefly reviews some of what is known about the perception of sound sources, speech production and speech perception, and music perception.

PERCEPTION OF SOUND SOURCES (SOUND SOURCE DETERMINATION)

It was pointed out that in order for the nervous system to process the peripheral neural code to determine the sources of sound, the information in that code must be similar in some ways, to allow for fusion, and different in other ways, to facilitate segregation. The following list suggests several cues that the central nervous system might use to aid in sound source determination.

1. Spectral separation
2. Spectral profile
3. Harmonicity/temporal regularity
4. Spatial separation
5. Temporal separation
6. Temporal onsets and offsets
7. Temporal modulations

SPECTRAL SEPARATION

We have already described the frequency-resolving capability of the auditory periphery and its many consequences (e.g., masking) for hearing. Figure 14.1 (see also Figure 9.16) clearly indicates that the different spectral components of a complex sound may be coded as separate neural events. Thus, for a relatively simple complex sound field, the frequency-resolving abilities of the nervous system may aid the system in distinguishing one sound source (e.g., one frequency) from another sound source (e.g., another frequency). However, for more complex sound fields, such as the one shown in Figure 14.1, where the spectral components from the sources are interlaced, frequency separation alone is not sufficient to allow the auditory system to differentiate one sound source from another.

SPECTRAL PROFILE

If one sound is more intense than another, the central nervous system might be able to determine the sources of the sounds based on their relative level differences. However, in order to accomplish this task, the nervous system must be able to differentiate the spectral profile of the sound. Consider, for example, differentiating a loud sound from that of a soft sound, as diagrammed in Figure 14.2. Most sound sources produce a particular amplitude spectrum that remains relatively constant in terms of its *spectral profile* as the overall level of the sound is changed. That is, the characteristics of the sound from a source are largely determined by the shape of the sound's amplitude spectrum. Making the sound louder or softer changes the overall level of the sound but usually not the shape of its spectral profile.

The auditory system is remarkably sensitive to small changes in the spectral profile of sounds. Consider an experiment in which listeners are asked to detect a small level increment of a signal tone when a number of other equal-level tones are simultaneously added to the signal tone. From Chapter 11 we know that the ability to detect a signal tone of one frequency is interfered with when tones with frequencies close to that of the signal are simultaneously presented. The other tones mask the signal if the signal and the maskers are close together in frequency, and there is little masking when the signal and the masker are very different in frequency. Figure 14.3 shows the experimental context for studying *profile analysis*; listeners are asked to determine which stimulus in a two-alternative, forced-choice task (see Appendix D and Chapter 11) contains the more intense signal tone. The key ingredient in the experiment is that the overall level of both complexes (the signal complex, with the signal-level increment, and the nonsignal complex, consisting of all tones presented at the same level) is randomly varied over a 40-dB range from observation interval to observation interval. Thus, regardless of the relative levels of the two sounds, the listener is to decide which presentation contains the signal stimulus with the middle signal tone's level incremented. There are at least three ways the auditory system might process these stimuli in order for the listener to perform this task: (1) The system could determine which stimulus is louder overall, because the signal stimulus could be more intense due to the signal-tone level increment that is added to the background tonal complex. However, given the 40-dB randomization of overall level, the signal tone would have to be incremented by a great deal (nearly 40 dB) to overcome this 40-dB random variation. (2) The auditory system might process the stimuli in only the critical band tuned to the frequency of the increment signal component, as was assumed for much of the discussion of masking in Chapter 11. However, even if only the signal component is processed by this critical-band filter, its level is still varying randomly by 40 dB, which in turn would require an extremely large increment in signal tone level for a listener to determine that the signal was incremented in level versus simply changed because of the 40-dB random variation in overall level. (3) The auditory system might be able to compare the level of the signal tone relative to that of the nonsignal, masking tones. That is, the levels of the nonsignal tones are all the same, but when the signal level is incremented it is an increase in level relative this constant background. The signal added to the constant background produces a spectral profile with a spectral bump that will always be a spectral bump no matter what the overall level is. Because this *relative* level difference remains constant as the overall level of the complexes is randomly varied over the 40-dB range, only a small increment in level might be required to detect the tonal signal increment.

Figure 14.4 shows the results from an experiment like that previously outlined for three conditions: four maskers flanking the 1000-Hz signal, 10 maskers flanking the signal, 20 maskers flanking the signal, and 42 maskers flanking the signal. In addition, the

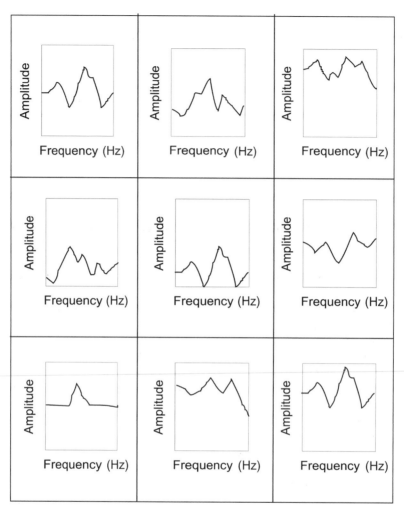

FIGURE 14.2 Schematic diagram of the spectrum of a complex sounds coming from different sources. Which spectra belong to the same sound source? The spectra along the diagonal from upper left to lower right are from the same sound source, but with the sound source producing different overall levels. The other spectra are from different sound sources. As the overall level of the sound increases, that is, as the sound from the source gets louder, the spectral profile of the source does not change. That is, the relative amplitudes of the frequency components remain the same as the overall amplitudes increase. Thus, a key to processing such stimuli is for the auditory system to monitor the relative differences of the amplitudes of the spectral components as the overall level changes.

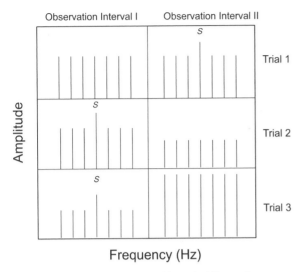

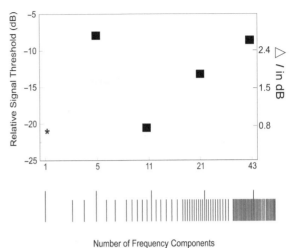

FIGURE 14.3 In a typical "profile analysis" experiment, two stimuli are presented per trial and the listener's task is to determine in which observation interval (I or II) the stimulus contains an level increment of the signal (S, the center frequency component). From trial to trial and from observation interval to observation interval the overall level of the stimulus is randomly varied over a 40-dB range. Thus, the listener would be correct if he or she indicated that the signal occurred in observation interval II for trial 1 and observation interval I for trials 2 and 3. Because of the overall level variation, a very large signal level increment would be required if the listener used either the overall level of the sound or the level at only the signal (center) frequency as the basis for his/her decision.

FIGURE 14.4 The results from a profile analysis experiment in which the number of masker frequency components surrounding a 1000-Hz signal component increased from 4 to 42. The thresholds for detecting an increment in the 1000-Hz signal component (the center component) are shown in decibels relative to that of the rest of the masker component intensity. The asterisk on the far left indicates the typical threshold for detecting a level increment of a single, 1000-Hz tone. Thresholds for the 10-masker condition are almost as low as those for the single-tone condition, and the thresholds first decrease and then increase as the number of masker components increases from 4 to 42. The level of the signal is expressed in terms of the signal-to-background level; see the section at the end of the book on Terms, Measurements, Equations, and Conversions. Figure 14.3 should be consulted for a description of the profile stimuli and the listener's task. Based on data from Green (1989), used with permission.

threshold for detecting a level increment for a 1000-Hz signal presented alone without any maskers is shown (data taken from Figure 10.7). As can be seen, the thresholds for detecting the signal-level increment when the maskers are present and the overall level is randomly varying is almost as low as that obtained for a single tone presented without maskers and without any level randomization. Also note that the thresholds are high for the 5-component stimulus, decrease for the 11-component stimulus, and then increase again for the 21- and 43-component stimuli.

Both the fact that the thresholds are low and the way in which they change as a function of the number and spacing of the components are consistent with the assumption that the auditory system uses the relative difference in level between the signal component and

the masker components as cues for detection [earlier option 3]. That is, the auditory system detects the peak in the spectral profile of the signal stimulus independent of the overall level of the spectrum. When there are a few widely spaced masker components, it is difficult to discern the difference in level across these widely spaced spectral components (see the spectral profiles along the bottom of Figure 14.4). When the components get closer together in frequency, the difference in the level of the signal component as compared to the constant level of the maskers becomes easier to discern; thus, thresholds decrease as the number of masker components increases from 4 to 10. However, as the spectral density of the number of components increases further, the masker components begin to interfere directly with the signal and with each other because they are close enough together in frequency to excite the same critical band, and, thus, the maskers begin to provide direct masking of the signal (see Figure 11.1). That is, as the number of masker components increases beyond 10, they directly mask the signal, making it more difficult to detect a signal-level increment. Data like these suggest that the auditory system is performing a profile analysis in order to make comparisons across the spectrum of a sound so that subtle spectral intensity changes can be detected. Such processing is advantageous for a system designed to determine the sources of sound.

HARMONICITY/TEMPORAL REGULARITY

In Chapter 13 the phenomenon of complex pitch was described, in which complex sounds with particular spectral or temporal structures are perceived as having a pitch, even when there are no apparent periodicities in the time-domain waveform envelope or energy in the amplitude spectrum that could be used to predict the perceived pitch (e.g., missing fundamental pitch). Such complex pitches are often obtained when the complex sounds consist of harmonics of some fundamental. Many sound sources in our world consist of spectral components that are harmonically related. Most musical instruments and voiced speech are typical examples of such harmonic sound sources. Thus, the ability to perceive these sound sources as having a unitary pitch is an excellent example of the auditory system's fusing the information from many spectral regions to produce a single auditory image, in this case described as a pitch. As such the pitch of a complex sound might be used as a cue for sound source determination.

However, we are often unable to perceive two or more pitches when a complex sound consists of two or more different harmonic series. For instance, a sound consisting of the harmonics of 200 and 333 Hz (e.g., 200, 333, 400, 600, 666, 800, 999 Hz) all presented at the same time would not usually be perceived as having two complex pitches (and therefore, perhaps, come from two sources) of 200 Hz (i.e., 200, 400, 600, and 800 Hz) and 333 Hz (i.e., 333, 666, and 999 Hz). The auditory system would in most cases *synthesize* (the auditory system is behaving *synthetically*) the entire sound into a single percept rather than *analyze* (auditory system behaving *analytically*) it into its two harmonic parts. In the example just given, the two complex pitches may be perceived if something else is done to help separate the sound sources. For instance, if the complex sound with the 333-Hz fundamental were turned on before that with the 200-Hz fundamental, then the two complex pitches of 200 and 333 Hz might be detected (see the later section "Temporal Onsets and Offsets"). Thus, although phenomena such as the "missing fundamental pitch" indicate one means by which the auditory system may synthesize spectral information to form a single percept, such pitch processing does not always appear to aid the auditory system in segregating different harmonic series into a multisource sounds.

As described in Chapter 13, if one of the tonal components of a complex harmonically related tonal complex is changed in frequency, it might be perceived as different in pitch from the fundamental pitch of the complex. That is, the detection of the mistuned harmonic as having one pitch in the presence of a harmonic series that produces another pitch is an example of a complex sound that produces two pitches, which might indicate some of the ways in which the pitch perception can aid sound source determination. Recall from Chapter 13 that sounds with harmonic spectral structure and/or temporal regularity can produce pitch sensations, and, therefore, both harmonicity and temporal regularity are potential cues for aiding sound source determination.

SPATIAL SEPARATION

In Chapter 12 the concept of the "cocktail party effect" was described. The cocktail party effect refers to the auditory system's ability to determine the sources of sounds when they are located at different places in space. A number of different experimental findings (e.g., the MLD results; see Chapter 12) indicate that the auditory system's ability to localize the sources of sounds aids it in sound source determination. Thus, interaural differences of time and level and aspects of the head-related transfer functions that we know are crucial for sound localization may also aid the auditory system in determining the sources of sound. However, our ability to localize sound sources cannot be the only way in which we determine sound sources. Consider a case in which a symphony is played by an orchestra and recorded through a single microphone and played back through a single loudspeaker (refer to Figure 1.1. There is very little, if any, information in this monaural recording about where the instruments of the orchestra are located, yet we have little difficulty in determining a large number of the instruments when we listen to the symphony (e.g., we can determine that there were violins, drum, horns, etc). That is, the single recording contains no interaural differences or HRTF structure, which is necessary for sound localization, yet we can determine many of the sound sources (instruments) in the orchestra.

There is also growing evidence that spatially separating sound sources as the only means to achieve sound source segregation may provide only a weak ability to determine the actual sound sources. Some have characterized this work as suggesting that cues other than spatial separation must be used to determine what a sound source is, and then spatial cues help determine where that source is located. Thus, although spatial separation in one means by which we can determine the source of a sound, it is not the only means.

TEMPORAL SEPARATION

Clearly, if two sources produce sounds at very different times, the separation in time would allow us to determine the sources. In Chapter 11 we described aspects of temporal masking (forward and backward masking) that indicate that when short target sounds precede or follow other sounds they may be masked. Thus, temporal masking will play a role in one's ability to determine the sources of sounds that appear close together, but separated, in time.

Many sounds that occur more or less concurrently are also intermittent sounds that go on and off. In many situations the sound from one source alternates with that from another source, yet we are more likely to perceive the sound as two sources occurring together at the same time rather than one source with an alternating percept. This is diagrammed in Figure 14.5. For instance, source A might be a tone of one frequency and source B a tone of a different frequency.

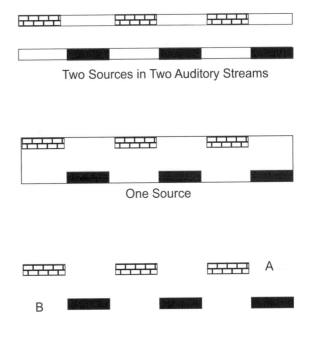

FIGURE 14.5 Schematic diagram indicating the type of procedure used in many streaming experiments. Two alternating sounds (e.g., two different frequencies alternating in time) are presented. Under the appropriate conditions, the listeners do not report hearing a single sound (i.e., from one sound source) that alternates in pitch, but rather they report hearing two sound sources (A and B, as if there were two streams), each with its own pulsating pitch.

Under the proper stimulus circumstances, listeners describe the stimulus as if there are two concurrent sounds, each with its own distinct pulsating pitch, rather than one sound that alternates in pitch. That is, the perception is not of one source that has an alternating pitch, but of two different sources, each with its own pitch that is going on and off. The perception of the two alternating tones is of two "streams of sound" running concurrently as if they were two sound sources. Understanding the conditions that lead to *auditory stream fusion* (the stimulus conditions that allow nonsimultaneous sounds to appear as one source) and *auditory stream segregation* (the stimulus conditions that lead to the perception of different sources when there is more than one alternating sound) is important for understanding how we determine the sources of sounds in multisource acoustic environments. Under the appropriate conditions, sounds differing in spectral content, temporal modulation pattern, level, and/or spatial dimensions and presented in an alternating pattern will be perceived as streams of simultaneously occurring sound. However, it is usually the case that sounds that differ in spectral content in one way or another produce the strongest stream segregation.

When complex sounds are generated from simple sounds, it is not always possible to predict how the complex sounds will be perceived based on what is known about how the simple sounds are processed. Consider the example shown in Figure 14.6. A temporal sequence of 10 tones is presented in a same–different psychophysical procedure such that the 10-tone pattern is presented twice per trial. On the second presentation, the frequency of one of the 10 tones is changed on half of the trials on a random basis. The listener is asked to determine for each trial if the two patterns are the same or different, and the responses are used to determine a frequency-difference threshold for tones presented at each of the 10 positions in the pattern. From trial to trial a different 10-tone pattern may be generated, but for any one test condition the test tone whose frequency might be changed remains at the same temporal location (e.g., the third tone is the one that might be changed in fre-

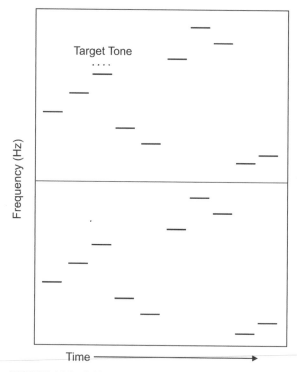

FIGURE 14.6   A 10-tone pattern (each short line represents one tone presented at a particular time in the pattern and with a particular frequency) typically used to study informational masking. The listener's task is to determine if the frequency of the target component was changed in a same–different task (i.e., the listener was presented either the same 10-tone pattern twice or a slight change in target frequency is introduced for the second presentation of the pattern, shown in the bottom pattern, in which the shift in the target frequency is indicated by the dotted line). In a high-uncertainty task the spectral components would vary from trial to trial. In a minimum-uncertainty task, the same 10-tone pattern would be presented on each trial, with the same target tone having its frequency altered in the same–different task.

quency) for the duration of the condition. When the frequencies in the 10-tone pattern are varied randomly from trial to trial, listeners have very high frequency-discrimination thresholds, with those tones coming at the beginning of the pattern having the highest threshold. In this case there is a lot of *uncertainty* about the stimulus structure from trial to trial and it is difficult to determine if one of the tone's frequencies changed, especially if that tone occurred at the beginning of the pattern. If a *minimal-uncertainty task* is used in which the same 10-tone pattern is presented on every trial (there is no randomization of the frequencies, thus little uncertainty about the frequency content of the 10-tone pattern), the frequency-difference thresholds are much smaller and the tones appearing at the beginning of the pattern no longer have the highest thresholds.

The elevation in frequency-discrimination thresholds just described is due to the amount of uncertainty in the stimulus, not to a physical aspect of the stimulus. Thus, this increase in threshold is referred to as *informational masking*, to differentiate it from the type of masking we discussed in Chapter 11, which is often referred to as *energetic masking*. That is, energetic masking in this context is masking or interference that is a direct result of auditory interaction of the sounds, while informational masking is masking in addition to energetic masking that is caused by uncertainty.

Another example of informational masking is a signal-detection experiment with a single tone to be detected in the presence of a masker complex that can be made up of many tones. In one example, the masker may consist of up to 100 tones added together. These 100 tones are chosen from a frequency range that brackets the signal frequency such that some tones in the masker may have frequencies higher and some lower than the signal frequency. The number of tones used for the masker may range from 2 to 100, and the choice of tones from the range of possible tones is made at random from trial to trial. Thus, in some conditions only two tones are added to make up the masker, while in other conditions 100 tones may be chosen. There is considerably more masking (as much 40 dB more) when the masker contains only two tones as opposed to when it contains 100 tones. That is, signal threshold is as much as 40 dB greater for a two-tone masker than for a 100-tone masker when the tones in the masker are chosen at random from trial to trial. This should appear surprising based on what you learned in Chapter 11. Many times when only two tones are chosen (at random) for the masker, the frequencies of these two tones will be very different from

that of the signal, and these masking tones should provide very little direct (energetic) masking. Even when the two masking tones are close in frequency to the signal frequency, why should two maskers produce more masking than when there are 100 tones making up the masker? The explanation deals with informational masking caused by the uncertainty about the masking spectrum that exists from trial to trial in this type of experiment. That is, the listeners need more information about the stimulus context than just what is happening in the spectral region near the signal, as implied by the work described in Chapter 11. This information appears to depend on the uncertainty the auditory system has about the stimulus context; the more uncertainty there is, the more informational masking there is. With only two tones, the variability in the masker from trial to trial is much larger than when 100 tones are used. In this sense, there is more uncertainty about the masker spectrum with two rather than with 100 tones.

In several studies of information masking, when informational masking occurs it has been found that spatially separating the signal from the masker significantly reduces informational masking, while the amount of energetic masking is not changed or only changed a little. Thus, spatial separation may play an important role in sound source determination when there is informational masking.

These and other data indicate that the nature of the listening task, especially those tasks involving complex sounds and uncertainty, may determine a great deal about the sensitivity of a listener in processing many complex sounds. Thus, in understanding sound source determination of complex sounds in real-world situations we need to understand both the stimulus context and the nature of the listening task.

TEMPORAL ONSETS AND OFFSETS

If the sound from one source starts after that from another source has already begun, then the differences in the onsets and/or offsets of the two sounds may be a cue for sound source determination. We have already studied situations in which the onsets of two sounds are different. In Chapter 11 we mentioned the fact that thresholds for detecting signals during the forward or backward temporal fringe of a masker may be higher than those measured more toward the temporal middle of the masker. In Chapter 12 we introduced the precedence effect, in which the ability to accurately locate a sound source depends to a large extent on the first wave reaching the ears, in that interaural information arriving after the first wavefront appears to be suppressed.

In many situations the characteristic quality of a sound (its timbre) may depend on how the sound is turned on or off. The *attack* and *decay* of the sound produced by many musical instruments provide most of the information that allows us to differentiate among different instruments. A major aspect of music synthesis and music synthesizers is to accurately simulate the temporal and spectral aspects of the attack and decay of a note played by the instrument being synthesized.

A powerful method to enhance the detection or discrimination of many complex sounds in the mixture of several sounds is to vary the onset of the stimulus of interest relative to that of background or competing stimuli. The immediate change from the background to the target sound of interest often provides a cue to highlight the target sound. For instance, the ability to hear out the pitch of a mistuned harmonic (see the earlier section "Harmonicity/Tempora Regularity") can be significantly influenced if the mistuned harmonic comes on before the rest of the harmonic sound.

TEMPORAL MODULATIONS

Many naturally occurring sound sources produce complex sounds that have a slow amplitude or frequency modulation (see Chapter 4). Thus, all the spectral components that constitute such a complex sound will have either their amplitudes or their frequencies slowly modulated in time in a coherent manner. Thus, the auditory system might be able to fuse spectral components that are modulated with the same tempo-

ral pattern as one means of grouping together spectral components of a source to aid sound source determination.

Stimuli that contain spectral components in different regions of the spectrum but that share a common pattern of temporal amplitude modulation produce some interesting auditory phenomena. Consider a masking situation in which a narrow band of noise (called the *target band*) is used to mask a tonal signal centered in the noise band. We know from Chapter 11 that such a noise will elevate the threshold of the signal and hence mask the signal. If another band of noise (called a *cue band*) with the same bandwidth as the target band is presented in a different frequency region simultaneously with the target band, we would not expect much additional masking unless the cue noise band was close in frequency to the target noise band. It turns out, however, that the amount of masking generated by the target band may depend on the cue band, even when the cue band is located in a spectral region far away from that of the target band. To understand the results you must first recall that a narrow band of noise has a strong slowly amplitude-modulated envelope, with the frequency rate with which the envelope amplitudes fluctuate being proportional to the bandwidth of the narrowband noise (see Chapter 4 and Figure 4.16).

It is possible to generate two narrow bands of noise in different frequency regions that have the same (coherent) amplitude-modulated envelopes or different (incoherent) amplitude-modulated envelopes. If the cue and target bands have incoherent envelopes, then the cue band does not alter the amount of masking of the signal provided by the target band. However, if the cue and target bands have the same (coherent) envelopes, then the masked threshold of the signal drops by 10 to 12 dB. That is, the signal is 10 to 12 dB easier to detect when the target and cue bands are modulated coherently (i.e., comodulated) than when they are modulated incoherently. The release in masking caused by the addition of the coherently modulated cue band is called *comodulation masking release* (CMR). Figure 14.7 describes both the basic stimulus paradigm (with schematic diagrams

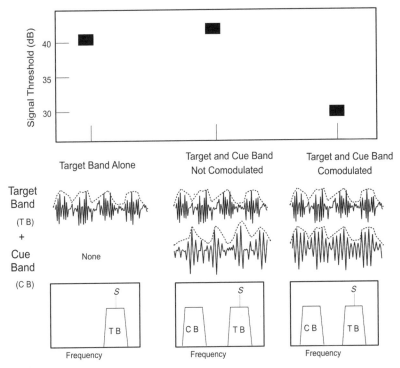

FIGURE 14.7 Both the basic comodulation masking release (CMR) task and results are shown. At the bottom the time-domain waveforms for the narrowband maskers (target and cue bands) and the amplitude spectra for the maskers and the signal are shown in a schematic form. The dotted line above each time-domain waveform depicts the amplitude envelope of the narrowband noises. The listener is asked to detect a signal (*S*) that is always added to the target band. In the target-band-alone condition, the signal is difficult to detect. When a cue band is added to the target band such that it is located in a different frequency region than the target band and has an amplitude envelope that is different from (not comodulated with) the target band, there is little change in threshold from the target-band-alone condition. However, when the target and cue bands are comodulated, the threshold is lowered by approximately 12 dB, indicating that the comodulated condition makes it easier for the listener to detect the signal. The waveforms are not drawn to scale. Based on data from Hall, Haggard, and Fernandes (1984), used with permission.

of the noise bands) and the results from a typical CMR experiment.

Although there is not a complete understanding of how the CMR effect occurs, CMR does show that the auditory system uses information from a wide region of the spectrum to aid in the processing of some complex sounds. Notice that because the amplitude of the noise is modulated, brief periods of time occur when the noise level is low, making the tone easy to

detect at that time. One possible explanation of the CMR effect is that the comodulated cue band provides additional information about when the noise band's level will be low, making it easier for the auditory system to detect the signal during these brief periods of low masker level.

The procedure and data shown in Figure 14.8 describe another form of interaction between stimuli that occur in different spectral regions but have common patterns of amplitude modulation. In this procedure, listeners are asked to detect a change in the depth of amplitude modulation provided for a probe tone (with a carrier frequency of 4000 Hz), using the same procedures that were used to obtain the TMTF

described in Chapter 10. This condition is referred to as the "probe-alone" condition. Next, another tone, with a different carrier frequency (the masker tone, which for the conditions of Figure 14.8 has a carrier frequency of 1000 Hz), is simultaneously added to the

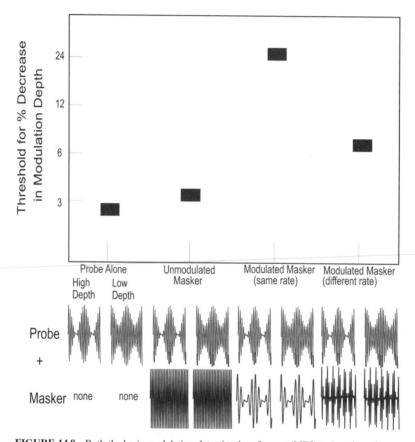

FIGURE 14.8   Both the basic modulation detection interference (MDI) task and results are shown. The basic task for the listener is depicted along the bottom of the figure. The listener is to detect a decrement in the depth of probe amplitude modulation (difference between low and high depths). When just the probes are presented, the task is relatively easy. When an unmodulated masker tone with a frequency different from that of the probe is added to the probes, thresholds for detecting a decrease in probe modulation depth are not changed much from the probe-alone condition. However, when the masker is modulated with the same rate pattern as the probe, the threshold for detecting a decrement in probe modulation depth increases greatly, indicating that modulation depth is difficult to detect when both the probe and the masker are comodulated. When the masker is modulated but with a different rate (shown as a faster rate in the figure) than the probe, then the threshold for detecting a modulation-depth decrement is lowered. The waveforms are not drawn to scale. Based on data from Yost (1992b), used with permission.

modulated probe tone in the "unmodulated masker" condition. Since the masker tone is far removed in frequency from the probe tone, there is little change in the threshold decrease in modulation depth for the probe tone. However, when the masker is modulated with the same pattern as the probe ("modulated masker" condition), the threshold decrease in modulation depth is much higher, indicating that it is difficult to detect the change in modulation depth when both the masker and the probe are comodulated. That is, the comodulated masker interfered with the detection of modulation of the probe, and hence the effect is referred to as *modulation detection interference* (MDI).

It has been argued that MDI reflects a process by which the common modulation pattern applied to the masker and the probe fuses them into one auditory image as if they had originated from the same modulated sound source. As such, it is difficult for the auditory system to process information about amplitude modulation for the individual components (the probe and the masker) of this image. If such an argument is valid, then one might predict that if the masker and the probe were modulated with different patterns (e.g., the probe and the masker were amplitude modulated at different rates), they would no longer be fused into a single auditory image, because a single sound source would not produce components with different modulation patterns. Thus, if the masker and the probe were amplitude modulated at different rates they would be treated as separate sound sources, and there would be less MDI. The data point on the far right of Figure 14.8 shows just such a result; that is, when the masker was modulated at a higher rate than the probe, the threshold for detecting a decrease in modulation depth returned closer to those obtained in the "probe alone" and "unmodulated-masker" conditions (i.e., there was less MDI).

While amplitude modulation has been shown to affect sound source determination and segregation, frequency modulation per se does not appear to provide a potent cue for sound source determination. The pitch shifts and other cues that covary when a sound contains frequency modulations appear to be the cues used in sound source determination and not the frequency modulation per se. Thus, coherent amplitude modulation, but probably not frequency modulation, can aid in sound source determination.

Thus, CMR and MDI results suggest that stimuli that share a common pattern of amplitude modulation can be processed across a wide range of the auditory spectrum. The work on profile analysis also shows that the auditory system is capable of using information from different regions of the spectrum to aid in performing a complex sound-detection task. Such across-frequency processing would appear to be a critical aspect of sound source determination, in that the complex sound field will usually contain spectral components from a number of sound sources, which are likely to cover a wide region of the spectrum. Similarly, research such as that on streaming shows how the auditory system integrates information across time when processing many types of complex sounds. If the auditory system is to use this widely spaced spectral and temporal information in sound source determination, then it must be able to make comparisons across wide spectral regions and across time. Thus, experiments such as those on profile analysis, CMR, MDI, streaming, and complex tonal pattern processing provide some insights into how these aspects of cross-spectral and cross-temporal processing might operate.

SPEECH

Speech represents the major complex acoustic stimulus used by most humans, and it is essential for language and language development. Understanding speech perception requires some knowledge of speech production and language as well as of how the auditory system functions. Much work has been devoted to understanding our ability to perceive speech; however, the speech waveform is extremely complex, and, hence, gaining knowledge about speech perception is a significant undertaking. Because humans rely to such a great extent on speech for communication, there are large areas of mutual interest among scientists working in audition and those investigating speech.

When speech is produced, air is pushed from the lungs into the throat by the *diaphragm*. Then the *vocal cords*, which reside toward the top of the throat, vibrate in response to the airflow from the lungs and under muscle control, and finally this vibratory vocal-cord waveform causes the *vocal tract* to resonate. The vocal tract consists of many *articulators*, such as the tongue, palette, lips, velum, and nasal cavity, that move or are used in different ways to form the sounds of speech due to the articulators' changing the shape of the vocal tract and hence its resonance properties (see Chapter 3).

The vocal cords vibrate at a somewhat periodic rate, with a frequency (called the *fundamental voicing frequency* or *fundamental frequency*, F_0) ranging from about 80 Hz for males to 320 Hz for children. The amplitude of the vocal cord waveform is somewhat random (*jitter*), as is its period/frequency (*vibrato*). That is, there is variation in how open or closed the vocal cords are from moment to moment (jitter), and the period of the vocal cords' opening and closing varies somewhat (vibrato) around the average value of F_0. The pitch of a voice (e.g., when one sings or the pitch difference between a female and a male speaker) is determined by F_0. Men have the lowest-pitched voices, women produce higher pitches, and children produce the highest pitches. The size of a person (and other things, such as hormones) affects the rate at which the vocal cords can open and close, such that the bigger the person, the more likely it is that the vocal cords are massive (relative to those of a smaller person) and, hence, vibrate more slowly, producing a lower pitch.

The vocal tract is responsible for the sounds of a speech utterance. The basic speech sound is the *phoneme*. Letters represent the basic units of written language, but a letter such as the vowel *a* is perceived differently in the word *head* than in the word *heart*. The different sounds that *a* can have in voiced speech are some of the phonemes of speech. The articulators of the vocal tract change in the manner (*manner of articulation*) in which they are used or in the location in which they are placed (*place of articulation*) to produce the phonemes of speech. So speech production is based on two crucial structures: the vocal cords,

which are responsible for voiced or sung pitch, and the vocal tract, which is responsible for the phonemes of speech.

The speech waveform that arrives at a listener has components that are related to the vocal cords and those that are related to the vocal tract. It is these *acoustic properties* of speech that are the basis for understanding the perception of speech. Figure 14.9 shows the time-domain waveform of the vowel /a/ uttered at two different values of F_0 due to the vocal cords' vibrating at different rates. The peaks represent the openings of the vocal cords and the valleys the closings. Note that each opening is not the same amplitude (jitter), nor does the time between openings or closings have the exact same period (vibrato). Also, the two utterances of the vowel /a/ have different frequencies, which are likely to be perceived as different voiced pitches, with that in the top of the figure being

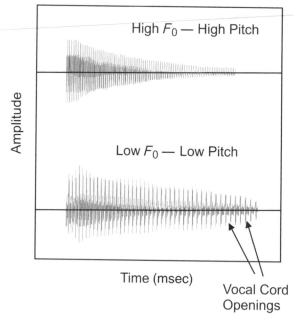

FIGURE 14.9   Time-domain plot of the utterance of the phoneme /a/. On top, the vocal cords are vibrating at a high rate (high F_0), producing a high-pitched vowel, while on the bottom the vocal cord rate (F_0) is low, producing a lower pitch. There is jitter and vibrato in the vocal cord openings and closings.

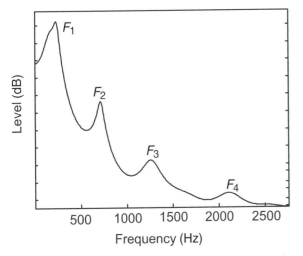

FIGURE 14.10 Smoothed amplitude spectrum at a moment in time of the vowel /a/ shown in the bottom of Figure 14.9. The various formant peaks (F_1, F_2, F_3, and F_4) represent the resonances of the vocal tract.

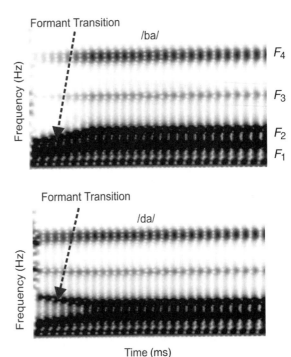

FIGURE 14.11 Spectrographs of the constant-vowel (CV) utterances of /ba/ (top) and /da/ (bottom). The bands of energy at the various frequencies represent the formants (F_1–F_4). Note that during the /a/ portion of both CVs there is no change in the formants (/a/ is a steady-state vowel), while at the beginning of the CV during the /b/ portion there is a formant transition for F_2, with F_2 starting low in frequency for /ba/ and then ending higher in frequency, while for /da/ F_2 starts high and ends low in frequency.

related to a lower perceived voiced pitch than the waveform shown in the bottom of the figure.

It is not apparent what aspects of the waveform in Figure 14.9 reflect the actions of the vocal tract. Figure 14.10 is the amplitude spectrum of an utterance of the same phonemic vowel /a/ at one moment in time in its production. The amplitude spectrum reveals regions of the spectrum (F_1, F_2, and F_3) where there are spectrally local increases in level. These spectral regions are the *formants* of speech (labeled from low to high frequency as F_1, F_2, F_3, . . .). The spectral location of formants, their relative amplitudes, and the width of a formant spectral region are based on the resonant properties of the vocal tract. That is, different vocal tract shapes, based on different manner and places of articulation, which lead to the different phonemes of spoken speech, produce different formants. Each phoneme of speech has a characteristic formant structure. Thus, F_0 and the formants (F_1, F_2, F_3, . . .) of speech are the basic acoustic properties of speech that are important for understanding speech perception.

A phoneme, like most vowels, is said to be *steady state* when the formants (and, hence, the vocal tract)

do not change as the phoneme is spoken. Consonants (e.g., /b/) require a change in the vocal tract (e.g., the lips are closed as the /b/ sound is started, but the lips open before it is finished). Changes in the vocal tract result in changes in the formants. In general, one or more formant frequencies change over time (there is a *formant transition*) when a consonant is uttered. Figure 14.11 shows three-dimensional spectrographs (see Chapter 4) of the consonant-vowel (CV) utterances /da/ and /ba/. Recall that a spectrograph plots frequency as a function of time, with the level of each frequency component indicated by the darkness of the plot (dark areas represent more intense levels than light or white areas). Note the formant transition for the second formant (F_2) at the beginning of the utterance and the fact that the transition is an increase in the frequency of F_2 for /da/ and a decrease for /ba/.

The study of speech perception involves an understanding of how the acoustic properties of speech (F_0, formants, and formant transition) influence our perception of speech and often how these perceptions are related back to the way in which speech is produced. For instance, the frequency differences between formants may be small, and thus the spectral difference may not be resolved by the auditory system. This leads to a question about the role of spectral resolvability by the auditory periphery in speech perception. The pitch of voiced speech is highly perceptible, even when the level of F_0 in the spectrum of the speech waveform is low. This is similar to the case of the missing fundamental pitch (see Chapter 13), so the role of pitch processing and its effects on speech perception are topics of investigation.

A major issue in speech perception is often referred to as problems of *perceptual invariance*. That is, despite what can be considerable variability in the acoustic properties of speech, we tend to have a constant or invariant perception. For instance, if several different people all utter the vowel /i/, it is highly likely that everyone would perceive the sound as the phoneme /i/. However, the actual formant structure of each person's utterance will be different, perhaps very different. Thus, how is it that one perceives a constant or perceptually invariant sound (e.g., the phoneme /i/) in light of a highly variable acoustic signal? Understanding how the nervous system solves problems of perceptual invariance is crucial for understanding speech perception, helping people who have difficulty understanding speech, and designing machines/computers that can automatically recognize speech.

An issue of speech perception related to the problem of perceptual invariance is the study of *categorical perception*. One example of categorical perception can be explained based on the spectrographs of /da/ and /ba/ shown in Figure 14.11. Note that the end of the two CVs contain about the same formant structure, so the main difference between /da/ and /ba/

occurs during the formant transitions at the beginning of the utterance. The formants start at different F_2 frequencies for each CV but end at about the same F_2 frequency at the end of the formant transition. One can generate artificial or computer speech that is perceived very much as natural speech. With the computer, one can produce different stimuli by varying the starting frequency of the formants in a continuum that starts with the beginning F_2 formant of /da/ and ends with that of /ba/. Thus, a series of utterances can be generated, each with a different F_2 transition due to the varying of the starting frequency of F_2. When these stimuli are played for listeners, it is common for the listeners to be aware of subtle perceptual differences in the various sounds, but they label the sounds as being either the CV /da/ or the CV /ba/, and these are rarely labeled anything other than /da/ or /ba/. There is a rather abrupt change in the label of the sound as the formant transition changes from one position on the continuum to the next. That is, as the formant transition begins to vary from the original /da/, listeners continue to label the sound as being /da/ until a formant transition is reached, when they switch to labeling the sound as /ba/ and then continue to label the sounds as /ba/ as the formant transitions continue toward that of the original /ba/. That is, there is a sharp boundary in the labeling function as the formant transitions are varied from stimulus to stimulus. When listeners are asked to discriminate between adjacent pairings of sounds with different formant transitions, their discrimination performance is poor, except if the two sounds being discriminated have formant transitions that are on each side of the labeling boundary. Thus, categorical perception is said to occur when there is a sharp boundary in a labeling function accompanied by increased discrimination performance when sounds on either side of the boundary are compared. Categorical perception is a tool that is used often in the study of speech perception.

A frequently used method for studying sound source segregation is the *two-vowel procedure*. In the two-vowel procedure, two vowels are produced (usually by a computer program) and played simultaneously. Then one of the stimulus parameters we discussed in the chapter (e.g., spatial separation) is used to determine if it will aid listeners in segregating the two sounds so that they perceive the two vowels. The logic of the experiments is that each vowel represents a different sound source. For instance, if two artificial vowels are computer generated such that they each have the same and completely periodic fundamental frequency representing perfectly periodic vocal cord openings and closings, the vowels presented in isolation will be perceived as the speech vowels, even though for real voices vocal cord function is not periodic (i.e., there is jitter and vibrato). When these computer-generated periodic speech sounds are played together, it is difficult to segregate the combined sound into the two vowel sources. Thus, even though the two vowel sounds have different formant structures, they cannot be perceptually segregated when played together, probably because they have the same periodic fundamental frequency. If the fundamental frequency of one vowel is made different than that of the other vowel, then it can be easier to identify the two vowel sounds when they are played simultaneously. This is an example of a change in harmonicity promoting sound source segregation, because changing the fundamental frequency changes the harmonic structure of each artificial vowel. There are many other experiments in which speech is used to study aspects of auditory perception in general.

MUSIC PERCEPTION

The study of the perception of music can be broadly divided into studies of the ability to discern melody, rhythm, and the various instruments that produce music. A great deal of melody perception has to do with pitch perception, which was covered in Chapter 13. However, melodies are more than just a series of pitches. Melody perception is also a study of what makes a series of pitches into a musical melody. What causes a musical interval to be dissonant or consonant (see Chapter 13)? Are the special relationships among pitches (e.g., octave or semitone relationships) based on auditory processing alone, or are they more

a function of experience and culture? Each musical note has a different fundamental frequency, so the pitch changes, but all musical notes played in the same position relative to the octave also are often said to have the same pitch (e.g., all A's on the piano keyboard have the same pitch). Changes in pitch that are associated with the actual frequency content of sound are sometimes referred to as *pitch (tone) height*, while notes that only differ by an octave are said to vary in *pitch (tone) chroma*. Music perception scientists also investigate differences in tone chroma and height.

The study of rhythm involves many questions. The ability to determine the order of temporal events is of interest to those who study music perception. How one detects or is able to play or tap out different beats in the rhythm of a musical piece is not completely understood. The detectability of different rhythm structures and the relationship of this detection to other abilities dealing with music and sound are of interest to those studying music perception.

The spectrum of most musical instruments, including the human voice, has a harmonic structure, with many harmonics (sometimes called *overtones* in music) of the fundamental frequency. The harmonic structure of the spectrum associated with most musical instruments is due to the resonance properties (see Chapter 3) of vibrating strings (e.g., violin), resonances associated with air moving in closed tubes (e.g., pipe organ), or the resonances of vibrating reeds in combination with closed tubes (e.g., clarinet). The pitch played by a musical instrument corresponds to the fundamental frequency in the spectrum of the sound. The timbre (see Chapter 13) of the instrument is determined by the resonance properties of the instrument as reflected in the sound's spectral structure. The levels of the different harmonics in the spectrum of most musical instruments vary considerably from instrument to instrument. There is considerable interest in music perception in understanding what it is about the spectral structure of an instrument that gives it its distinct timbre. As mentioned earlier in this chapter the onset (attack) and sometimes the offset (decay) of playing an instrument contains a great deal of information about the instrument's timbre as compared to the perceived timbre occurring during the ongoing portions of the sound. Thus, understanding the perceptual aspects of attack and decay is of interest in music perception research. While those who study music perception are sometimes unconcerned with the details of understanding hearing, many scientists interested in understanding music perception are extremely knowledgeable about hearing, and their research provides valuable data and insights about hearing.

SUMMARY

After the basic acoustic attributes (frequency, intensity, and time/phase) of a complex sound field are coded by the auditory periphery as a property of sensation, the neural information is further processed in order to assist in auditory perception. Seven possible physical variables may aid in sound source determination: spectral separation, spectral profile, harmonicity/temporal regularity, spatial separation, temporal separation, onsets and offsets, and temporal modulation. Experiments studying profile analysis, CMR, MDI, and streaming indicate that the auditory system processes information across a wide frequency and time range. In conditions of stimulus uncertainty, informational masking can be involved in complex-sound processing. The speech utterance can be described by its phonetic units, speech production mechanisms (manner and place of articulation), or acoustic properties (fundamental frequency, formant frequency, formant transitions). Perceptual invariance, categorical perception, and the two-vowel task are examples of how speech can be used to study auditory perception. Music perception involves melody, rhythm, and the timbre of musical instruments. Tone height, tone chroma, and overtones are some of the aspects of sound that are studied in the field of music perception. The fundamental frequency in the spectrum of an instrument's sound determines the pitch played by the instrument, while the instrument's spectral structure determines its timbre, often during the attack or decay part of playing the instrument.

SUPPLEMENT

Additional information on the topics of this chapter can be found in the books by Yost and Watson (1987), Handel (1989), Bregman (1990), Warren (1999), and Yost, Fay, and Popper (2006), in the articles by Yost (1992a and 1992b), and in Chapters 7 and 8 in the book by Moore (1997), Chapters 11 and 13 in the book by Rosen and Howell (1991), and the chapter by Yost and Sheft (1993). Bregman (1990) describes sound source segregation as *auditory scene analysis*, in which auditory perception is viewed as processing an auditory scene of sound images representing different sound sources. Bregman (1990) is most responsible for the work on auditory stream fusion and segregation.

Dave Green's (1989) book *Profile Analysis* covers a range of topics related to profile analysis and intensity perception. The topic of auditory perception has often been relegated to a discussion of speech and music perception. There is a growing recognition that sound source determination, or auditory image perception, is a global topic of auditory perception that can encompass special acoustic waveforms such as speech and music. The chapter by Yost and Sheft (1993) provides a review of the seven variables that might support sound source determination.

A phenomenon similar to streaming occurs in which two alternating sounds are presented, one soft and one loud (the sounds usually also differ spectrally); under the appropriate conditions the softer sound appears to be steady, even though it is pulsating. One can adjust the level of the sound until it is just perceived to be pulsating (or conversely, steady). In this case one is estimating the *pulsation threshold* of the sound. Many phenomena that have been studied using masked thresholds have also been studied using pulsation thresholds (or *auditory induction*, as it has also been called; see Warren, 1999).

Informational masking has been studied by Watson and colleagues (Watson, 1976, 2005) in their work on

10-tone pattern recognition. Neff and Green (1987) have also investigated properties of informational masking in a manner similar to that described in this chapter. The article by Durlach et al. (2002) provides a review of the concept of informational masking as opposed to energetic masking.

Carlyon (1991) has demonstrated that frequency modulation per se probably does not support sound source segregation. Darwin and colleagues have studied the role of interaural and spatial differences in sound source segregation as well as the use of onset cues (Darwin and Ciocca, 1992). Several investiga-tors, including Darwin (1981) and Summerfield and Assmann (1991), and have used the two-vowel pro-cedure to study sound source segregation.

Textbooks on speech, such as those by Borden and Harris (1980), Zemlin (1981), Rabiner and Juang (1993), and Greenberg et al. (2004), cover speech pro-duction and perception. The Sensimetrics Series in Human Communications: *Speech Production and Per-ception* (1997) provides an informative CD-ROM for understanding the fundamentals of speech production and perception. Reviews of music perception can be found in Deliege and Sloboda (1992) and Revesz (2001).

15

The Central Auditory Nervous System

As explained in Chapter 1, the majority of this book (Chapters 2–14) is devoted to understanding how the basic attributes of sound are coded within the auditory periphery and the sensory and perceptual consequences of this coding. Chapters 1 and 14 also explained that hearing involves more than neural coding of frequency, intensity, and time (e.g., auditory perception). A great deal of this additional processing takes place in neural centers that lie in the auditory brainstem and cortex. In addition, because localization and other binaural perceptions depend on the interaction of information arriving at the two ears, we need to study central auditory centers, since neural information from the two cochleas interact only in the brainstem and cortex. This chapter deals briefly with the structure and function of the *central auditory nervous system* (CANS) as it receives information from the cochlea. A review of Appendices E and F will be helpful in understanding many of the topics in this chapter.

ANATOMY OF THE CENTRAL AUDITORY PATHWAYS

Figure 6.1 depicted the general anatomy and physiology of the auditory system but not the anatomy of the central auditory nervous system. Figure 15.1 illustrates in schematic form the principal connections of the *ascending* (from the cochlea toward the cortex), or *afferent,* auditory system. A glance at this figure demonstrates the intricacies of the system. The flow of neural information starts in the auditory nerve and then travels to the *brainstem* and then to the *auditory cortex.* Neural fibers (*axons*) high in the system (above the auditory nerve) are grouped in many pathways, called *tracts,* some traveling *contralaterally* (to the opposite side of the brain) and others remaining *ipsilateral* (on the same side). Furthermore, some fibers may leave one neural point and go directly to the next, whereas others may bypass the obvious next point and travel to a higher location. Still others will send *collaterals,* or branches, to one point as the main tract travels past that point to terminate at a higher location. Because of the complexity of this intricate system of pathways connecting one point to another, it is often convenient to label the fibers within a tract according to the number of connections (*synapses*) that occur earlier than the region under discussion. The fibers of the auditory nerve that leave the cochlea are the *primary,* or *first-order, fibers*, all of which make connections, or *synapse*, in the cochlear nucleus. The fibers that leave the cochlear nucleus after one synapse

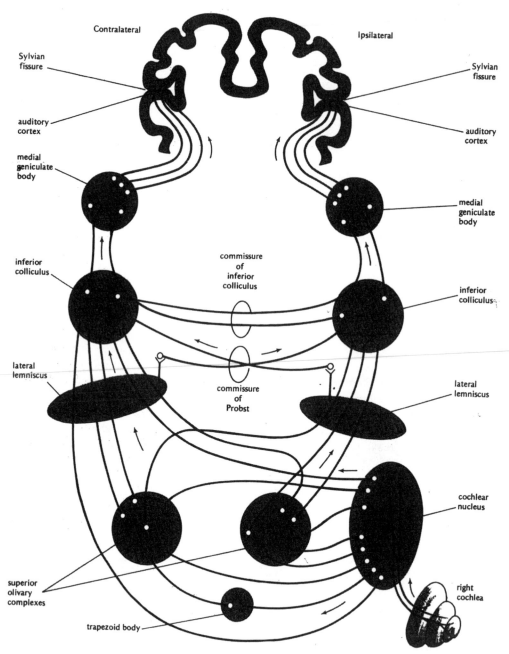

FIGURE 15.1 Schematic diagram of the ascending (afferent) pathways of the central auditory system, from the right cochlea to the auditory cortex. No attempt is made to show the subdivisions and connections within the various regions, cerebellar connections, or connections with the reticular formation. Based on similar diagrams by Ades (1959), Whitfield (1967), Diamond (1973), and Harrison and Howe (1974a, 1974b).

are *higher-order fibers* (e.g., second-order fibers, third-order fibers, and so on). Within the central nervous system are *nuclei,* which are groupings of nerve cell bodies. Within these nuclei lie *interneurons,* which interconnect various nerves within the nuclei but do not carry information between the nuclei. Sometimes a nerve fiber will pass through a nucleus without making a synapse with any units in the nucleus; these are called *fibers of passage.* Afferent pathways can provide either excitatory or inhibitory inputs to the neural units within the nuclei that they innervate. These inputs cause the cells with a nucleus to process the neural information it receives, and then the cells send the processed information on to the next nucleus in the ascending auditory pathway. Nuclei that receive auditory inputs along with inputs from other sensory systems have been excluded from the figure. Other information not elaborated in Figure 15.1 involves cerebellar connections, the innervation pattern within the various auditory nuclei, and the various types of cell bodies and their synaptic interconnections within auditory nuclei.

Figure 15.2 is another simplified schematic illustration, this one showing that the main tracts and nuclei above the cochlear nucleus are stimulated *binaurally* (that is, by both ears). By studying Figure 15.2, we can trace the general pathway of the neural signal from the cochlea to the cortex. After the neural impulses leave the cochlea, they travel to the *cochlear nucleus,* where the first synapse is made. From the cochlear nucleus, tracts lead to both the ipsilateral and contralateral *olivary complex,* so most bilateral representation occurs at this point and above. From the superior olive, neural impulses are transmitted to the *inferior colliculus* through and/or around the *lateral lemniscus,* from there to the *medial geniculate body,* and finally to the auditory cortex. These are the major nuclei of the central auditory nervous system, although other nuclei exist. Figures 15.1 and 15.2 are tremendous oversimplifications. It is not our purpose, however, to present a detailed account of the anatomy of the central auditory system, but rather to stress the importance of the major nuclei shown in Figure 15.2 and to bring an

awareness of the complexity of the auditory nervous system shown in Figure 15.1.

Descending (efferent) fiber tracts, shown in Figure 15.3, may arise in the auditory cortex or in a variety of nuclei and terminate at lower nuclei, e.g., in the cochlear nucleus or in the olivary complex. Chapter 8 has already discussed part of this system, which consists of the olivocochlear bundle arising in the olivary complex and terminating in the cochlea. Those fibers appeared to have an inhibitory action on electrophysiological responses of the cochlea, although their exact function is as yet unknown. All descending pathways cannot be considered as simply inhibitory neural networks. For instance, electrical stimulation of a particular segment of the superior olive can cause an increase in discharges in certain cochlear nucleus neurons. Thus, both excitatory and inhibitory connections might exist within this descending system. Therefore, rather than considering this system as only one that limits the passage of information from "lower" to "higher" levels of the ascending system through inhibition, a more general view is that the efferent (descending) auditory pathways represent a control system (or a modulator) that varies the routing of the sensory input and helps shape the neural input.

The anatomy of individual neural units (*morphology*) within the CANS can vary considerably. Figure 15.4 shows some of the various forms of neural cell types found within the cochlear nucleus and inferior colliculus. Similar diversity exists throughout the other neural centers of the CANS. These anatomical differences probably have significant physiological consequences. *Bushy cells* with their large dendritic trees with multiple synapses may process neural information from many different input axons. If these axons come from nerves with different frequency tuning (i.e., different CFs), bushy cells may play a role in integrating spectral information such as might be required for processing changes in the spectral profile of complex stimuli. When the cells are seen in a neural circuit such as shown in Figure 15.4D, one sees an organization of cells with axons going from top to bottom in layers (i.e., the *banded cells*—a and b) and cells that cut across the circuit, like the *stellate cells*

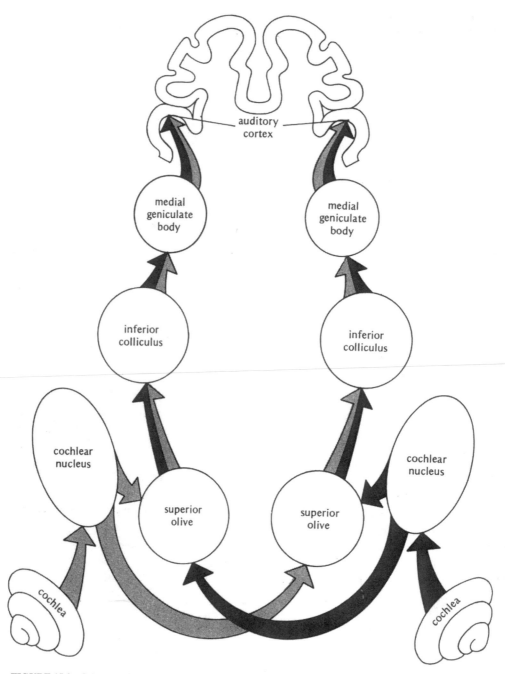

FIGURE 15.2 Schematic diagram of the bilateral central auditory system; the main pathways and nuclei are shown for both cochlea. Bilateral representation from binaural stimulation occurs at the superior olive and in all regions above. Based on a similar diagram by Lindsay and Norman (1972).

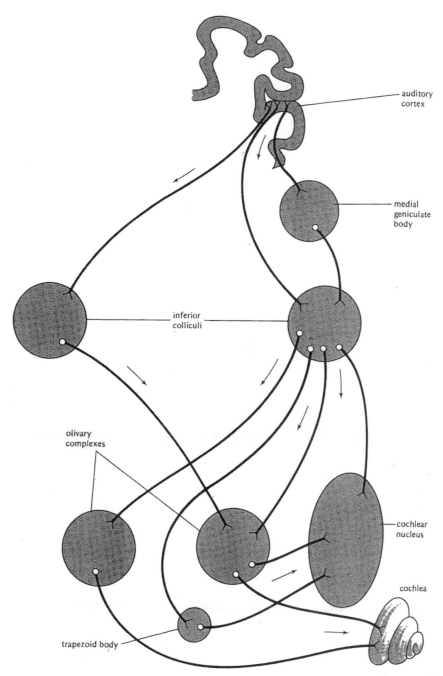

FIGURE 15.3 Schematic diagram of the descending pathways of the central auditory system from one side of the auditory cortex to the right cochlea. No attempt is made to show the subdivisions and connections within the various regions. The complex crossing and bilateral innervation shown for the ascending system in Figure 8.1 is also present in this system. Based on a diagram by Harrison and Howe (1974b).

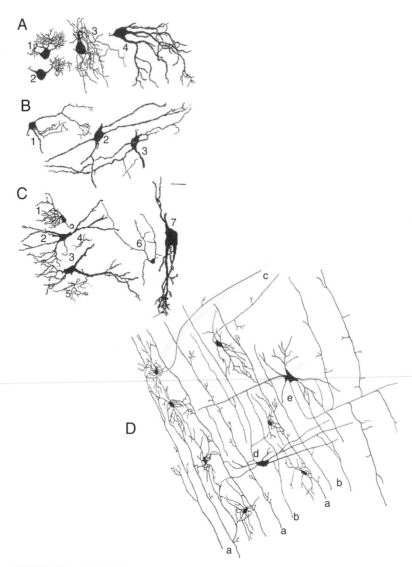

FIGURE 15.4 **(A–C)** Cell types in the cochlear nucleus. **(A)** 1 and 2 = *spherical bushy cells*, 3 = *globular bush cells*, **(B)** 1–3 = *multipolar cells*, **(C)** 1 = *cartwheel cells*, 2 and 3 = *fusiform cells*, 4 and 5 = *granule cells*, 6 = *stellate cells*, 7 = *giant cells* (scale bar = 1 μm). From Cant (1992), with permission. **(D)** Part of a neural circuit in the inferior colliculus (central nucleus of the inferior colliculus). a and b = *banded cells*, d and e = *stellate cells*. From Oliver and Huerta (1992), used with permission.

(d). The stellate cells may help integrate neural information in the layers of cells and axons flowing from top to bottom. Other neural cells may receive inputs from axons connected to each ear (*bipolar cells*) and as such may provide a way to process binaural information. Exact structure–function relationships have been established for some but not most cell types. Some of these properties will be described later, in the section "Single-Fiber Responses."

STRATEGIES FOR STUDYING THE CENTRAL AUDITORY SYSTEM

TOPOGRAPHICAL ORGANIZATION

In Chapters 7, 8, and 9 we discussed the concept of frequency as being represented by a particular place along the basilar membrane, the place being determined by the location of maximum displacement of the basilar membrane in response to a particular frequency of stimulation. Fibers with high characteristic frequencies innervate the base of the cochlea, and those with low CFs innervate the apex. The maintenance of this neural spatial representation of frequency throughout the auditory nerve and the nuclei of the central auditory pathways is referred to as *tonotopic organization*. The test for tonotopic organization is to determine where within a nucleus there is an orderly neural spatial representation of fibers with various CFs. In order to determine how a nucleus is tonotopically organized, the tuning curves for nerve fibers in the nucleus are measured and their characteristic frequencies determined. The organization of CFs in terms of the fiber's anatomical location within the nucleus usually determines the tonotopic organization of the various parts of the CANS (e.g., perhaps the CFs of the neural fibers increase from the medial to the lateral part of the nucleus). However, the enormous variation in the ways in which CANS nerves respond to sound often makes the determination of tuning curves and CFs a more difficult task in the CANS than at the periphery. All neural centers have a tonotopic organization, although the neural map for frequency in some nuclei is quite complex.

In most other sensory systems, the response of neural units in the central nervous system is systematically organized in terms of a number of different features of the stimulus that drives these units. In the CANS, investigators search for similar *topographical organizations*. For instance, are there fibers that respond best when sound is presented from a particular spatial location? If so, then cells that may be "tuned" to the spatial location of a sound source might provide a <u>neural map for auditory space</u>. There is evidence that parts of the inferior colliculus and auditory cortex may be topographically organized to process amplitude modulation, in that neural units fire selectively for different rates of amplitude modulation. Based on what happens in other sensory systems, spatial maps or modulation rate–processing might occur in conjunction with a tonotopic organization, providing a two-dimensional topographic organization. Topographical organization for features of sound other than frequency, and perhaps space and modulation, have been found in a few species (e.g., owl and bats), but a number of emerging data hint that such neural organization exists in the CANS of many other species.

EXCITATION AND INHIBITION

The ability of a single neuron or a circuit of neurons to process information important for auditory perception depends to a large extent on how inputs to the synapse of the neurons interact. The interactions can be reinforcing (additive) or canceling (subtractive). Thus, the excitatory and inhibitory properties of neural transmission across a synapse are valuable pieces of information for understanding neural processing.

The transfer of a neural event across a synapse is crucial for the integration of information within the central nervous system. The basic circuitry that exists in the CANS is caused by nerves that interact with each other in either an excitatory or inhibitory manner. That is, two nerves may converge on the synapse of another cell and the combined excitation of the input nerves may produce a firing pattern in the target nerve as if it were adding the information from the two input nerves. If one input nerve is excitatory and one inhibitory, the target nerve may serve as if it were differencing the information between the inputs. In some circumstances these cells are referred to as *E–E* or *E–I*, in terms of how the inputs to the cells interact in an excitatory (*E*) or inhibitory (*I*) manner.

Chemical structures like *acetylcholine* (ACh) are believed to act as excitatory neurotransmitters at the synapses, while *amino acids* such as *gamma-aminobutyric acid* (GABA) and *glycine* may act as inhibitory neurotransmitters. By studying the concentrations of these and other neural chemicals, the excitatory or inhibitory function of a neural site or part of a neural site can be inferred (see Appendix F). Quite often, other chemicals are used in experiments to *block* the generation or flow of these types of neurotransmitters. These attempts to change the normal chemical activity in a neural structure can help determine how information is transmitted from one neuron or group of neurons to other neurons. For instance, if one blocks the inhibitory action of GABA on a neural unit, one might be able to determine how the inhibitory action effects the processing provided by the neural unit.

SINGLE-FIBER RESPONSES

Measures of single-fiber responses used to characterize the discharge patterns of auditory nerve fibers are also useful for studying the central pathways. In auditory nerve fibers, spontaneous activity varies greatly in discharge rate from fiber to fiber. The interval histograms of spontaneous activity of various auditory nerve fibers, however, are essentially unchanged regardless of the CF of the unit and its discharge rate. In the central auditory system, this regularity of interval histograms of spontaneous activity is not maintained. Interval histograms of spontaneous activity at these higher levels are more variable, changing as a response to a variety of nonauditory events, such as the state of alertness.

Single auditory nerve fibers were shown to have rate-level functions that produced an increased discharge rate with an increase in level over a 20- to 50-dB range. Single fibers from the central pathways generally have a smaller dynamic range than those of the auditory nerve. Furthermore, central neurons may show a decrease in discharge rate with an increase in stimulation at high levels. Thus, the rate-level function of a central neuron may be similar to that of an auditory nerve fiber, or it may be shaped like an inverted U, showing an increase in discharge rate with an initial increase in stimulus level and then a decreasing neural rate at higher levels. Such rate-level functions can be further changed by acoustic stimulation of the opposite ear.

As discussed in Chapter 9, single-unit responses of the auditory nerve show phase locking to the period of a stimulating sinusoid. Phase locking to individual cycles of the tone also occurs in many units of the cochlear nucleus for the low-frequency stimuli. In addition, synchronous responses to low-frequency stimuli have been observed in the trapezoid body, the inferior colliculus, and the superior olive. As we investigate higher in the system, however, we find that the relationship between the neural discharges and the period of low-frequency stimuli is less clear. When phase locking does occur in the CANS, it often only occurs for very low frequencies or low rates of stimulation.

In Chapter 9, we showed that PST histograms to tone bursts were essentially the same for all fibers of the auditory nerve. In the central auditory system, however, PST histograms to tone bursts may illustrate any number of patterns, as seen in Figure 15.5. The higher-order fibers may respond in the same manner as the primary fibers; they may produce *"on" responses*, *"off" responses*, or *"on–off" responses*; or they may exhibit more complex responses, such as those called *pausers* or *choppers*. Not all of these patterns can be recorded from every nucleus within the system. On the other hand, one pattern may be recorded from one region within a nucleus and another from a different region within the same nucleus. In addition, one neuron may have different response pat-

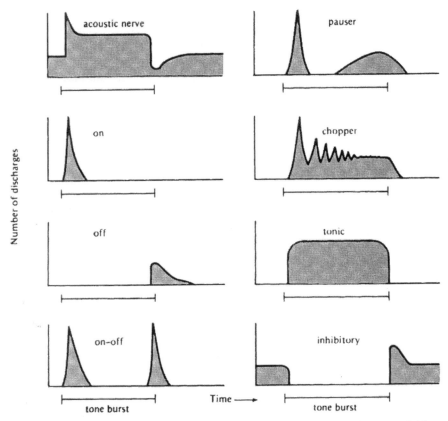

FIGURE 15.5 Idealized post stimulus time (PST) histograms to a variety of tone bursts recorded from the central auditory system. The time patterns of responses of the central system are thought to reflect the wide variety of tasks that it must accomplish.

terns, depending on the type of stimulation (e.g., the PST histogram may appear different for a CF than for a non-CF tone). Usually, neural units with the same morphology exhibit about the same physiological properties (see Figures 15.4 and 15.16) while units with different anatomical structures often have different physiological properties.

Presumably these different neural response patterns help process information about sound. For instance, the chopping response seen in the PST histograms of chopper cells probably results from some intrinsic property of the cell that causes it to discharge at a par-

ticular rate. If the rate of envelope fluctuations of an amplitude-modulated stimulus drives a chopper cell at a rate that is similar to its intrinsic chopping rate, then this chopper cell may respond best to this particular modulation rate. As such, chopper cells may encode or be tuned to the rate of amplitude modulation.

As the neural impulse ascends the auditory pathways, it is delayed relative to stimulation at the cochlea. A measure of the delay time can be used as an indicator of a variety of physiological events. For instance, if two cells in the same region of the central nervous system receive information at different times, one can assume that the neuron with the later-arriving information is fed by pathways that involve more synapses than the other neuron. A convenient way to investigate the timing information of a neuron is to obtain a PST histogram to a click. The time between the onset of the click and that of a neural discharge is an indicator of the travel time from the cochlea to the neuron under study.

Poststimulus time (PST) histograms to click stimulation for auditory nerve fibers demonstrate either a single peak or multiple peaks, depending on the interaction of the stimulating frequency and the fiber's CF (recall Figure 9.10). For higher-order fibers, PST histograms to click stimuli may have a variety of patterns. These patterns are not, however, related to the CF of the fiber, as they are at the periphery. The typical PST histogram of low-CF fibers to click stimulation recorded from the auditory nerve fibers is not as prevalent in the responses of higher-order fibers even as "low" in the system as the cochlear nucleus. The lack of the multiple peaks related to the CF of the unit (that is, peaks at times equal to 1/CF) is interesting because this temporal information is evidently not usually transmitted beyond the cochlear nucleus. Figure 15.6 shows a comparison of PST histograms

from low-CF fibers in both the auditory nerve and the cochlear nucleus in response to click stimulation. Such data imply that a simple relaying of information from one low-CF nerve to another does not occur in this part of the cochlear nucleus.

NEURAL CIRCUITS

The study of neural circuits in the CANS is difficult. Almost all electrophysiological research involves measuring from one nerve fiber at a time. Studies of the activity of several neurons in the intact animal measured at the same time are very hard, given the difficulties in developing *multi-electrode recording techniques*. One way to study neural circuits is to use what is called the *slice preparation*. This technique involves excising a segment of neural tissue from an animal and placing it in a Petri dish with the appropriate chemicals that allow the neural tissue to continue to physiologically function. While this is a difficult procedure, segments of different neural centers can be preserved and studied using the slice preparation technique. While "sound" cannot be delivered to such tissue slices, various neural fibers within the slice can be electrically stimulated and/or their function altered by chemical means. And one can record neural activity from other fibers in the slice preparation. Thus, one fiber can be stimulated and neural responses can be recorded from other fibers to help determine how the nerves in this section of tissue process information. While such *in vitro* (in glass) experiments have provided important information about the function of the CANS, caution must always be exercised in making generalization to the *in vivo* state (in the living organism).

There is one type of neural circuit that might play an important role in the central processing of sensory information. This circuit, or network, is called a *lateral inhibitory network*. A schematic diagram of a simple lateral inhibitory network is shown in Figure 15.7. Fibers that are adjacent or lateral to an excitatory fiber send inhibition across the network as shown in Figure 15.7. One important consequence of a lateral

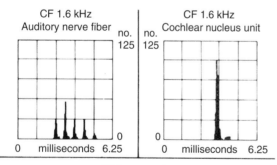

Click rate: 10/sec

FIGURE 15.6 Comparison of post stimulus time (PST) histograms to click stimulation for two fibers of the same characteristic frequency (1.6 kHz): auditory nerve fiber (left) and cochlear nucleus fiber (right). Low-CF fibers in the cochlear nucleus typically do not show the modulated pattern related to 1/CF that is characteristic of auditory nerve fibers. The click is presented at time equal to 0. Adapted from Kiang (1965), with permission.

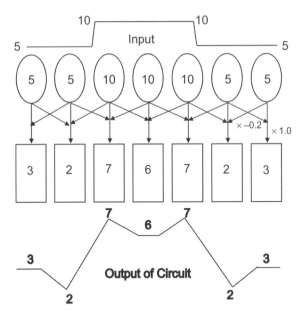

FIGURE 15.7 Schematic diagram of a lateral inhibitory network. Input neurons, shown as ovals, send information to output neurons, shown as rectangles. The input neurons send an excitatory signal (×1.0) to the output neuron directly below it and inhibitory signals to the output neurons to the left and right (× −0.2). The excitation is equal to the activity in the input neuron (i.e., multiply the input activity times 1, ×1), while the inhibition is equal to negative 0.2 times the activity in the input neuron (i.e., multiply the input activity by −0.2, × −0.2). The amount of neural activity in an output neuron is the sum of the excitation and the two paths of inhibition. An input stimulus is shown along the top such that the stimulus increases in magnitude from 5 to 10 and back to 5 across the neuronal array. Consider the output neuron on the left: It receives 5 units of excitation from the input neuron, −1 units of inhibition (−0.2 × 5) from the right and −1 units of inhibition from the left (assuming the network continues to the left). The result is 3 units of excitation for this output neuron (5 − 1 − 1 = 3). Similar mathematics will yield the units of output activity shown along the bottom. Note that the input contrast change at each edge of the input stimulation is made more obvious in the output due to this lateral inhibitory network.

inhibitory network is that it sharpens the information presented at the input to the network. That is, contrasts in the neural excitation that occur in the input are amplified by the lateral inhibitory network, making the changes in contrast that occur across the network more noticeable. For instance, a change in the amplitude

between one region of the spectrum and another region (as occurs for the formants of speech; see Chapter 14) might be enhanced and made more obvious if the spectral information is processed by a neural network that had lateral inhibitory properties. That is, in Figure 15.7, the input stimulus might be the amplitude spectrum of a sound, which changes in amplitude from 5 to 10 at one frequency region and back to 5 at another frequency region. If each input neuron was tuned to a particular frequency and each input neuron fed its outputs to this lateral inhibitory network, the spectral contrast might be enhanced, allowing for the neural coding of subtle spectral changes.

EVOKED POTENTIALS

In our discussion of the CANS, we stressed that many CANS locations (e.g., the cortex) are relatively inaccessible and that discrepancies in the data from various investigations can often be attributed to differences in anesthesia. This being the case, responses from the auditory cortexes of awake-behaving animals (especially humans) become extremely significant to the contribution of knowledge about how we hear. A method of recording CANS activity that can be used with awake adult humans is to place electrodes on the scalp and to record variations in electrical activity that occur in conjunction with the presentation of an auditory stimulus. When responses are recorded in this manner, the electrical activity of interest, called the *auditory-evoked response* (AER), is often quite small relative to other recorded activity. This activity reflects changes in the *electroencephalogram* (EEG) that are related to acoustic stimulation. By a method known as *signal averaging* (see Appendix E), the desired responses, which appear in conjunction with the presentation of an auditory stimulus, can be separated from the unwanted or uncorrelated activity. These potentials are usually recorded from the scalp at a position at the center of the top of the head, known as the *vertex*. The AER, a complex response, occurs at the abrupt onset or termination of an acoustic signal.

Its waveform has a negative peak about 100 msec after presentation of an appropriate stimulus and a later positive peak. The response often increases in amplitude and decreases in latency (time between stimulus onset and response onset) with increases in stimulus level. Different cortical locations have been postulated to account for the early (about 50 to 100 msec) and later (about 300 msec) components of the waveform. Correspondingly, it has also been suggested that the earlier AER components are more affected by variations in the acoustic stimulus, whereas the later components are more affected by nonacoustic variables, such as attention, expectancy, significance, decision, and contingency.

The waveform in Figure 15.8 shows the auditory-evoked response to a 1000-Hz, 300-msec tone presented at 20, 40, and 60 dB SL. The AER was obtained by presenting the tone 64 times. The EEG activity fol-lowing each stimulus presentation was then summed over the 64 presentations. This method of signal averaging tends to cancel any parts of the EEG activity that are random (not correlated) with respect to the signal and to enhance any EEG activity correlated with the signal. The peaks and valleys are referred to as P_1 (positive peak 1), N_1 (negative peak 1), P_2 (positive peak 2), and N_2 (negative peak 2), etc. These peaks almost always occur in the AER, but their amplitude and time of occurrence (latency from stimulus offset) can vary as a function of the stimulus variable (e.g., level) or the variables dealing with the attention of the subject.

In Chapter 8, we discussed the recording of the AP from humans. The AP has a latency from stimulus onset of about 1 msec, depending on the level of the stimulus. The AERs just discussed have latencies of 50 msec or more, depending on which particular

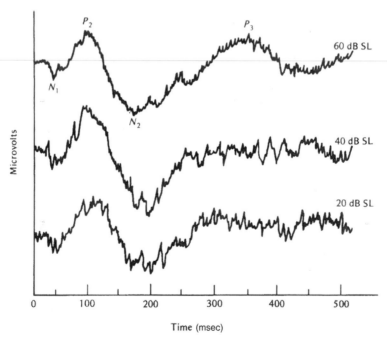

FIGURE 15.8 Auditory-evoked response (AER) to 64 repetitions of a 1000-Hz, 30-msec tone burst presented at 20, 40, and 60 dB SL. Points N_1, P_2, N_2, and P_3 refer to par-ticular points in the waveform (see text). Figure courtesy of Dr. Donald C. Teas, University of Florida, Gainesville.

response is being measured. The AP is known to be generated by the synchronous firing of primarily high-frequency cochlear nerve fibers, and the AER is thought to be a cortical response. Are there electro-physiological responses with intermediate latencies that involve brainstem auditory pathways that can be recorded from humans? The answer appears to be yes. The recording of these responses is accomplished with a vertex electrode. These responses are called *brainstem-evoked responses* (BSERs) because they are thought to be generated predominantly by nuclei of the brainstem. Figure 15.9 shows a brainstem-evoked potential in response to a click stimulus presented binaurally. The latencies of these responses are from 1 to 8 msec. The responses are low in voltage and require signal averaging (often over 1000 recordings are averaged) to make them "stand out" from the background electrical activity. The source of the first wave, wave I, is the auditory nerve. The places where the other potentials originate are thought to be generated at the different sites in the ascending auditory pathways of the brainstem, with wave V most likely arising from the inferior colliculus.

There are also evoked potentials that can be measured with latencies between those of wave V (approximately 5 to 7 msec after stimulation, which may represent inferior colliculus activity) and the N_1 of the AER (approximately 60 to 90 msec after stimulation). These potentials are often referred to as *middle-latency* potentials. For the AER, BSER, and the middle-latency potentials, both the amplitude of the evoked response and its latency are used to relate the response to the stimulus or the state of the listener. Figure 15.10 shows the decrease in the latency of wave V that occurs with increasing the level of the click stimulus. Given the very short latencies of these responses, a click stimulus or short tone burst must be used to evoke the BSER. A change in the latency of wave V implies a change in the speed with which the neural information reaches the site of generation of wave V (presumably the inferior colliculus). The latency of wave V may also vary as a function of changing the spectral content of the click.

Because normative data are established for these responses and the neural source or sources for each wave identified, deviations from these norms can be used to detect possible deficiencies in the auditory pathways of the brainstem. Thus, the study of the electrophysiology of the auditory pathways is producing data for the study and diagnosis of human hearing, from the cochlea to the cortex.

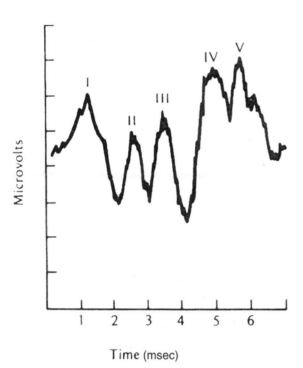

FIGURE 15.9 Brainstem-evoked potential response (BSER) to a click presented 1000 times binaurally. The response was recorded from the vertex referenced to the right mastoid. Roman numerals represent the labeling of the peaks according to Jewett and Williston (1971; see text). Recording courtesy of Dr. Donald C. Teas, University of Florida, Gainesville.

BRAIN IMAGES

Brain images can also be used to determine the structure and function of the human CANS. An X-ray provides an image of our internal organs. Similarly, various imaging techniques (see Appendix F) can be

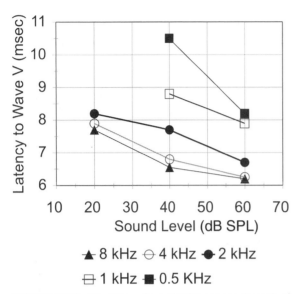

FIGURE 15.10 The latency from stimulus onset to the peak of wave V of the brainstem-evoked response is shown as a function of level and frequency content of the click stimulus. The latency decreases with increases in stimulus level and as the frequency content of the click is restricted to higher and higher frequencies. The frequency content of the click was controlled by filtering a brief acoustic transient with the center frequencies shown in the figure legend. From Klein and Teas (1978), used with permission.

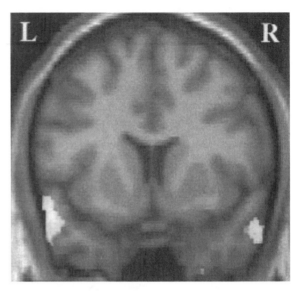

FIGURE 15.11 Positron emission tomography (PET) image showing increased brain activity (light areas) in the left and right superior planum areas at the level of the primary auditory cortex in response to iterated rippled noise, which produces a complex pitch (see Chapter 13). From Griffiths et al. (1998), with permission.

used to image the brain. Some image techniques provide an anatomical view of the brain (e.g., computed axial tomography, or CAT, scan). Other imaging techniques can provide a functional image, that is, an image that represents which neural circuits were active during particular stimulus events. Figure 15.11 displays a PET (*positron emission tomography*) image of the cortex of a human when the subject was presented a stimulus like that shown in Figure 13.10 (the stimulus, iterated rippled noise, produces a complex pitch perception, whose pitch strength can be systematically varied). PET images result from the way in which cells of a neural circuit that are actively discharging while processing information take up a glucose that is bonded to a radioactive marker that has been injected into the subject. Only those cells that are highly active while the stimulus is present will have a high concentration of glucose and its radioactive

marker, since glucose (a sugar) is required for the metabolic function of the nerve cell. The cell's metabolism increases (glucose use increases) when a neuron is discharging action potentials. The PET scanner forms an image of the brain allowing one to see where this high concentration of the radioactive marker is found. Computer and statistical methods are used to make sure that the cortical area of high concentration results from the stimulus presentation and is not just a result of random neural activity. The image in Figure 15.11 suggests that a particular cortical region (in this case, in the left and right *temporal planum* area of auditory cortex) is active when this stimulus is present and that its activation is enhanced when the strength of the pitch associated with the stimulus increases. This implies that this region of the cortex plays a role in processing pitch strength for these types of complex sounds.

The technique used most often to study the function of the central nervous system in human subjects is *functional magnetic resonance imaging* (fMRI). "Brain mapping" using fMRI is achieved by setting up an advanced MRI scanner (see Appendix F) in a special way so that increased blood flow to the activated areas of the brain shows up on fMRI scans. This "blood oxygenation level–dependent," or "*BOLD,*" effect can be observed by noninvasive magnetic resonance imaging in high magnetic fields. Basically the MRI scanner detects changes in the hemoglobin content in blood. Neurons need a blood supply for their metabolism; the more the neurons "work," the more blood is needed and the larger the fMRI signal. The fMRI signal is measuring the BOLD effect, which in theory is related to neural functioning. Figure 15.12 shows fMRI recordings from different MRI slices representing the area of different nuclei in the ascending auditory pathway. The responses represent statistically significant BOLD-signal differences between silence and sound presentation as measured in different fMRI slices taken in the region of the cochlear nucleus, infe-

rior colliculus, and medial geniculate body. The figure indicates that the particular sound is being processed by most of the nuclei in the ascending auditory pathway of this human subject.

DEVELOPMENT AND PLASTICITY

The structure and function of the nervous system change during development and as result of experience. While a great deal, but not all, of the human peripheral auditory system is fully developed at birth, the central nervous system continues to develop after birth. For instance, the myelin sheath (see Appendix E) that covers most central nerve fibers continues to grow and to develop after birth. This development means that neural conduction time increases after birth. The various parts of the auditory system develop under the genetic control provided by the DNA code. How the various neural structures develop from the

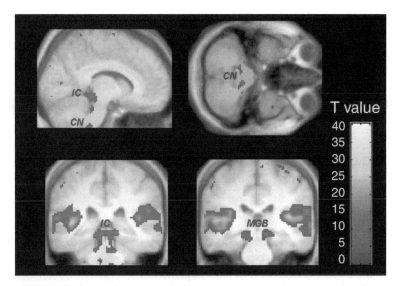

FIGURE 15.12 Functional magnetic resonance imaging (fMRI) images of different MRI slices indicating different brainstem areas that were responsive to a particular sound (CN = cochlear nucleus, IC = inferior colliculus, MGB = medial geniculate body). The shades of darkness and the scale on the right indicate the statistical significance (*T* value) of the fMRI images, which reflects a difference between the blood oxygen level–dependent (BOLD) response to no sound and that to sound. From Griffiths et al. (2001), with permission.

embryonic to the mature state is important for a functioning normal auditory system. For instance, understanding how a nerve fiber develops such that it connects one nucleus to another provides valuable information on how neural circuits function. Several hearing disorders (see Chapter 16) occur when normal development of the auditory pathways is arrested due to genetic mutations. Understanding auditory neural development can potentially aid in understanding many aspects of normal and abnormal auditory function. For instance, in Chapter 16 we will learn that damaged hair cells do not regenerate in mammals, but they do in birds and fish. By understanding how hair cells develop in mammals as opposed to birds may reveal mechanisms that could make it possible for mammalian (including human) hair cell regeneration.

Neural structure and function can also change based on the experience of the organism. Such neural change based on experience is called *neural plasticity*. In Chapter 16 we will learn that there is considerable evidence of auditory neural plasticity in listeners with impaired hearing who have been successfully fitted with a cochlear implant. Figure 15.13 indicates a form of plasticity that occurs following an altering of the pinna in such a way that HRTFs (see Chapter 12) of subjects are significantly changed. Recall that the pinna diffracts high-frequency sound in such a way as to alter the spectrum of the sound arriving at the outer ear canal, and these spectral alterations (the HRTF) are probably responsible for the capability of locating sound sources in the vertical dimension. The pieces of plastic were placed in the pinna in order to change the diffraction pattern, and hence the HRTFs were also changed. The data in Figure 15.13 indicate that immediately after being fitted with the plastic pinna pieces, listeners were unable to localize sounds in the vertical direction, presumably because they were receiving HRTF information that they were not used to. However, after several weeks of wearing the plastic pinna pieces, the subjects were able to use the new HRTF information to successfully localize sound sources. Immediately after removing the plastic pieces, the subjects were nearly back to their baseline (before the experiment began) ability to successfully

localize sound sources in the vertical dimension. This change in localization performance over time is an example of auditory neural plasticity, and this experiment suggests that both the new neural function that developed to deal with the altered HRTFs exists along with the original neural anatomy and physiology that processed the normal spectral information provided by the listeners' normal HRTFs. Research involving the barn owl has shown similar forms of neural plasticity for spatial alterations, and this work also shows how new dendritic fields develop after the animals adapt to the new (altered) spatial information, indicating that such plasticity may actually involve a "rewiring" of the auditory nervous system.

We will now turn to a discussion of several neural centers in the ascending CANS. The various strategies discussed previously are being used to better understand the role each center plays in auditory processing.

COCHLEAR NUCLEUS

Figure 15.14 shows schematically the projection of the cochlear location and cochlear nerve fibers in the cochlear nucleus. Upon entering the cochlear nucleus, each nerve fiber separates and goes to three separate regions within the cochlear nucleus: the *anteroventral cochlear nucleus* (AVCN), the *posteroventral cochlear nucleus* (PVCN), and the *dorsal cochlear nucleus* (DCN). From this diagram we can see that in each division of the cochlear nucleus the cochlear partition is completely tonotopically represented, from the base to apex. Electrophysiological investigations of the cochlear nucleus confirm this representation by demonstrating that the CFs of fibers within each region duplicate the CFs expected on the basis of the auditory nerve innervation of that region. An example of an electrode penetration from one such investigation is given in Figure 15.15. This figure shows how the CFs of the various units are arranged in a tonotopic manner from low CF to high CF in both the AVCN and the DCN.

Figure 15.16 summarizes many of the physiological findings from different neuronal types in the dif-

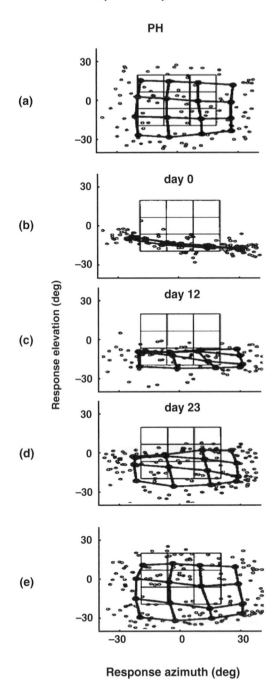

Response elevation (deg)

Response azimuth (deg)

ferent regions of the cochlear nucleus. The center portion of Figure 15.16 shows the variety of cell types and schematic diagrams of the neural cell morphology (see Figure 15.4) spherical bushy cell (SB), stellate cell (St), globular bushy cell (GB), multipolar cell (M), octopus cell (O), globular cell (G), and fusiform cell (F), reading from the left to the right of the figure. These different neuronal types are distributed in the different subareas of the cochlear nucleus, and the arrows heading upward depict the fact that these neurons send information up the brainstem to other nuclei in the CANS. The nerve coming in from the bottom of the figure is an auditory nerve fiber (a.n.). The typical tuning curve, rate-level functions, period histogram, and PST histogram for auditory nerve fibers are shown at the bottom from left to right, respectively. Notice how these various physiological measures vary from neuronal type to neuronal type within the cochlear nucleus. Additional explanation is provided in the figure caption. This diagram suggests the enormous variation and complexity that exist in the anatomy and physiology of the cochlear

FIGURE 15.13 Localization responses of a listener (PH) whose head-related transfer functions (HRTFs) were altered by the insertion of small pieces of plastic into and around each pinna. The subject was asked to look at (point the eyes at) a sound source that was located in a 4 × 4 array of four vertical locations (shown along the *y*-axis) by four azimuth locations (shown along the *x*-axis) (the center of each of the 16 squares bounded by the light lines indicate the location of the sound source). An eye tracker recorded the position of the eye when the subject indicated that he or she was looking at the sound source. The dark dots connected by dark lines indicate the mean eye position for each of the 16 sound-source locations. The top panel (a) indicates the subject's pretty good ability to locate each sound source before the plastic pieces were inserted. Panels b–d indicate the subject's performance immediately following the insertion of the plastic pieces (b) and two time periods later (c and d). Immediately after the plastic pieces were inserted (b), the subject could no longer accurately localize in the vertical direction, but could in the horizontal/azimuth direction. By day 23 (d) of wearing the plastic pieces, the subject had recovered an ability to accurately vertically localize. Immediately after the plastic pieces were removed (panel e) the subject's localization responses were very similar to that achieved before the plastic pieces were used (a). From Hofman et al. (1998), with permission.

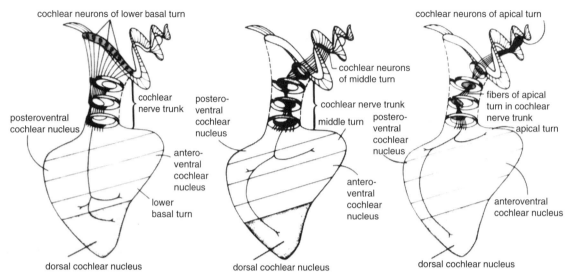

FIGURE 15.14   Schematic diagrams showing that basal turn (left), middle turn (center), and apical turn (right) auditory nerve fibers innervate different areas of the three main regions of the cochlear nucleus. The spatial separation of frequency from base to apex in the cochlea is reflected in the characteristic frequencies of the fibers that leave the cochlea and is maintained within each of the three main regions of the cochlear nucleus. Based on a similar diagram by Schuknecht (1974), with permission.

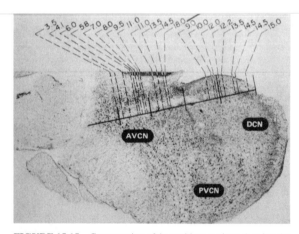

FIGURE 15.15   Cross section of the cochlear nucleus showing the track made by an electrode penetration. The characteristic frequencies of neurons recorded from various points within the anteroventral cochlear nucleus (AVCN) and dorsal cochlear nucleus (DCN) show that the spatial separation of frequency is maintained within those two divisions of the cochlear nucleus. PVCN = posteroventral cochlear nucleus. This tonotopic organization is maintained throughout the central auditory system. Adapted from Rose, Galambos, and Hughes (1959), with permission.

nucleus. Similar complexity exists at each level of the CANS.

Although it isn't yet clear what function the cochlear nucleus plays in auditory processing, the large interconnections and the complex physiology suggest that the cochlear nucleus is refining the code for sound provided by the auditory periphery. The fibers coming from the cochlear nucleus appear to innervate most of the other nuclei in the auditory brainstem. The neural circuits of the cochlear nucleus appear capable of making neural comparisons between neurons that are tuned to approximately the same frequency as well as among fibers that have different CFs. There is also evidence that many cells in the dorsal cochlear nucleus react in a manner that suggests a lateral inhibitory network. Comparisons among fibers with different CFs might aid in processing the spectral profile of complex stimuli. The presence of a lateral inhibitory network could help sharpen the neural representation of spectral information that is present in a complex sound field, as discussed earlier.

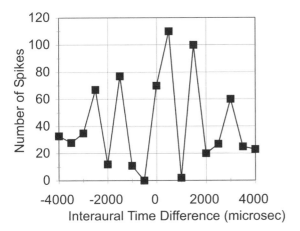

FIGURE 15.18 Response (number of spikes) of a neuron in the inferior colliculus with a low-frequency center frequency responding to a wideband noise presented with different interaural time differences (in μsec). Adapted from Yin and Chan (1988), used with permission.

lus is to combine information from different processes that occur lower in the brainstem, such as combining interaural information with spectral information to provide processing of sound in two or three dimensions (see Chapter 12).

Figure 15.18 displays the neural output of an inferior colliculus (IC) unit in response to a broadband noise stimulus presented with interaural time delays ranging from −4000 μsec (4-msec sound leading to the contralateral ear) to 4000 μsec (4-msec sound leading to the ipsilateral ear). This IC cell with a low-frequency CF has a peak number of neural responses that occur as a periodic function of the interaural time delay. The peak closest to zero ITD is at approximately 400 to 500 μsec, which may be the interaural time difference that this IC cell is signaling. Such cells may be part of a neural circuit in the IC that helps process interaural time differences.

AUDITORY CORTEX

As shown schematically in Figure 15.1, the human *auditory cortex* is located in a deep groove, or convo-

lution, in the brain called the *fissure of Sylvius*. The inaccessibility of the auditory cortex in the primate brain makes it difficult to study. In the cat brain the auditory cortex is more accessible, and therefore the cat brain is often used in research involving the cortex. The cat cortex is often subdivided into various areas, as illustrated in Figure 15.19, which compares the cortexes of cat and monkey. The human auditory cortex is more like the monkey's. The bottom diagram is drawn with the Sylvian fissure opened to expose the auditory cortex. The projections to the cortex contain bilateral information. Thus, each cochlea has an input to each hemisphere.

Early studies of the tonotopic organization of the auditory cortex revealed that frequency maps of the cortex could be made by stimulating small portions of the exposed cochlea and demonstrating a point-to-point projection of the cochlea onto the primary cortex (tonotopic organization). Frequency maps of the cortex could also be made by using tone bursts and recording the resulting activity at the cortex. The studies were made with the animal under deep anesthesia; in some cases *strychnine* was applied to various areas of the cortex to raise the excitability of these cortical areas. Later studies showed that under reduced or no anesthesia, less well-defined tonotopic organization could be obtained in the cortex. However, more recent studies using monkeys have produced consistent results from both anesthetized and awake animals. From studies of both anesthetized and awake animals, evidence now exists that the cortex is organized in columns of cells. Each column is perpendicular to the surface of the cortex and has cells of similar CF. The tuning curves for cortical neurons vary in shape, some being as narrow as those found in the auditory nerve and others being broader. This type of cortical organization might allow the auditory system to arrange information for complex auditory pattern recognition. There is considerable evidence of inhibitory connections in the auditory cortex, such that many cortical neurons often exhibit inhibitory sidebands like those seen in the tuning curve of auditory nerve fibers for two-tone suppression (see Figure 9.11).

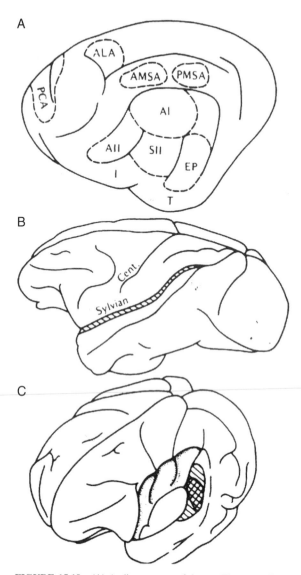

FIGURE 15.19 **(A)** Auditory cortex of the cat. The cat auditory cortex, which is easily accessible, is often subdivided into the various regions indicated. The primary auditory regions are AI, AII, SII, and EP. Other areas that receive auditory input are shown. **(B)** The auditory cortex of the monkey, which, like the human one, lies within the Sylvian fissure. **(C)** The monkey auditory cortex is shown by opening the Sylvian fissure. Adapted from Elliott and Trahiotis (1972), used with permission.

The time pattern of responses of cortical neurons seems to be especially sensitive to changes in stimulation. One-third of the cortical neurons can be stimulated only by tones of changing frequency or by more complex dynamic sounds. Very few units maintain a discharge rate above the spontaneous level for the duration of the stimulus, as was seen in auditory nerve discharge patterns. Figure 15.20 shows PST histograms illustrating various discharge patterns of cortical neurons to stimuli at their CFs and at various levels of intensity. Sinusoidal tone bursts are *not* often the appropriate stimuli to investigate the response patterns of many cortical neurons, since many cortical units respond poorly to tonal stimulation.

By using stimuli that vary in their frequency content as a function of time (frequency modulation; see Chapter 4, interesting response patterns have been detected. Some neurons will respond only to an increase in frequency, others only to a decrease in frequency, and still others only to an increase in frequency of low-frequency stimuli and to a decrease in frequency of high-frequency stimuli. Units in the auditory cortex and other neural centers can also be investigated using amplitude-modulated stimuli. *Neural temporal modulation transfer functions*, like those acquired psychophysically (see Chapter 10) can be obtained in which neural discharge rate is determined as a function of stimulus modulation rate. Although some units respond in a manner similar to the psychophysical results, others appear to respond best to certain modulation rates, as if these units were tuned to a particular amplitude modulation rate. Figure 15.21 displays the neural response of an auditory cortical with a CF of about 10 kHz when a 10-kHz tone was sinusoidally amplitude modulated (100% depth of modulation) at different rates (from 1 to 30 Hz). The vector strength of this cell was greatest for modulation rates of approximately 5 Hz, as if this unit might be tuned to low modulation rates of approximately 5 Hz. Vector strength is a measure of how well the unit's discharge rate is synchronized to the period of the modulation envelope (see Chapter 9). A vector strength of 1.0 means that the neural unit only produces spikes at one phase (e.g., at the peak) of the

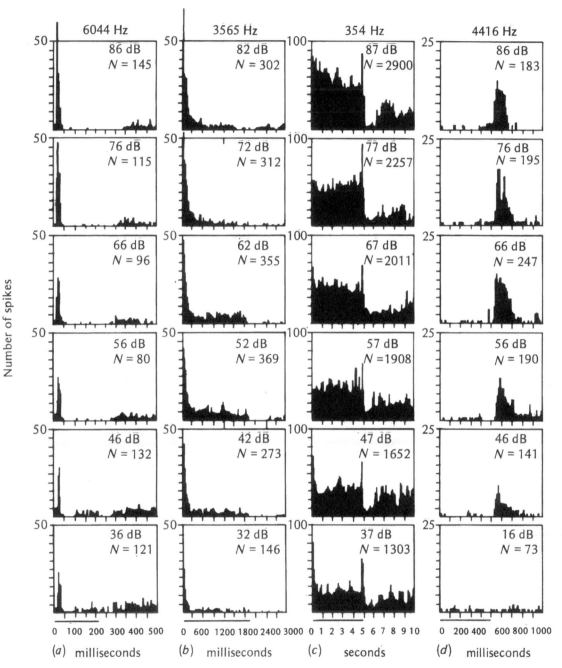

FIGURE 15.20 Post stimulus time (PST) histograms to tone bursts recorded from cortical units. Bar at bottom of each column = duration of the tone burst. Columns = variations in the patterns caused by changes in frequency. Rows = changes in level. Note that most of the units respond to changes (at onset or offset) in stimulation, rather than to the total duration of the stimulus. Adapted from Brugge and Merzenich (1973), with permission.

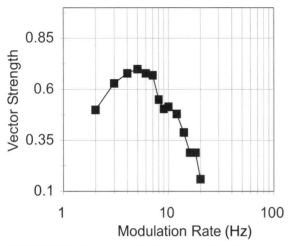

FIGURE 15.21 Vector strength of a neuron in the auditory cortex to a sinusoidally amplitude-modulated, 10-kHz carrier tone. The CF of the neuron was approximately 10 kHz. Vector strength is a measure of the ability of the neuron to phase lock to the modulated envelope of the amplitude-modulated sound (see Chapter 9). A vector strength of 1.0 indicates maximal phase locking. This neuron appears to phase lock best to a modulation rate of approximately 5 Hz. Adapted from Schreiner and Langner (1988), with permission.

modulation envelope. Low modulation rates are those that produce the largest amount of MDI and CMR (see Chapter 14). Thus, cortical amplitude and frequency modulation–sensitive neurons might underlie the perception of some of the more complex stimuli to which we are sensitive (see Chapter 14) like those that exist in studies of MDI and CMR.

As the PET data in Figure 15.11 suggest, there are regions of auditory cortex that appear to be involved with processing the pitch of complex sounds, especially the pitch of complex sounds with temporal regularity. The cortical region near the auditory cortex called *Heschl's gyrus* in humans (only humans have a Heschl's gyrus) and a *homologous* (meaning having a similar structure and position) region in the monkey auditory cortex seem to be very responsive to complex sounds that produce the perception of pitch.

Another method of studying the function of the auditory system is to cut, remove, or render unresponsive part of the system and to observe differences

in an animal's ability to process acoustic stimulation. Typically, animals are trained to make a response that indicates they have detected or recognized some auditory stimulus; a part of the cortex is then removed or altered, and the animal is retested to see whether there is a change in its ability to perform the original task. If so, the missing part of the cortex is assumed to be responsible for the animal's ability to analyze the stimulus for this auditory task. Experiments utilizing such *lesions* and behavioral techniques are difficult to summarize because of differences in the site and size of the lesions, the testing techniques, and the nature of the stimulus. Generally, simple tasks are less affected by cortical lesions than are more complex tasks. Pure-tone intensity and frequency discrimination tasks (see Chapter 10) may be disrupted after the lesion, but they can be relearned. More difficult tasks based on patterns (such as order of presentation or localization of a sound in space) suffer more after lesion of the auditory cortex than do simpler tasks. Thus, it appears probable that failure on different types of tasks reflects different deficits in central processing of the stimulus. On the other hand, failure to find a deficit, temporary or permanent, does not necessarily indicate that the lesioned structure did not take part in analysis of the stimulus tested in the normal animal. The animal behavioral studies, in agreement with the electrophysiology, appear to indicate that the cortical centers are organized more to process complex stimulus situations than to encode the basic parameters of the stimulus.

SUMMARY

In this chapter, we have attempted to describe briefly the anatomy and physiology of the central auditory nervous system. The anatomical description was limited to the main nuclei of the bilateral ascending and descending pathways of and to the auditory cortex in general. Both pathways were shown to have complicated innervations and bilateral representation at almost every nucleus. The interconnections within each nucleus were not discussed in detail, but their existence is evident. There is a wide variety in the neural morphology of CANS neurons, which most likely leads to a variety of physiological responses. Neural circuits within each nucleus appear to operate on excitatory and inhibitory interactions. Neural circuits may be studied using the slice preparation technique, and such circuits may exhibit properties such as lateral inhibition. The major nuclei of the central auditory nervous system are the cochlear nucleus (subdivided into the DCN, PVCN, and AVCN), superior olive (subdivided into the MSO and LSO), inferior colliculus (subdivided into the central nucleus, dorsal cortex, and paracentral nuclei), and auditory cortex (subdivided into AI, AII, SII, and EP). Tonotopic organization was said to be maintained at every level of the system, and tuning curves retained their sharpness for most neurons at all levels. The descending pathways perform a control function of both an excitatory and inhibitory nature on the incoming information. Time patterns of neurons in the central auditory system, both in the nuclei and the cortex, reflect the anatomical complexities of the nuclei, the pathways, and the cortex. Cells in the olivary complex and higher (e.g., the inferior colliculus) in the CANS discharge differentially to changes in interaural differences. Auditory-evoked responses and brain images are means of obtaining information concerning central auditory processing. The development of the auditory nervous system from its embryonic state and the plasticity of the central auditory nervous system can reveal important information about neural processing.

SUPPLEMENT

A great deal of the material in this chapter is covered in Chapters 6, 7, and 8 of the book by Pickles (1988), in books by Webster et al. (1992), Fay and Popper (1992), Altschuler et al. (1989), Jahn and Santos-Sacchi (2001), and Oertel et al. (2002). Information about neural development can be found in

Rubel et al. (1997), and information about plasticity is found in Parks et al. (2004). Work on development and plasticity can also be found in articles by Brugge et al. (1981) and Lippe and Rubel (1983) and in edited books by Ruben et al. (1986) and Werner and Rubel (1992). Information about plasticity in the barn owl can be found in the work of Knudsen (2004).

Two nuclei that were not discussed in any detail in this chapter were the lateral lemniscus and medial geniculate body (see Figure 15.1). Descriptions of both nuclei can be found in Oertel et al. (2002). Neurons in the lateral lemniscus appear to respond primarily to monaural stimulation, often with great temporal precision. There is speculation that it plays a role in determining the spectral and temporal patterns of complex sounds. The medial geniculate body is a multisensory nucleus receiving ascending and descending inputs from several sensory systems and as such presumably plays a role in integrating information about sound with that from other sensory systems.

The functional study of the CANS is in its infancy, with the major effort being devoted to describing the basic anatomical structures and physiological properties of these structures. As has been pointed out many times, both the anatomy and the physiology are complex, making it difficult to determine the functional role of any particular neural site. With few exceptions (e.g., the MSO and LSO), the functional role of the auditory nuclei are largely unknown. That is, very little is known about exactly what features of sound and sound sources are processed by each nucleus. Most of what we know about CANS function comes from studies of animals such as the bat (Suga, 1988) and the barn owl (Konishi et al., 1988). Articles by Wickesberg and Oertel (1990; see also Oertel et al., 2002) and Neti, Young, and Schneider (1992; see also Oertel et al., 2002) provide insights into some possible functional properties of the cochlear nucleus. Langer (1992) provides a similar review of modulation processing in the CANS. Shamma (1985) should be consulted for a review of one role that lateral inhibition might play in auditory processing. In addition to the brain-imaging work using human subjects

(Griffith et al., 1998, 2001), the work with monkeys on pitch processing by Bendor and Wang (2005) should be consulted.

The details about the various anatomical subareas of a nucleus often change over time as more is learned about its structure. This applies especially to the infe-rior colliculus, where the subareas defined in this chapter are based on the work of Morest and Oliver (1984). Auditory brainstem electric responses have proven to be useful tools in clinical assessment of the auditory system. Interested students might read text-books by E. J. Moore (1983) and by Glattke (1983).

16

The Abnormal Auditory System

The previous chapters have dealt with the structure and function of the normal auditory system. Over one's lifetime, these normal systems can become abnormal for many reasons. In these cases one may experience a hearing loss and, in extreme cases, deafness. While knowing about the normal auditory system is crucial for understanding the causes of hearing loss, it is also important to understand the abnormal auditory system. In addition, knowledge about the abnormal system can provide valuable information about the normal auditory system. Many things can be done to reduce the likelihood that the auditory system will be damaged, and a variety of sensory aids and rehabilitation strategies are available to help people who have a hearing loss. Medical interventions exist that can eliminate or reduce the severity of a hearing loss. Chapter 1 provided a general description of the clinical fields of *otology* and *audiology* and the practitioners in these fields. This chapter does not cover in any detail the treatment of hearing loss, but it does provide an overview of some of the things that can happen to the structure and function of the auditory system when it is damaged.

DAMAGE TO THE AUDITORY SYSTEM

In general, hearing loss can be caused by: *sound exposure*, *ototoxic drugs* (drugs and chemicals that are poisonous to auditory structures), *aging*, *diseases and infections*, *heredity*, and *accidents* (e.g., trauma to the head). Most is known about how the inner ear can be damaged, and a great deal of this knowledge is based on studies of *noise-induced hearing loss* (NIHL), which refers to changes in normal auditory function that occur as a consequence of exposure to intense levels of sound. In this context, sound at these high levels is considered unwanted because it causes hearing loss. *Noise* is used as a general term (as opposed to the more specific definitions provided in Chapters 4 and 11) to refer to any sound that is unwanted. In addition to causing a hearing loss, sound can become unwanted (a noise) because it interferes with work or play, interferes with communication, interferes with sleep, or is annoying.

EFFECTS OF NOISE ON THE INNER EAR

In Chapters 7 and 8, we discussed the important role of the hair cells and their stereocilia in converting or transducing the mechanical and hydrodynamic forces within the cochlea into neural impulses in the auditory nerve. Obviously, damage to the hair cells would drastically affect the transduction processes and change the ability to hear. Unfortunately, hair cells appear to be most vulnerable to overstimulation.

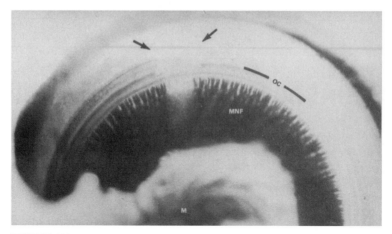

FIGURE 16.1 Low-power light micrograph of a large portion of the cochlea. The curvature of the cochlea is obvious. The innervation of the organ of Corti (OC) by the myelinated nerve fiber (MNF) leaving the modiolus (M) is clearly seen. The arrows indicate an area in which the organ of Corti is missing due to a lesion caused by acoustic overstimulation, that is, a loud sound. Chinchilla photographs courtesy of Dr. Ivan Hunter-Duvar, Hospital for Sick Children, Toronto.

The amount of inner ear damage is related to the exposure level of the noise, among other factors. Exposure to a very high level of noise can cause the type of inner ear destruction illustrated in Figure 16.1. In this example, the noise destroyed the entire organ of Corti in one section of the cochlea. It appears that the primary cause of inner ear damage is that the elastic limits of the organ of Corti were exceeded, and it was virtually torn apart. Noises with very high levels can also cause middle ear damage, such as rupture of the tympanic membrane. For lower levels of noise exposure, the outer hair cells may remain in place, but their stereocilia may swell, fuse, or otherwise be distorted, as shown in Figure 16.2. The stereocilia, tectorial membrane, and basilar membrane may all be structurally changed if the noise exposure is sufficiently intense. Because each of these structures plays an important role in the normal transduction of sound to neural impulses, their damage from noise exposure can produce significant hearing loss.

The effects of noise on hearing may be temporary or permanent. In mammals, if the hair cells are severely damaged, they will not recover or be replaced by new hair cells (see "Hair Cell Regeneration"). If hair cell damage is slight, hair cells can recover and hearing will return to normal. Mechanical destruction of the organ of Corti caused by exceeding its elastic limits will result in permanent loss of the hair cells. However, less severe hair cell damage is probably caused by various physicochemical processes, such as those associated with the metabolic activity (which takes place in the stria vascularis; see Chapter 8) of the overexerted hair cell. It is also possible that moderate noise exposure alters the sensitive biomechanical connections of the inner ear; especially those that might be maintained by the motile responses of the outer hair cells (see Chapter 8).

HEARING LOSS DUE TO NOISE EXPOSURE

Hearing may be affected in several ways by exposure to noise. One that has received the most attention is a change in hearing sensitivity, or threshold. An increase in auditory thresholds because of exposure to

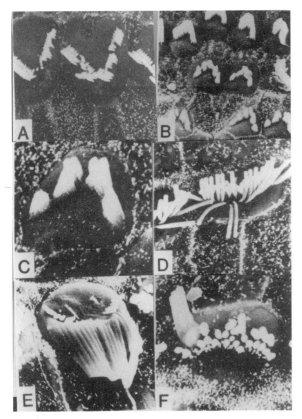

FIGURE 16.2 Various types of stereocilia distortion due to noise exposure. Micrographs A–C are outer hair cells (OHCs) and D–F are inner hair cells (IHCs). **(A)** Missing OHC stereocilia a few days after a pure-tone exposure. The remaining stereocilia are erect. **(B)** Three rows of OHCs showing various degrees of fusing of stereocilia due exposure. **(C)** Higher magnification of fused OHC stereocilia from B. **(D)** Floppy IHC stereocilia due to pure-tone exposure. This situation is probably not reversible. **(E)** Fused inner hair cell bundle (IHC). **(F)** IHC with many stereocilia missing and some remaining stereocilia fused due to noise exposure. This situation is not reversible. Chinchilla photomicrographs courtesy of Dr. Ivan Hunter-Duvar, Hospital for Sick Children, Toronto.

noise is called a *noise-induced threshold shift* (NITS). If over time, be it minutes, hours, or days, the threshold returns to its preexposure level (i.e., there is no NITS), it is called a *noise-induced temporary threshold shift* (NITTS) or simply *temporary threshold shift* (TTS). If, however, the threshold does not return to its

preexposure value, it is called a *noise-induced permanent threshold shift* (NIPTS) or simply PTS (*permanent threshold shift*). In many situations, the amount of TTS reaches a limit at an asymptotic value; in these cases the term *asymptotic threshold shift* (ATS) is used to describe the upper limit of TTS. In order to measure TTS or PTS, the threshold (see Appendix D and Chapter 10) is measured twice, once before the exposure and then again after the exposure.

After exposure to noise, the amount of hearing loss depends greatly on when the postexposure measurement is made. For most situations in which the noise exposure is moderately high, some hearing will be restored as time passes after the exposure is terminated. For many laboratory TTS studies, threshold measurements are made about 2 or 4 minutes after the exposing noise is terminated (labeled TTS_2 or TTS_4; the subscript refers to the time in minutes after the noise offset). This is done because it takes some finite amount of time to measure a threshold by most psychophysical techniques, especially when animals are the test listeners. Figure 16.3 shows how TTS_2 increases as the time of exposure and level of the exposing noise increase.

Even in PTS studies, after the exposure has ceased, some hearing is restored. Thus, measures of hearing loss made immediately at the end of an exposure may consist of two components, a temporary component that will recover to some degree (that is, TTS) and a permanent component that remains for a lifetime (that is, PTS). A hearing loss that combines TTS and PTS is called a *compound threshold shift*, or CTS.

TEMPORARY THRESHOLD SHIFT AS A FUNCTION OF LEVEL, DURATION, SPECTRAL CONTENT, AND TEMPORAL PATTERN

Several exposure stimulus factors affect the amount of TTS or PTS: <u>level, duration, spectral content, and temporal pattern</u>. Also, individual differences among people and species differences greatly affect the

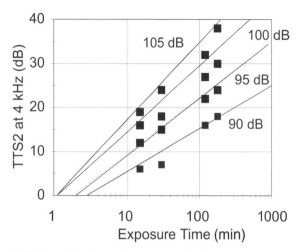

FIGURE 16.3 Growth of temporary threshold shift measured after 2 minutes (TTS$_2$) at 4 kHz after exposure to a bandpass noise (1200 to 1400 Hz) as a function of exposure time. Growth functions are shown for four different noise-exposure levels. Data of Ward et al. (1959), with permission.

magnitude of the threshold shift. The relationship between hearing loss and each of these factors is complex because no one factor can be considered apart from the others.

For continuous exposures of moderate intensities (approximately 75 to 105 dB SPL) lasting less than 8 hours, hearing loss (in decibels of threshold shift) as reflected in TTS measurements grows approximately linearly with increases in sound pressure level of the exposure stimulus. For low intensities, below about 70 or 75 dB SPL, there is no measurable TTS. At very high intensities, above about 130 dB SPL, the effects on hearing loss are more erratic as a function of varying sound level.

For moderate noise levels (80 to 105 dB), TTS is approximately proportional to the logarithm of the exposure time up to 8 or 12 hours, after which the amount of TTS appears to remain relatively constant. For instance, if a 15-minute exposure produces a TTS$_2$ of 10 dB and a 30-minute exposure produces a TTS$_2$ of 15 dB, then a 1-hour exposure will result in a TTS$_2$ of 20 dB (that is, for this example each doubling of the exposure time results in 5 dB of TTS$_2$).

Figure 16.3 illustrates the growth of TTS$_2$, measured at 4000 Hz, as a function of the duration of the exposure to a 1200- to 2400-Hz bandpassed filtered noise of various intensities.

A number of "rules" have been suggested to establish the amount of threshold shift that a noise might generate as a function of exposure duration. One rule, called the *equal energy rule of noise exposure*, states that sounds of the same energy produce the same threshold shift. Thus, for each doubling of a sound's duration, the sound power can be reduced 3 dB (see Chapters 3 and 10) to maintain the same energy and thus the same amount of TTS (thus, the equal energy rule is sometimes called the *3-dB rule*). Some data suggest that the sound power needs to be decreased by 5 dB or 4 dB for each doubling (the *5-dB* or *4-dB rule*) of duration to produce a constant amount of TTS.

The amount of measured TTS also depends on the frequency spectrum of the fatiguing sound and on the frequency at which the threshold is being measured. For exposure levels of less than 80 dBA or for short exposure durations that produce thresholds shifts lasting less than 2 minutes, the maximum TTS occurs at test frequencies that are equal to those of the exposure stimulus. TTS decreases equally along the spectrum on both sides away from the exposure frequency that produces the maximum TTS. For higher-level exposures (greater than 80 dBA) that produce longer-lasting TTS, the maximum effect does *not* occur at the frequency of the exposure sound. Also, TTS is not produced equally for exposure stimuli of different frequencies even though the level of the exposure may be the same at all frequencies. In general, more TTS is produced at higher frequencies, at least up to approximately 4 to 6 kHz. Thus, when the exposure stimulus is a broadband noise, maximum TTS is found at frequencies between 3000 and 6000 Hz (Figure 16.4). When the exposure is a pure tone, TTS is found to increase as the frequency of the exposure tone increases. Furthermore, maximum TTS occurs at frequencies above the exposure frequency, with progressively higher frequencies showing the maximum TTS as the level of the exposure is increased. For high levels of exposure to a pure tone, the maximum TTS is

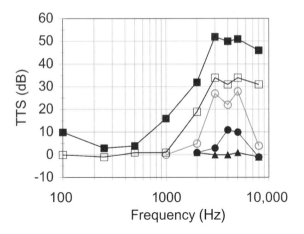

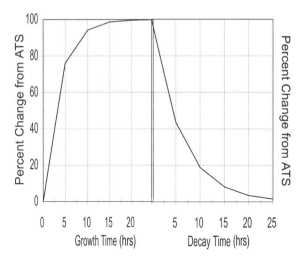

FIGURE 16.4 Amount of hearing loss in dB as a function of signal frequency with a 20-minute, 115-dB SPL, white, broadband Gaussian noise as the exposure stimulus. The curves represent temporary threshold shifts (TTS) measured at various times after the noise was turned off. Some hearing loss is still evident 24 hours after exposure to the noise. Adapted from Postman and Egan (1949), by permission.

FIGURE 16.5 Growth and decay of temporary threshold shift (TTS) as a function of exposure time and time after exposure. The amount of TTS is plotted in terms of percentage of asymptotic threshold shift (ATS), that is, a percentage of the maximum amount of TTS. The curves are a fit to a wide variety of data. The growth curve is fit by the equation $y = D(1 - \exp(-t/T))$ and the decay curve by $y = C \exp(-t/T)$, where D and C are constants, T is the growth or decay constant, t is the exposure time or time after exposure, and "exp" is the exponential argument. Adapted from Melnick (1991), with permission.

produced one-half to one octave above the exposure frequency (sometimes called the *half-octave shift*). The spread of TTS to higher test frequencies is also seen for bands of noise where the maximum TTS is produced one-half to one octave above the upper cutoff frequency of the exposing noise band. The exact relationship between the frequency region of maximal TTS (or PTS) and the parameters of the exposing stimulus is complex and depends on the details of the situation in which the exposure takes place.

The relation between hearing loss and the temporal pattern of the exposure stimulus is extremely complex, and a detailed explanation is beyond the scope of this text. For instance, when an exposure is intermittent, hearing may recover somewhat during the time the noise is turned off or increase when the noise comes on again, or it may stimulate the middle ear reflex (helping to reduce the effect of the noise on the inner ear; see Chapter 6). The situation is further complicated if the exposure stimulus has high peak

levels of short duration (e.g., the sound of a gunshot). Such stimuli are called *impulses*, and their effects on hearing are difficult to study because they can vary in many ways, such as peak pressure, pulse duration, rise and decay time, direction of the pressure change (rarefaction or condensation), repetition rate, and the number of impulses in a given exposure period.

RECOVERY OF HEARING AFTER NOISE EXPOSURE

In many cases, hearing loss will disappear after the exposing noise is turned off. Figure 16.5 shows how the threshold shift builds up (growth) as the duration of the noise exposure increases and then decreases (decay) as the time after the cessation of the noise increases. The functions shown in the figure caption represent curves fit to data from several studies. As

the influence of genes on the development of the auditory system and hearing disorders is the use of *transgenetic* mice (see Appendix F).

RELATION BETWEEN INNER EAR DAMAGE AND HEARING LOSS

We have seen that noise or drug exposure or other variables can lead to inner ear damage and its resultant hearing loss. We might therefore expect that measuring threshold shift would indicate the amount of inner ear damage. Several studies have investigated this proposition, using animals that can be trained to respond to the presence or absence of a sound. Threshold sensitivity curves can be measured with these animals by various psychophysical techniques (see Appendix D). After their normal hearing has been assessed, the animals are exposed to the noise or some other agent that can cause hearing loss; then their hearing recovery curves are calculated, and the amount of PTS is determined. Once PTS is established across the frequency range, the inner ears are prepared for histological observation via various microscopic techniques (see Appendix F). The histological examination assesses the condition of the organ of Corti along the whole length of the basilar membrane, with particular attention to the condition of each hair cell. The orderly arrangement of the hair cells allows the investigator to count the existing hair cells and also those that are missing. Such plots are called *cytocochleograms* or simply *cochleograms*; one is shown at the bottom of Figure 16.6. The top of Figure 16.6 shows PTS for this animal as a function of the frequency tested. Note the correspondence between the way in which the hearing loss is distributed from low to high frequencies and the way the outer hair cell loss is distributed from apex to base along the cochlea. Such a correspondence supports the place theory of frequency encoding (Chapter 8), which states that each place along the cochlear partition codes for a particular frequency.

The correspondence between hair cell loss and threshold shift is not always as straightforward as Figure 16.6 suggests. The amount and pattern of hair

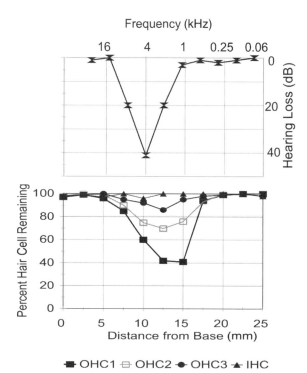

FIGURE 16.6 A cochleogram is shown (**bottom**) for an animal exposed to a signal with frequencies in the 4000-Hz region of the spectrum. As can be seen, between 10 and 15 mm from the base there are missing outer hair cells (OHC1, 2, and 3 for the three rows) but few missing inner hair cells. Permanent threshold shifts (**top**) were measured in a spectral region from 1 to 16 kHz. The figure shows the typical correspondence between the frequency region of a hearing loss and a localized region of outer hair cell loss. Adapted from Moody, Stebbins, and Hawkins (1976), with permission.

cell damage caused by the same noise, drug exposure, or other insult can vary greatly between individuals. Also, the hearing loss and hair cell damage do not always correspond with each other. A further complication is that different animal species differ in susceptibility to acoustic overstimulation, drug dose, etc. Thus, it is difficult to generalize from research on animals to the effects on humans.

As reviewed in Chapters 8 and 9, the inner and outer hair cells have different functions. Thus, it is reasonable to assume that the consequences of damage to each type of hair cell will differ. Figure 16.7a shows a normal tuning curve (solid line) and a neural tuning curve after the outer hair cells were destroyed but the inner hair cells remained relatively intact (dotted line). Figure 16.7b shows a similar comparison, but for when the inner hair cells have received more damage than the outer hair cells. Figure 16.7c shows a comparison of tuning curves when both the outer and inner hair cells are damaged.

As can be seen, the loss of outer hair cells (Figure 16.7a) results in a significant loss in neural sensitivity in the region of the "tip" of the tuning curve, that is, in the frequency region to which the nerve fiber is tuned. There appears to be a shift toward higher frequencies for the lowest sensitivity (CF) of the tuning curve after outer hair cell damage. There is a small change in the low-frequency "tail" of the tuning curve after outer hair cell damage, and the difference in the "tip-to-tail" sensitivity changes by about 40 dB after outer hair cell damage. Inner hair cell loss (Figure 16.7b) tends to preserve the general shape of the tuning curve but results in a 40- to 50-dB overall loss in the sensitivity of the nerve. When both types of hair cells are damaged (Figure 16.7c), the shape of the tuning curve is altered, as it was for the condition when just the outer hair cells are damaged, and there is a very large decrease (75 to 90 dB) in neural sensitivity. Changes in the sensitivity and shape of the tuning curves suggest that both hearing sensitivity and frequency resolution would be severely altered when outer hair cells are destroyed. Damage to just the inner hair cells would probably result in hearing loss as measured by threshold shift, but since the shape of the tuning curve is not significantly altered, frequency resolution may not be affected as much.

Other changes occur in the function of the auditory nerve following hair cell loss. For instance, when outer hair cells are damaged, the nonlinear (compressive) input–output relationship between sound level input and either basilar membrane displacement (see Chapter 7, Figure 7.19) or auditory nerve discharge rate (see Chapter 9, Figure 9.2) becomes much more linear, especially for signals whose frequencies are near the CF of the fiber. The loss of the compressive

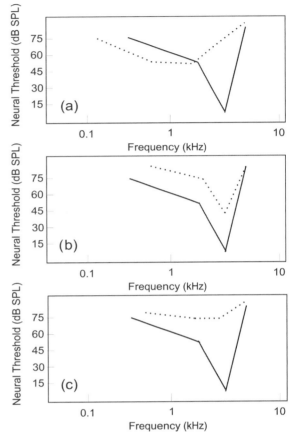

FIGURE 16.7 A comparison of a normal auditory nerve tuning curve (solid dark line) with its tip at CF and low-frequency tail with tuning curves from animals with severely damaged or missing hair cells (dotted curve). **(a)** Comparison when outer hair cells are severely damaged, showing the loss of the highly tuned tip of the tuning curve, loss of sensitivity, and movement of the tip toward high frequencies. **(b)** Comparison when inner hair cells are severely damaged, showing that the tuning curve maintains its overall shape but that there is an overall loss of sensitivity. **(c)** Comparison when both inner and outer hair cells are severely damaged, showing a major loss in sensitivity and a significant change in the shape of the tuning curve.

nature of coding sound level is probably responsible for several manifestations of hearing impairment. For instance, loudness recruitment (see Chapter 13, Figure 13.2) can be partially explained by the loss of nonlinear compression due to outer hair cell loss.

The loss of hair cells may occur in isolated and different regions of the cochlea. Recall that the cochlea transduces sound in a frequency-specific manner, so a loss of hair cells in one region of the cochlea means that one region of the spectrum will probably not be coded in the auditory nerve, potentially leading to a hearing loss for those frequencies. Measuring thresholds and other frequency-specific perceptions at particular frequencies can expose where *dead zones* may be. These perceptual dead zones at particular frequencies often represent regions of the cochlea of hair cell damage.

HAIR CELL REGENERATION

As mentioned previously, mammalian hair cells do not regrow (*regenerate*) after they have been damaged. As a result, damaged hair cells lead to a permanent loss of hearing. However, in some species (birds, fish, and amphibians) hair cells appear to regenerate after being destroyed from exposure to intense noise or ototoxic drugs. In birds it has been shown that not only do hair cells regenerate after damage, but they appear to regain their physiological function of generating nerve impulses. In some bird species, auditory thresholds recover to near-normal levels after intense noise or ototoxic drug exposure. Thus, for birds (and perhaps fish), hair cells can regenerate, and as a result these species may not experience permanent hearing loss due to noise or ototoxic drug exposure. Figure 16.8 shows a *basilar papilla* from a bird (zebra finch) immediately after a major noise exposure and the basilar papilla 90 days following the exposure. The basilar papilla is the sensory receptor surface in birds that contains auditory hair cells. The basilar papilla 90 days later is near normal, indicating that the hair cells have regenerated.

Why the hair cells of fish and birds regenerate and those of mammals do not is incompletely understood. The inner ear of birds and fish is different from that of mammals. For instance, neither species has the coiled cochlea that characterizes mammalian inner ears. It is also the case that the hair cells that exist in

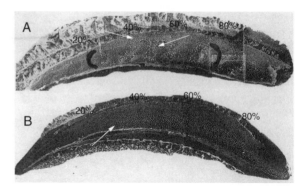

FIGURE 16.8   **(A)** The basilar papilla from a bird (zebra finch) obtained immediately after 24 hours of exposure to an intense sound. A large area of abnormal or missing hair cells is noted in the region bracketed by the black parentheses and highlighted by the arrows. **(B)** The basilar papilla from a bird exposed to the same sound but allowed to recover 90 days before the basilar papilla was studied. The hair cells appear normal or near normal throughout the entire basilar papilla, suggesting that the hair cells have regenerated after damage. From Ryals et al. (1999), with permission.

fish and in most birds are not excited by a membrane that vibrates with traveling wave properties. The arrangement of the hair cells also differs in birds and fish from that found in most mammals. Several other differences in the basic anatomy and the genetic makeup of the hair cells of birds and fish offer suggestions as to why hair cells may regenerate in birds and fish but not in mammals. Recent studies of a gene (*Atoh1*) that controls hair cell growth during development have been manipulated in the guinea pig both to slow down and to increase the generation of hair cells in this mammal. Inserting *Atoh1* into the inner ear of the guinea pig that had had its hair cells destroyed with ototoxic drugs yielded the growth of new hair cells and the return of some normal physiological cochlear function. Thus, such genetic treatment offers the promise of a method of regenerating hair cells in mammals.

There is also growing evidence that the hair cells and maybe neurons higher in the auditory system can be protected from overstimulation or ototoxicity. Providing certain drugs appears to protect the hair cells of some animals from being damaged by ototoxic drugs or acoustic overstimulation. It also appears that presenting a moderate level of noise prior to presenting an intense, potentially damaging noise level can reduce the amount of TTS and PTS in some animals.

AUDITORY CENTRAL NERVOUS SYSTEM CHANGES

While most is known about the effects of noise and other agents on the inner ear, several important changes have also been studied in the brainstem and cortical regions responsible for auditory processing. An important concept in investigating central nervous system changes that result as a function of exposure to environmental conditions is plasticity, as discussed in Chapter 15.

The *cochlear implant* offers another example of the possible plasticity of auditory function. The cochlear implant, or prosthesis, is a wire containing up to 22 electrodes that is inserted into the cochlea (following surgery) of people with significant hearing loss that is of a cochlear origin. A sound transducer translates sound into electrical current that stimulates the different electrodes, which in turn can stimulate surviving auditory nerve fibers. Each electrode carries information about a specific frequency region of the sound according to the way in which the transducer operates. Since each electrode is at a different place along the cochlea, presumably the frequency information is distributed in the cochlea in a manner similar (but by no means identical) to way the normal cochlea operates. The current follows the approximate amplitude envelope of the sound. Many patients fit with a cochlear implant can learn to function very well with sound, often gaining significant ability to understand speech and even music. In many cases, people who have had no or little ability to hear throughout most of their life learn to use sound when fitted with a cochlear implant. This suggests that the auditory system can "learn" to process this new form of information. If so, then the auditory system is exhibiting strong evidence for neural plasticity. Recently brainstem implants have been successfully used to stimulate the cochlear

nucleus of patients with tumors that have rendered the auditory nerve inoperative. There is some promise that bilaterally implanting patients with a cochlear implant in both ears may restore better sound localization and speech perception in noisy environments. If so, then it is likely that some form of neural plasticity occurs in patients successfully implanted with such bilateral devices that enable them to use acoustic information they previously were unable to use.

Amplification hearing aids are the more widely used form of hearing aids. In principle, amplification aids are simple devices that amplify sound as an aid for people with mild to moderate hearing loss. Most modern hearing aids amplify sound in a frequency-specific manner so that sound in the region of the spectrum where the patient has a hearing loss (usually in the high frequencies) is amplified and sound in spectral regions where the patient has better hearing is amplified less or not amplified at all. Recall from Chapter 13 that recruitment occurs for most patients with a hearing loss, meaning that amplifying loud sounds will make such sounds uncomfortably loud. Thus, some aids contain technology (compression electronics) that allows soft sounds to be amplified more than loud sounds so as to limit the overstimulation that results from recruitment. The use of digital technology offers other advantages for many hearing aids, such that their users can receive amplification for sounds that are the most challenging for them to perceive.

SUMMARY

Intense sounds, aging, ototoxic drugs, disease and infections, accidents, and heredity may lead to an abnormal auditory system. Hearing loss caused by high sound levels can be permanent (causing PTS) or temporary (causing TTS). The level, duration, spectral content, and temporal pattern of the exposing sound all influence the amount of PTS and TTS and the way in which TTS decreases after cessation of the exposing sound. Ototoxic drugs (such as kanamycin, neomycin, and streptomycin)

damage different tissues of the auditory system, often in a selective manner. Other drugs (such as salicylate and quinine) can cause tinnitus or hearing loss. Hearing loss due to aging (presbycusis) progresses from high to low frequencies as we age. Many diseases or conditions can lead to hearing loss (e.g., otitis media, otosclerosis, Meinere's disease, tumors). Many forms of hearing loss are also inheritable. Cochleograms reveal the relationship between hair cell loss and the frequency region of PTS. Auditory nerve tuning curves change in different ways, depending on whether inner or outer hair cells are damaged. While the hair cells of mammals do not regenerate, those of many birds and fish appear to regrow, and perhaps regain their function, after being damaged or destroyed. The anatomy and physiology of the central auditory nervous system often change (plasticity is demonstrated) as a result of insult, injury, or other forms of alterations in how acoustic input reaches the central nervous system. Cochlear implants and amplification hearing aids can benefit people with impaired hearing.

SUPPLEMENT

The book by Moore (1995), *Perceptual Consequences of Cochlear Damage*, provides a thorough review of the existing data on inner ear damage and its effects on hearing. Van de Water, Popper, and Fay's (1996) book covers material related to clinical issues, including aspects of the genetic causes of hearing loss. Pickles (1988) provides a good overview of many ototoxic drugs, especially how they are used to better understand auditory structure and function. The website of the National Institutes on Deafness and Other Communication Disorders (NIDCD) of the National Institutes of Health (NIH) (www.nih.gov/nidcd) often provides up-to-date material on clinical issues in hearing and how they relate to the basic hearing sciences.

Interest in the effects of noise on hearing had resurgence during World War II, and research on the subject has continued since then. As a result, there is a large body of literature and several published summaries. Two texts, one edited by Henderson et al. (1976) and the other edited by Hamernik et al. (1982), and a series of articles in volume 90 (issue 1) of *The Journal of the Acoustical Society of America* (1991) represent an outstanding collection of research relevant to the effects of noise on hearing.

As a result of noise exposure studies on humans and animals, criteria have been established for the levels and durations of exposures likely to cause PTS. Called *damage risk criteria* (DRC), these data show the combinations of duration and level that can be expected to cause permanent hearing loss if we are exposed to them on a regular basis, such as at work. The damage risk criteria were first developed by the Committee on Hearing, Bioacoustics, and Biomechanics (CHABA) of the National Research Council, the action organization of the National Academy of Sciences. Recent standards developed by the Environmental Protection Agency (EPA) and the Occupational Safety and Health Agency (OSHA) recommend that people not be exposed in the workplace to sound levels that exceed 85 dBA in any 8-hour day. Other standards for permissible noise level exist for community noise, airport noise exposure, and noise in the workplace (see Harris, 1991).

A major goal of the work on TTS was to use TTS to predict what might lead to PTS. For obvious reasons, studies of PTS are difficult to do in humans, yet it is crucial to understand what noise exposure conditions might lead to PTS. By studying TTS and ATS, it was hoped that reliable predictions for PTS could be obtained. The CHABA DRC were largely based on TTS data and assumptions concerning the ability of TTS to predict PTS. A great deal of data suggest that many of these assumptions are not valid, indicating that caution is required in using TTS and ATS measures as predictors of PTS (see Melnick, 1991). Clark (1991a) provides a review of the damaging effects of everyday sounds. Impulse noise (brief but intense noise) presents several special problems for the accurate assessment of noise and its effects on hearing. These short-duration sounds have a broad spectrum (see Chapter 4), and both the level of the sound and its spectral content determine the amount of threshold shift (see Patterson, 1991).

Understanding why fish and bird hair cells regenerate and those of mammals do not is an important area of study. If a way can be found to regenerate hair cells, then many forms of hair loss might be overcome by whatever intervention causes hair cell regeneration (see, for instance, Salvi et al., 1996). The recent work involving an adenoviral vector to deliver the gene *Atoh1* into the inner ear of the guinea pig was done by Izumikawa et al. (2005).

Canlon et al. (1988) have studied the neural "toughening" that is thought to occur following moderated exposure to sound. Also see Campbell (2002) for information on druglike treatments that might protect hair cells from overstimulation. Fan-Gang et al. (2004) and Miller and Spelman (1990) should be consulted to learn more about the cochlear prosthesis. The book by Sandlin (2000) can be consulted for some of the literature regarding amplification hearing aids. Animals have been used in noise and hearing research since Pavlov's work in the 1920s. Most systematic current studies using animal models can trace their origins to the study of Miller et al. (1963), which used the cat as the animal model. In 1963, Miller introduced the chinchilla as an animal for use in hearing research. Later studies by Miller (1970), Carder and Miller (1972), and Clark (1991b) indicate that the chinchilla is a widely used animal model for hearing. The work of Fay (1988) should be consulted to learn more about other animal models used to study hearing.

Appendix A: Sinusoids and Trigonometry

In addition to describing harmonic motion or vibration, sinusoids describe the relationship between sides and angles of triangles. The sinusoidal function is one of many *trigonometric functions*. Figure A.1 is a triangle with sides A, B, and C and angles a (opposite side A), b (opposite side B), and c (opposite side C). The following equations describe some of the trigonometric relationships among sides and angles:

$$\sin a = A/B, \quad \cos a = C/B, \quad \tan a = A/C, \quad (A.1)$$

where sin is the sine function, cos the cosine function, and tan the tangent function.

Another way to view these three trigonometric relationships is presented in Figure A.2. The circle is a *unit circle* (radius of 1); "sin a" describes how far the point P has moved along the circumference of the unit circle from the zero (or starting) position in the vertical direction, and "cos a" describes how far point P has moved along the unit circle from the zero (or starting) point in the horizontal direction. Note that the sine function starts at 0, goes to 1, and back through 0 to -1, then to 0 again as angle a increases from $0°$ to $360°$. The cosine function, however, starts at 1, goes to 0, then to -1, back to 0, and then to 1 as angle a increases from $0°$ to $360°$.

The tangent function is formed from the sine and cosine functions:

$$\tan a = \sin a / \cos a. \quad (A.2)$$

This can easily be seen from equation (A.1):

$$
\begin{aligned}
A = B\sin a \quad &\text{and} \quad C = B\cos a, \\
&= \tan a = A/C = (B\sin a)/(B\cos a) \quad (A.3) \\
&= \sin a / \cos a
\end{aligned}
$$

Given equation (A.2), we see that the tangent takes on values from minus infinity to positive infinity as the angle a is varied.

Some of the relationships among the trigonometric functions that provide powerful tools in analyzing acoustic signals are as follows:

$$\sin a = \cos(90° - a) \quad \text{or} \quad \cos a = \sin(90° - a) \quad (A.4)$$

$$\sin^2 a + \cos^2 a = 1. \quad (A.5)$$

Equations (A.4) and (A.5) can be derived directly from the unit circle shown in Figure A.2.

Other relationships are:

$$\sin(a \pm b) = \sin a \cos b \pm \cos a \sin b \quad (A.6)$$

$$\cos(a \pm b) = \cos a \cos b \pm \sin a \sin b \quad (A.7)$$

$$\sin a + \sin b = 2\{\sin[(\tfrac{1}{2})(a+b)] \times \cos[(\tfrac{1}{2})(a-b)]\} \quad (A.8)$$

$$\sin 2a = 2\sin a \cos a \quad (A.9)$$

$$\sin a \sin b = (\tfrac{1}{2})[\cos(a-b) - \cos(a+b)]. \quad (A.10)$$

Many more relationships can be derived from those just listed. For instance, we can derive $\cos 2a$ from equation (A.7):

$$
\begin{aligned}
\cos 2a = \cos(a+a) &= \cos a \cos a - \sin a \sin a \\
&= \cos^2 a - \sin^2 a.
\end{aligned}
$$

Rearranging equation (A.5), we get

$$\sin^2 a = 1 - \cos^2 a.$$

And substituting for $\sin^2 a$ in the equation for $\cos 2a$ we obtain

$$\cos 2a = \cos^2 a - (1 - \cos^2 a) = 2\cos^2 a - 1. \quad (A.11)$$

USING SINUSOIDS TO DESCRIBE ACOUSTIC EVENTS

These few ideas concerning sinusoids and trigonometry can help solve and describe a great variety of acoustic situations, e.g., (1) to determine the instantaneous amplitude of a sinusoid at different times and for different frequencies and starting phases, and (2) to investigate nonlinearities.

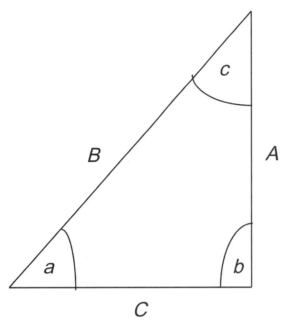

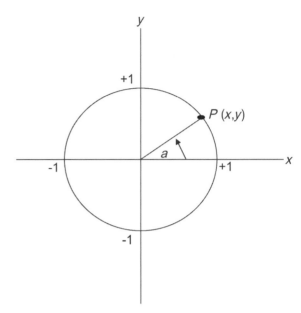

FIGURE A.1 Trigonometric functions are derived from the relationships among the sides A, B, and C and angles a, b, and c of a right triangle.

FIGURE A.2 The sine and cosine functions can be viewed as the distance point P moves along the unit circle.

Suppose there is a 100-Hz sinusoid with a peak amplitude A and a starting phase of $0°$ and that we would like to know the instantaneous amplitude one and a quarter thousandths of a second (1.25 msec) after the sinusoidal vibration begins. We can use the equation for a sinusoid (A.12) to obtain this result. The equation $y = A \sin(2\pi ft + \theta)$ is the definition of a sinusoid when the sinusoidal terms are expressed in radians. We can change the equation for terms expressed in degrees by using the following:

$$y = A\sin(360° \times 1/T \times t + \theta), \qquad (A.12)$$

where T is the period of the sinusoid in seconds ($1/T$, of course, equals f), θ is the starting phase, A is the peak amplitude, and y is the instantaneous amplitude. In our example, $T = 1/100$ sec (10 msec), $t = 1.25/1000$ sec (1.25 msec), and $\theta = 0°$. Thus,

$$y = A\sin(360° \times 1/(1/100) \times 1.25/1000 + 0)$$
$$= A\sin(360° \times 1.25/10) = A\sin 45°.$$

The sin of $45°$ is 0.707, so 1.25 msec after a 100-Hz vibration begins, the instantaneous amplitude is $0.707A$ in magnitude. Thus, if the peak amplitude was 100 micropascals of pressure, the instantaneous amplitude at 1.25 msec would be 70.7 micropascals.

If θ were $30°$ instead of $0°$, then the equation would be

$$A\sin(45° + \theta) = A\sin(45° + 30°)$$
$$= A\sin 75° = A \times 0.97,$$

or, in our example, where A is 100 micropascals, the instantaneous amplitude of a 100-Hz vibration with starting phase of $30°$ would be 97 micropascals at 1.25 msec after it started.

NONLINEARITY

A linear system, as we stated in Chapter 5, is one described by a straight-line relationship between the input to the system and its output. The general equation for a straight line is

$$y = mx + b,\qquad\text{(A.13)}$$

where m = slope constant, b = intercept constant, x = input, and y = output.

A nonlinear system is one described by a relationship between an input and output that is not represented by a straight line. One such simple nonlinear equation is

$$y = x + x^2.\qquad\text{(A.14)}$$

If we assume that the input to the system is the sum of two sinusoids, $A \sin 2\pi f_1 t + A \sin 2\pi f_2 t$, then, according to equation (A.14),

$$x = A \sin 2\pi f_1 t + A \sin 2\pi f_2 t.$$

(Throughout this discussion, we shall assume that all phase angles θ are zero.)

Since $y = x + x^2$, the value of y is as follows:

$$
\begin{aligned}
y &= A \sin 2\pi f_1 t + A \sin 2\pi f_2 t \\
&\quad + (A \sin 2\pi f_1 t + A \sin 2\pi f_2 t)^2 \\
&= A \sin 2\pi f_1 t + A \sin 2\pi f_2 t + [A^2 \sin^2(2\pi f_1 t) \\
&\quad + 2A^2(\sin 2\pi f_1 t)\sin 2\pi f_2 t + A^2 \sin^2(2\pi f_2 t)]
\end{aligned}
$$
$$\text{(A.15)}$$

Let us look at the last three terms of equation (A.15) and use trigonometric identities.

First, using equation (A.10), we get

$$
\begin{aligned}
A^2 \sin^2(2\pi f_1 t) &= A^2(\sin 2\pi f_1 t \sin 2\pi f_1 t) \\
&= (A^2/2)[-\cos(2\pi(2f_1)t) + \cos(2\pi(0)t)] \\
&= (A^2/2)[-\cos(2\pi(2f_1)t) + 1] \\
&= -(A^2/2)\cos(2\pi(2f_1)t) + A^2/2 \\
&= A^2/2 - (A^2/2)[\cos(2\pi(2f_1)t)].
\end{aligned}
$$
$$\text{(A.16)}$$

Second, using equation (A.10), we get

$$
\begin{aligned}
2A^2 \sin^2 2\pi f_1 t \sin 2\pi f_2 t \\
= A^2\cos(2\pi(f_1 - f_2)t) - A^2\cos(2\pi(f_1 + f_2)t).
\end{aligned}
$$
$$\text{(A.17)}$$

Third, using equation (A.16) but substituting f_2 for f_1, we get

$$A^2\sin^2(2\pi f_2 t) = A^2/2 - A^2/2[\cos(2\pi(2f_2)t)].$$
$$\text{(A.18)}$$

By combining these three parts with the results of equation (A.15), we have

$$
\begin{aligned}
y &= A \sin 2\pi f_1 t + A \sin 2\pi f_2 t - A^2/[2\cos(2\pi(2f_1)t)] \\
&\quad - A^2/[2\cos(2\pi(2f_2)t)] + A^2\cos(2\pi(f_1 - f_2)t) \\
&\quad - A^2\cos(2\pi(f_1 + f_2)t)A^2.
\end{aligned}
$$
$$\text{(A.19)}$$

This in turn means that when f_1 and f_2 are the input frequencies of x, the following frequencies described in equation (A.19) constitute the output y if the output y is from the nonlinear system described in equation (A.15). These frequencies are $f_1, f_2, 2f_1, 2f_2, f_1 - f_2$, and $f_1 + f_2$. They may be the aural harmonics $(2f_1, 2f_2)$ and combination tones $(f_1 - f_2, f_1 + f_2)$ described in Chapters 5, 7, 8, 11, and 13.

VECTORS

In the previous examples, sinusoids of different frequencies were added together. In adding sinusoids of the same frequency, both the amplitudes and the starting phases of the sinusoids must be considered. Notice the example shown in Figure A.3. The two original sinusoids (A_1 and A_2) have the same frequency and amplitudes, but the starting phases are different. The resultant sinusoid has a different phase from either of the original starting phases, and the resultant amplitude is not the simple algebraic sum of the original two amplitudes.

An easy method of calculating the resultant amplitude and starting phase uses *vector addition*. In vector addition each unit to be added has two values: a magnitude and a direction, or phase value. For the addition of sinusoids the peak amplitude is the magnitude of the vector, and the starting phase is the direction or phase of the vector. Thus, for the example shown in Figure A.3, the vector diagram in Figure A.4 may be used to determine the sum or resultant peak amplitude

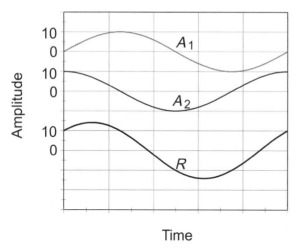

FIGURE A.3   The sum of two sinusoids (A_1 and A_2); see text.

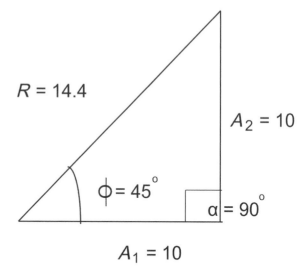

FIGURE A.4   Vector diagram for the condition shown in Figure A.3. The lengths of the vectors are the amplitudes of the two sinusoids, and the phase, α, is the starting phase difference between the two sinusoids. The resultant amplitude and phase can be determined from this right triangle or from equations (A.20) and (A.21).

and starting phase. The vector diagram of Figure A.4 is constructed by first plotting the amplitude of the sinusoid with the smallest starting phase angle as a horizontal line with a length proportional to its peak amplitude (A_1). A line representing the other sinusoid is drawn at angle α to the line A_1 and with a length proportional to its peak amplitude (A_2). The angle α is the difference in the starting phases between the two sinusoids. The resultant vector is determined by completing the triangle. Thus, the resultant sinusoid has a peak amplitude R and a starting phase of θ, as shown in Figure A.4. Rather than having to construct vector diagrams, some *trigonometric identities* may be used to solve for the resultant vector's magnitude (peak amplitude) and phase (starting phase):

$$R^2 = A_1^2 + A_2^2 + 2A_1A_2 \cos\alpha, \qquad (A.20)$$

and

$$\theta = \cos^{-1}[(R^2 + A_1^2 - A_2^2)/2RA_1], \qquad (A.21)$$

where A_1 and A_2 are the peak amplitudes of the two sinusoids being added together, such that A_1 represents the sinusoid with the small starting phase angle, α is the difference in the starting phases of these two sinusoids, R is the resultant peak amplitude, θ is the resultant starting phase, and $\cos^{-1}$ means the angle whose cosine

equals the ratio $(R^2 + A_1^2 - A_2^2)/2RA_1$. Equations (A.20) and (A.21) are called the *law of cosines*.

For example, in Figure A.3 and the vector diagram of Figure A.4, the resultant peak amplitude and starting phase using the law of cosines are:

$$R^2 = 10^2 + 10^2 + 2 \times 10 \times 10 \cos 90°$$
$$= 100 + 100 + 200 \times 0 = 200;$$

so

$$R = \sqrt{200} = 14.14.$$

And

$$\theta = \cos^{-1}[(14.14^2 + 10^2 - 10^2)/(2 \times 14.14 \times 10)]$$
$$\theta = \cos^{-1}(200/282.80)$$
$$\theta = \cos^{-1}(0.707)$$
$$\theta = 45°.$$

To find the inverse cos, or $\cos^{-1}$, or arccos, using a calculator or a computer program, look for keys or values that say arc, or $\cos^{-1}$, or arccos; enter the number (e.g., 0.707) and then the appropriate key or key sequence. On some calculators and programs, you may need to make sure that the calculator is in the "degree" rather than in the "radian" mode.

Vector diagrams and the law of cosines are useful tools for obtaining the magnitude (amplitude, R) and phase (starting phase, θ) in situations involving values of objects having both a magnitude (amplitude) and a direction component (starting phase).

The following table presents some values of $\sin a$, where a is an angle in degrees.

a (degrees)	$\sin a$	a (degrees)	$\sin a$	a (degrees)	$\sin a$	a (degrees)	$\sin a$
0	0.0						
15	0.26	105	0.97	195	−0.26	285	−0.97
30	0.50	120	0.87	210	−0.50	300	−0.87
45	0.707	135	0.707	225	−0.707	315	−0.707
60	0.87	150	0.50	240	−0.87	330	−0.50
75	0.97	165	0.26	255	−0.97	345	−0.26
90	1.0	180	0.0	270	−1.0	360	0.0

Appendix B: Logarithms

The logarithm is the solution to the following equation for x; that is, if

$$y = 10^x, \qquad \text{(B.1)}$$

then

$$x = \log_{10} y. \qquad \text{(B.2)}$$

In other words, $\log_{10} y$ (for simplicity, $\log y$) is the logarithm to the base 10 of the number y. Thus, x is the number to which 10 must be raised in order to obtain the answer y. A set of simple relationships between x and $\log y$ can be demonstrated:

$$
\begin{aligned}
0 &= \log 1, &&\text{since } 1 = 10^0 \\
1 &= \log 10, &&\text{since } 100 = 10^1 \\
2 &= \log 100, &&\text{since } 100 = 10^2 \\
3 &= \log 1000, &&\text{since } 100 = 10^3
\end{aligned}
\qquad \text{(B.3)}
$$

So, for instance, $\log 1{,}000{,}000$ is $\log 10^6 = 6$.

Two simple rules concerning logarithms are used to solve most problems.

Rule 1:

$$\log xy = \log x + \log y \qquad \text{(B.4)}$$

Rule 2:

$$\log x/y = \log x - \log y \qquad \text{(B.5)}$$

A special case of Rule 1 is Rule 1a:

$$\log x^n = n \log x,$$

since

$$\log x^n = \log(xxx \ldots, n \text{ times})$$
$$= \log x + \log x + \ldots, n \text{ times} = n \log x.$$

These two rules are useful in dealing with problems in which x is not a whole number or y is some integer multiple of 10. For instance, what is the log of 412? And what is $10^{0.63}$?

Tables of logarithms usually have the logarithms of numbers between 1 and 10; so if you use these tables to find $\log 412$, you are really looking up $\log 4.12$, which is 0.615. Any answer such as 0.615, when found in the logarithm tables, is called a *mantissa*. Rules 1 and 2 can help determine logarithms of numbers besides those from 1 to 10, such as 412: $\log 412 = \log(4.12 \times 100) = \log(4.12) + \log(100) = 0.615 + 2 = 2.615$ (remember from equation (B.3) that $\log 100 = 2$). The number 2 here is called the *characteristic* of the logarithm.

Here are some additional examples.

$\log 2.6 = 0.335$
 (obtained directly from a logarithm table)
$\log 2165 = \log(2.165 \times 1000)$
$\quad\quad = \log 2.165 + \log 1000 = 0.335 + 3 = 3.335$
$\log 0.31 = \log 3.1/10 = (\text{using Rule 2}) \log 3.1 - \log 10$
$\quad\quad = 0.491 - 1 = -0.509$
$\log 0.0031 = \log 3.1/1000 = \log 3.1 - \log 1000$
$\quad\quad = 0.491 - 3 = -2.509$

To solve the equation $y = 10^{0.63}$, we simply go backward through the table. That is, $\log 4.26 = 0.63$, so $10^{0.63} = 4.26$; thus $y = 4.26$.

DECIBELS

The primary use for logarithms in audition is in working with decibels.

To find decibels from a ratio r:

1. If the ratio is one of pressure, then $dB = 20 \log r$.
2. If the ratio is one of intensity, power, or energy, then $dB = 10 \log r$.

To find the ratio from a decibel number:

1. Determine if the ratio is pressure or intensity/power/energy.
2. If the measurement is pressure, divide the decibel number (dB) by 20; if it is intensity,

power, or energy, divide the decibel number by 10 (let's call this number z, i.e. $z = $ dB/20 or dB/10).

3. Then the ratio equals 10^z.

Recall that for ratios between 0 and 1 (measured value is less than the reference value), the decibel result will be a negative number. And for negative decibels, the ratios will be between 0 and 1.

Abbreviated Log Table

y	$\log y$
1	0
2	0.301
3	0.478
4	0.602
5	0.699
6	0.778
7	0.845
8	0.903
9	0.954
10	1.000

Examples:

1. What is a pressure ratio of 5000 in decibels?

$$\begin{aligned} \text{dB} &= 20\log 5000 \\ &= 20\log(5 \times 1000) \\ &= 20(\log 5 + \log 1000) \\ &= 20(0.699 + 3) = 20 \times 3.699 = 73.98 \text{ dB.} \end{aligned}$$

2. What is a power ratio of 0.005 in decibels?

$$\begin{aligned} \text{dB} &= 10\log 0.005 \\ &= 10\log 1/200 \\ &= 10(\log 1 - \log 200) \\ &= 10[\log 1 - \log(2 \times 100)] \\ &= 10(\log 1 - \log 2 - \log 100) \\ &= 10(0 - 0.301 - 2) = 10 \times -2.301 = -23.01 \text{ dB.} \end{aligned}$$

3. What is 40 dB as a pressure ratio?

$$p = 10^{(40\,\text{dB}/20)} = 10^2 = 100.$$

4. What is −60 dB as an energy ratio?

$$E = 10^{(-60\,\text{dB}/10)} = 10^{-6} = 0.000001.$$

Appendix C: Fourier Analysis

The complete description of the acoustic stimulus requires it to be defined in both the time and frequency domains. The auditory system is also capable of processing sound in both domains. We introduced the concept of Fourier analysis of time and frequency domains in Chapters 2 and 4. In these discussions, the reconstruction of the time-domain waveform was described from a complete description of the phase and amplitude spectra (see Figure 4.2 for an example of this description). Appendix A also shows how, with the use of trigonometric identities, the equations for summing sinusoidal functions would be written and solutions obtained. We have not described how the frequency-domain description can be derived from the time-domain waveform. We did point out in Chapter 5 that filters can be used in practical situations to estimate the amplitude spectrum of a sound. However, an analytic definition for equating the frequency domain to the time domain has not been presented. This appendix is intended to help the student, in a general way, to understand Fourier analysis. From this discussion the student should learn something about the processes by which the spectrum of a waveform can be derived from a definition of the stimulus in the time domain.

In general, $f(t)$ will represent the time-domain waveform. For instance, for a pure tone,

$$f(t) = A\sin(2\pi ft).$$

We will use $f(w)$ as our representation of the frequency-domain description, where $w_o = 2\pi f$, f is frequency in hertz, and t is time in seconds.

The equation for the *Fourier series* (C.1) is

$$f(t) = (1/2)a_o + \sum_{n=1}^{\infty} a_n \cos nw_o t + b_n \sin nw_o t, \qquad \text{(C.1)}$$

where n are integers from 1 to ∞ that represent the different frequencies in the frequency domain. Notice that the equation states that $f(t)$, the time-domain

description, is equal to a sum of sinusoidal terms [recall that $\cos x = \sin(90° - x)$, so cos is a sinusoidal term]. This is the essence of *Fourier's theorem*, that the time-domain waveform can be constructed from a sum of sinusoidal components.

To use equation (C.1), we need to know the values of a_o, a_n, b_n, and w_o. They are defined as follows:

$$a_o = 2/T \int_{T/2}^{T/2} f(t)dt \qquad \text{(C.2)}$$

$$a_n = 2/T \int_{T/2}^{T/2} f(t)\cos(nw_o t)dt \qquad \text{(C.3)}$$

$$b_n = 2/T \int_{T/2}^{T/2} f(t)\sin(nw_o t)dt \qquad \text{(C.4)}$$

$$w_o = 2\pi/T \qquad \text{(C.5)}$$

T (in seconds) is the period of the waveform in the time domain. This version of Fourier analysis is therefore limited to periodic time-domain waveforms, and, as can be seen in equation (C.1), this means that the spectra are discrete (only an integer number of frequencies exist in the spectra). The sinusoidal components in the frequency domain of the waveform consist of the *fundamental frequency* (w_o, or $2\pi/T$) and any of the higher harmonics (integer multiples of the fundamental frequency) that are present after equations of (C.2) through (C.5) are solved. The fundamental frequency is the frequency at which the periodic time-domain waveform repeats (with a period of T).

The $\int$ is the symbol for integration. In general, it means to find the total area under the function over the limits shown on the integration sign. In other words, it is the continuous sum of the magnitude of the value of the function over the limits of integration. Thus, in equations (C.2) through (C.4), we are to find the magnitude of the functions from minus half a period $(-T/2)$ to plus half a period $(T/2)$ of the periodic time-domain function.

By using trigonometric identities (see Appendix A), equation (C.1) can be rewritten as

$$f(t) = C_o + \sum_{n=1}^{\infty} C_n \cos(nw_o t - \theta_n), \qquad (C.6)$$

where $C_o = (1/2)a_o$ and

$$C_n = \sqrt{a_n^2 + b_n^2}, \qquad (C.7)$$

$$\theta_n = \tan^{-1}(a_n/b_n). \qquad (C.8)$$

The term C_n plotted as a function of nw_o is used to define the amplitude spectrum of the waveform, and plotted θ_n as a function of nw_o is used to define the phase spectrum of the waveform. The term C_o is often referred to as the dc (for direct current) term of the Fourier series. It indicates the amount of asymmetry the time-domain waveform has about the zero-amplitude value. It is also sometimes called the amplitude of the zero-hertz component in the amplitude spectrum.

To solve for these spectra, one usually performs the following steps. The time-domain waveform is defined. Then equations (C.2) through (C.5) are solved. The resulting vales of a_o, a_n, and b_n are used in equations (C.3) through (C.8). The relationship between C_n and nw_o is plotted as the amplitude spectrum, and the relationship between θ_n and nw_o is plotted as the phase spectrum, such as in Figures 4.8b and 4.8c.

Let us consider the waveform (a square wave) shown in Figure 4.8. This is a complex waveform, because it is not a sinusoid and it is periodic with a period of T msec. Thus, we can obtain its spectra following the steps outlined earlier.

The time-domain description is

$$f(t) = \begin{cases} 0, \text{ for } -T/2 \le t \le 0 \\ 10, \text{ for } 0 < t \le T/2. \end{cases} \qquad (C.9)$$

The time-domain waveform defined over an time interval of T sec duration is zero from $-T/2$ to 0 and is then 10 from 0 to $T/2$, and this function repeats itself. We now solve for a_o:

$$a_o = 2/T \int_{-T/2}^{T/2} f(t)dt = 5 \qquad (C.10)$$

This is the average amplitude of the square wave (0 for half a period and 10 for a full period).

The solution for a_n is

$$a_n = 2/T \int_{-T/2}^{T/2} f(t)\cos(nw_o t)dt$$
$$= 2/T \left[\int_{-T/2}^{0} -\cos(nw_o t)dt + \int_{0}^{T/2} \cos(nw_o t)dt \right] = 0,$$
$$\qquad (C.11)$$

as long as n is not equal to zero. Thus, <u>all the a_n are zero</u>, since all the integrals (areas) are zero.

The solution for b_n is

$$b_n = 2/T \int_{-T/2}^{T/2} f(t)\sin(nw_o t)dt$$
$$= 2/T \left[\int_{-T/2}^{0} -\sin(nw_o t)dt + \int_{0}^{T/2} \sin(nw_o t)dt \right] \qquad (C.12)$$
$$= 2(1 - \cos n\pi)/n\pi.$$

Thus, $b_n = 0$ when n is an even number and $b_n = 4/n\pi$ when n is an odd number (recall that the cosine of π and of its even integer multiples is 1, while the cosine of π and of its odd integer multiples is -1). Thus, only the odd harmonics of the fundamental exist in the spectrum of the square wave.

For equation (C.1), we have the Fourier series for the square wave:

$$f(t) = (4/\pi)(\sin w_o t + 1/3\sin 3w_o t + 1/5\sin 5w_o t + \ldots). \qquad (C.13)$$

Now we combine these to obtain C_n and θ_n:

$$C_n = \sqrt{a_n^2 + b_n^2} = \sqrt{b_n^2} = b_n = (4\pi)/n \qquad (C.14)$$

for $n = 1, 3, 5, 7, \ldots$ and $a_n = 0$ for all n, and

$$\theta_n = \tan^{-1}(a_n/b_n) = \tan^{-1}(0) = 90°, \qquad (C.15)$$

since $a_n = 0$ and the tangent of 90° is zero.

The amplitudes (C_n) of the odd harmonics ($n = 1, 3, 5, 7, \ldots$) of w_o are $4/\pi, 4/3\pi, 4/5\pi, 4/7\pi$, etc. All phases are 90°. Only odd harmonics of the fundamental frequency, $w_o = 2\pi/T$, exist. Figures 4.8b and 4.8c show the amplitude and phase spectra of this waveform.

A similar set of equations is used to solve for the spectra of time-domain waveforms that are not periodic. The Fourier series is replaced by the *Fourier integral*, which involves the use of *complex numbers*. A complex number is defined as $a + bi$, where $i = \sqrt{-1}$. Because the square root of -1 does not have a solu-

Appendix D: Psychophysics

In its broadest sense, *psychophysics* is the study of the relationship between the psychological (subjective or perceptual) and physical aspects of a stimulus. Historically, the methods of psychophysics have developed via two general approaches. One approach focuses on *discrimination*. The listener is presented with two or more stimuli—for instance, sinusoids of two different intensities—and then is asked whether the stimuli are different. The discrimination procedures are viewed as an "indirect" means of obtaining an answer to the question: What can the listener respond to? The late S. S. Stevens believed that an experimenter could obtain a direct estimate of what the listener does respond to and, often, what the listener can respond to. Thus, the second general class of psychophysical procedures involves directly asking the listener about the stimulus. These are usually called *scaling procedures.*

In discrimination tasks, the experimenter is interested in obtaining an estimate of the smallest differences in a stimulus parameter (e.g., sound level) to which the auditory system is sensitive. That is, to what difference in sound level can the listener respond? However, an experimenter who is not careful will find out only to what difference the listener does respond when asked to make the discrimination. Another way of stating the problem is that the experimenter is interested in the listener's *sensitivity* to the stimulus change and not in the ability to respond in the experimental situation (*response proclivity* or *response bias).* The listener might have a particular *bias* toward responding one way, and the experimenter does not want this bias to influence the measure of the auditory system's sensitivity. Discrimination tasks are designed to estimate sensitivity and minimize the effects of response bias.

The *scaling* procedures are generally designed to obtain information about various subjective or psychological aspects or dimensions. For instance, as the

level of a sinusoidal sound is changed, what does a listener report? If one responds that its loudness is changing, then scaling procedures attempt to measure how loudness changes.

CLASSICAL PSYCHOPHYSICS

Many psychophysicists are interested in measuring the smallest value of some stimulus parameter that a listener can detect (*absolute limen,* or *absolute threshold).* In addition to investigating the absolute threshold, investigators study the *difference limen,* or *difference threshold*, i.e., the smallest difference between two values of a stimulus dimension. Two of the *basic* classical methods were the *method of limits* and the *method of constant stimuli*, used to estimate absolute and difference thresholds. A variation of the method of limits, the *method of adjustment,* was also used.

Many of the classical methods, like the method of constant stimuli, were designed to obtain a *psychometric function* directly from a listener's responses. The experimenter may choose 5 to 10 values of a stimulus parameter, for instance, seven values of level between 12 and 18 dB SPL, of a 1000-Hz tone, and then presents each value approximately 100 times (in the example this would make 700 total trials). The listener is asked to indicate on each trial "Yes, I detected the tone" (Y) or "No, I did not detect the tone" (N). The experimenter then tabulates the proportion of times the listener said "yes" for each stimulus value. These data are then used to plot a psychometric function, as in Figure D.1. In general, a psychometric function relates a measure of a listener's performance (such as proportion of "yes" responses) to a value of the stimulus (such as sound level in decibels).

The estimate of either the absolute or difference threshold is obtained from a point on a psychometric

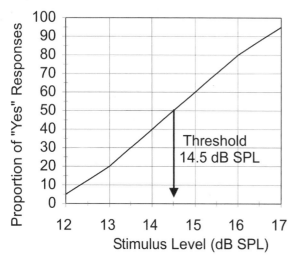

FIGURE D.1 Psychometric function relating proportion of "yes" responses to a stimulus value (intensity in dB SPL in this example). A threshold is obtained by noting the particular intensity (14.5 dB SPL) that yields 50% "yes" responses.

function, as shown in Figure D.1. Some arbitrary value of the proportion of "yes" responses is chosen. Usually this value is 50% of the total range possible for the proportion of "yes" responses. The psychometric function is then used to obtain that value of the stimulus parameter that would yield the 50% value for the proportion of "yes" responses. In Figure D.1 that value is 14.5 dB SPL, and thus 14.5 dB SPL is labeled the *absolute threshold* or *absolute limen.*

The method of constant stimuli has an advantage over the method of limits in that the experimenter can get an estimate of the listener's bias in the experiment by including "catch" or "blank" trials in the sequence. That is, occasionally the experimenter presents no stimulus (or no differences) to the listener. The listener does not know this has happened, and so the response is still either "yes" or "no." If there is a bias toward either response, then the proportion of "yes" responses on the blank trials will reflect this bias.

All of the classical procedures are, however, still affected by response bias. In most experimental contexts, instruction, experience, and feedback can be used

to control the effect of bias to some extent. However, bias can significantly influence a threshold estimate using any of the classical methods. If a listener has a bias to use the "yes" response a lot more than the "no" response, then the listener is much more likely to say "yes" even when the tone might not be detectable. As a result, the threshold might be significantly lower than it would be if the listener did not have the "yes" bias. The same is true in the opposite direction if the bias is to use the "no" response a lot. Thus, two listeners with exactly the same auditory sensitivity might have very different thresholds due to their response biases. We next study a psychophysical procedure in which a measure of sensitivity is obtained that does not change as a function of the listener's response bias or criterion.

THEORY OF SIGNAL DETECTION (TSD)

The TSD procedure is similar to the method of constant stimuli. The experimenter might present 100 trials to the listener; 50 trials contain a tone and 50 trials contain nothing (i.e., "catch" trials). The listener responds on each trial either "Yes, a tone was presented" or "No, a tone was not presented." Of course, only half the trials contained a tone.

There are four possible combinations of stimulus presentations and listeners' responses: The stimulus is presented and the listener can say "yes" (a *hit*); the stimulus is presented and the listener can say "no" (a *miss*); the stimulus is not presented and the listener can say "yes" (a *false alarm*); and the stimulus is not presented and the listener can say "no" (a *correct rejection*). The proportion of times the listener had a hit, false alarm, miss, and correct rejection is entered in a *response table,* as shown in Table D.1. In the theory of signal detection, the values of the stimulus parameters remain constant for all trials; then another block of trials is presented in which another value of a stimulus parameter (for example, sound level) is used. In one experiment there might be four or five response tables, each one representing the results from presenting a different level.

TABLE D.1   Four Stimulus–Response Tables[a]

A: High intensity, "yes" bias

	"Yes"	"No"
Signal	Hit 90	Miss 10
No signal	False alarm 30	Correct rejection 70
$P(C) = 80\%$		

B: High intensity, "no" bias

	"Yes"	"No"
Signal	Hit 70	Miss 30
No signal	False alarm 10	Correct rejection 90
$P(C) = 80\%$		

C: Low intensity, "yes" bias

	"Yes"	"No"
Signal	Hit 75	Miss 25
No signal	False alarm 45	Correct rejection 55
$P(C) = 65\%$		

D: Low intensity, "no" bias

	"Yes"	"No"
Signal	Hit 55	Miss 45
No signal	False alarm 25	Correct rejection 75
$P(C) = 65\%$		

[a]Tables A and B show data for a case when a tone was high in intensity and therefore easy to detect. These two tables differ in the response bias of the listener. Tables C and D show data for a case when a tone was low in intensity and therefore hard to detect. These two tables again differ in the response bias of the listener. The ROC curves for these data are shown in Figure D.2. The entries are the number of responses and, because they are based on 100 trials, also percentages.

The more intense the stimulus, the easier it is for the listener to detect the tone, and so the hit proportion will increase and the false alarm proportion will decrease (correct rejections must increase). That is, the listener will detect the tone more often when it is presented and correctly state "no" when the tone is not presented. The listener might be told to change

response bias. That is, in case 1 t. told to say "yes" only when abso. tone was heard; in case 2 the listen say "yes" even if the tone is not cle. situation the tone will not become "ei the listener will say "yes" more in ca. ... than in case 1. The hit proportion will be larger in case 2 than in case 1 because the listener is simply saying "yes" more often in case 2. The false alarms must also be larger in case 2 than in case 1 because the false alarms also represent the "yes" responses. Therefore, changes in sensitivity when the response criterion of the subject does not change increase (or decrease) hits and decrease (or increase) false alarms, whereas changes in bias when sensitivity does not change increase (or decrease) both hits and false alarms. Four examples of these types of stimulus–response tables are shown in Table D.1.

We can illustrate these effects in what is called a *receiver operator characteristic* (ROC) curve, as shown in Figure D.2. Each data point in the ROC curve is taken from the corresponding hit and false alarm proportions of Table D.1. If we vary (or the listener varies) the bias, then the data points will fall along curves like the two shown in Figure D.2. Notice that as you follow one curve from the lower left to the upper right the false alarms and hits increase. This is what should happen if bias is being altered and sensitivity has not changed. The difference between the two curves represents the listener's sensitivity to the difference in the level of the tone. For any two similar points on the two curves, the hit rate for the upper curve is greater than that for the lower curve. In general, changes in response criterion will move the hits and false alarms along one curve, whereas changes in sensitivity will yield a point on another curve in the ROC space. Therefore, the ROC curve enables us to separate bias effects from sensitivity effects. Notice that the area under the upper curve is larger than the area under the lower curve, and this area cannot change as a function of bias. Thus, the area under any ROC curve is a measure of sensitivity, which is unaffected by response bias.

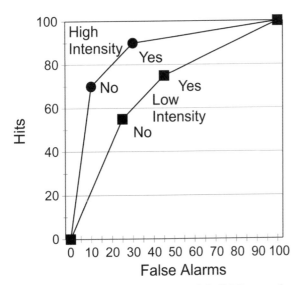

FIGURE D.2 Receiver operator characteristic (ROC) curves for the data of Table D.1. The upper curve shows the two bias conditions (A and B) when the tone's intensity was high (Tables D.1A and D.1B), while the lower curve shows the two bias conditions (C and D) when the tone's intensity was low (Tables D.1C and D.1D). The area under the upper curve is greater than that under the lower curve.

Another measure of sensitivity is computed by using this equation:

$$P(C) = \text{(hit proportion)}$$
$$\times \text{(proportion of times signal presented)}$$
$$+ (1 - \text{false alarm proportion})$$
$$\times \text{(proportion of times signal not presented)}$$

If the signal is present half the time and no signal is present the other half, then

$$P(C) = \frac{p(\text{hit}) + [1 - p(\text{false alarm})]}{2}$$

That is, percent correct ($P(C)$) is similar to the area under the ROC curve, although $P(C)$ is slightly affected by response bias. Other measures are derived from the TSD procedure that depend only on sensitivity and not on response bias. One such measure is d' (*d prime*). d' is a measure of sensitivity based on an assumption that the underlying decision is formed

from normal distributions of the likelihood that a signal-plus-noise was presented in combination with the assumed distribution that the noise was presented. The value of d' is the normalized distance between the means of these two normal distributions (difference in means divided by a common standard deviation). It can be computed by finding the *z-score* associated with the hit rate (Z_{hit}) and subtracting from it the z-score associated with the false-alarm rate (Z_{fa}): $d' = Z_{\text{hit}} - Z_{\text{fa}}$. The value of a z-score (Z) as a function of proportions or probabilities can be found in a table of statistical relationships and in most statistics book.

A psychometric function can then be derived using the area under the ROC curve, $P(C)$, or d'. For each value of a stimulus parameter (such as sound level) we obtain a response table; the response table is used to compute an ROC area, $P(C)$, or d'. As the stimulus level changes, the area under the ROC curve and $P(C)$ will vary between 50% and 100% (d' will vary between 0 and ∞), and the psychometric function will be similar to that obtained with the other psychophysical methods. We can then use the midpoint of this psychometric function ($P(C)$ or area = 75% or $d' = 1$) to estimate a threshold in the same way as in the method of constant stimuli (see Figure D.1).

In all three psychophysical procedures, the first and most important function obtained is the psychometric function. After the psychometric function is derived, an estimate of the threshold is obtained. The value of the threshold is arbitrary because the choice of a value of the listener's performance, such as $P(C)$, was arbitrary. The thresholds are, therefore, a function of both the stimulus and the listener's performance.

DIRECT SCALING

Magnitude estimation, ratio comparison, and *cross-modality matching* are three scaling techniques in which the listener is asked to judge the magnitude of a subjective attribute such as loudness, timbre, space, volume, and the like. From the techniques, a *scale* relating the perceived magnitude (e.g., loudness) to the physical stimulus value (e.g., level in decibels) is obtained to describe a scale for that subjective attribute.

These procedures are usually reliable and valid. When the data are plotted as the logarithm of the magnitude of the subjective measure versus the logarithm of the stimulus value, the data are almost always fit by a straight line. The fact that a straight line fits data that are plotted on log–log coordinates means that the magnitude estimate is related to the stimulus dimension by a *power function*.

The power function is given by

$$P = kS^n, \qquad (D.1)$$

where P is the subjective unit, S the physical unit, k the proportionality constant, and n the *power constant*. By knowing the power function we can compute such information as the number of decibels required to double the loudness of a tone (see Chapter 13). That is, P might be the perceived loudness of a tone in units ranging from 1 to 100 and S might be the physical level of the sound in decibels.

Notice that if in equation (D.1) we take the logarithm of both sides of the equation (see Appendix B for the use of logarithms), we have

$$\log P = n \log S \pm \log k. \qquad (D.2)$$

In equation (D.2), $\log k$ is still a constant and $\log P$ is now linearly related to $\log S$. That is, if we plot $\log P$ versus $\log S$ we generate a straight line, as exists over a large portion of what is shown in Figure 13.2. The slope of this line is the number n, or the *power constant*. The power value is often used in relating the psychological aspects to the physical aspects of any stimulus.

MATCHING PROCEDURES

In the matching paradigm two stimuli are presented to the listener, who is asked to match their equality along some stimulus attribute, such as loudness. With the matching procedures the two waveforms to be matched usually differ in many physical dimensions, and the subject is asked to adjust one of these physical dimensions to make a subjective match (e.g., two tones of different frequencies are compared and the level of one tone is adjusted so that the subjective loudness of this tone is the same as the subjective loudness of the other tone).

The matching procedures allow the experimenter to decide which aspect of a stimulus makes it appear equal, according to some subjective attribute, to another stimulus. Thus, although tones of different frequencies might have equal physical intensities, they may not be judged equal in loudness (e.g., a 200-Hz tone presented at 50 dB SPL might be perceived as being lower in subjective loudness than a 1000-Hz tone also presented at 50 dB SPL). In Chapter 13, we show how matching procedures allow us to determine the phon scale and equal-loudness contours as well as to measure subjective pitch.

Appendix E: Neural Anatomy and Physiology

ANATOMY

Anatomy is the science that studies the structure of the animal body and the relationship among its parts. In order to discuss the relationship among various parts of the body, it is necessary to develop an appropriate vocabulary. For instance, terms such as *upper* and *lower* are relative and, hence, meaningless unless you know in what position the animal is placed. Figure E.1 illustrates how confusing this situation can be when attempts are made to compare the anatomy of an upright two-legged animal with that of a horizontally oriented four-legged animal. The anatomist has developed a vocabulary that differs for animals carried in the horizontal versus the vertical position. For illustrative purposes, consider the humans and the dog shown in Figure E.1. The head of the human is the *superior* end, whereas that of the dog is termed the *anterior* end or *rostral* (which literally means "having a beak") end. The terms *cephalic* and *cranial* may be applied to the head end of an animal carried in either position. The terms *superior* and *anterior* have additional meanings: *Superior* is often used as a relative term meaning a structure occupying a higher position than another structure. For example, if you are standing, your nose is superior to your mouth; but if you are lying on your back, your nose is superior to your ear. *Inferior* is the opposite of superior and, thus, is used to describe a structure occupying a lower position than another structure. *Anterior* refers to the forward part of an organ or body; thus for horizontally oriented animals it is the head end, but for vertically oriented animals it refers to the belly surface of the body. The more general use of the term *anterior* is to describe a structure that is situated in front of another structure. *Ventral* means "toward the belly" and is, therefore, synonymous with *anterior* for humans. *Posterior* can also refer to the tail end of a horizontally oriented animal. *Dorsal* refers to the back side and is,

therefore, the upper side of horizontal animals and is the same as the posterior of humans.

Other anatomical terms do not have these dual meanings. In the text we have made an attempt to use these less ambiguous terms and to define them when they appear for the first time. For quick reference, the following definitions should be helpful.

Medial means the middle, or toward a line drawn lengthwise through the middle of the body (midline).
Lateral means the sides of the body (right and left) or away from the midline.
Peripheral means at or near the surface.
Central means situated near the middle or center of the body. In this text, it is often used to mean the part situated toward the center of the head or cortex.
Proximal means near and is, therefore, used with a particular structure as a reference.
Distal means away from some reference structure.
External means toward the outer surface.
Internal means toward the inner surface.

The auditory anatomist is mainly concerned with *microanatomy*—that is, the details of the structures as seen through the microscope—rather than the relationship of the structures to the body as a whole. When studying the structures of the ear with a microscope, one often concentrates on the minute structure of the tissue. This is called *histology*. The histologist may study normal or abnormal tissues with any of a number of microscopic techniques.

NEURAL ANATOMY

The auditory system, like other sensory systems whose sensory transducers are in the head (e.g., vision), consists of the sensory receptors (e.g., hair cells), a cranial nerve (e.g., VIIIth nerve), which connects the receptors to the neural centers in the brain-

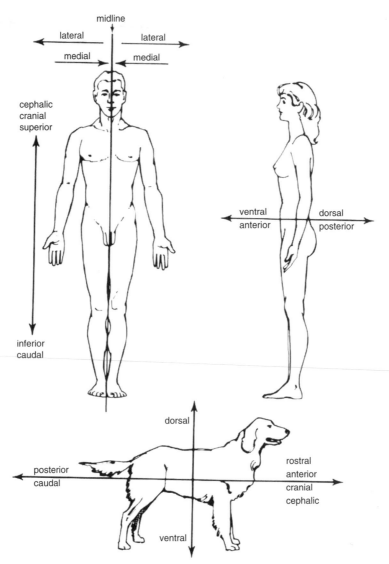

FIGURE E.1 Basic anatomical terminology. Terms as used for vertically and horizontally oriented animals.

stem, and then the cortex. The anatomy of the auditory system central to the cochlea (brainstem and cortex) consists of neurons and neural centers.

The branch of anatomy that investigates the nervous system and nerve tissue is *neuroanatomy*. There are many kinds of neurons: *receptor neurons,* which receive stimulation from sensory receptor cells (such as hair cells) and in turn excite other neurons; *interneurons,* which receive stimulation from one neuron and pass it to the next; *motor neurons,* which receive stimulation from a neuron and in turn stimulate a muscle; and various other neurons depending on the method of classification. For our present purposes, it will suffice to consider the receptor neuron in Figure E.2 to illustrate the general anatomy of a neuron.

The neuron consists of three main parts: the *cell body,* or *soma,* the *dendrites,* and the *axon.* The wall of the cell body is called the *cell membrane.* Inside the cell body is the *nucleus.* The nucleus is surrounded by an intracellular fluid called *cytoplasm* and is responsible for the metabolic activities of the cell. The dendrites are specialized for receiving excitation from another cell, receptor cell, or nerve. The axon usually is elongated and is specialized for transmitting the excitation out of the cell toward the dendrites at the end of the axon. Most neurons have several dendrites to receive stimulation and only one axon to deliver neural impulses. Axons may, however, have several branches, called *collaterals,* and they may also have many endings, called *telodendria.*

Transmission of stimulation from one neuron to another takes place across an interspace between neurons called a *synapse.* When observed by direct electron microscopy, the end of the axon or dendrite contains *vesicles* and a thickened cell membrane. These synaptic vesicles, which appear as little round sacs, contain chemicals, *neurotransmitters,* used in transmitting stimulation across the synaptic gap, or junction, to the next neuron. That is, the neurotransmitters allow the neural signal to be transmitted across the synapse to the receiving neuron. Axons may be covered with two coverings, or sheaths: the *neurilemma* and the *myelin sheath.* The neurilemma is a very thin sheath found on the outside of the peripheral nerve fibers that aids the axon in regeneration when it is injured. Neurons in the central nervous system generally do not have a neurilemma. Myelin sheath is a relatively thick, fatty substance that surrounds the axon and serves as sort of an insulator. This myelin sheath is interrupted at regular intervals called the *nodes of Ranvier.* These nodes assist the neuron in the transmission of neural impulses called *action potentials.* The myelin sheath does not cover the cell body. Groups of neural cell bodies in the central nervous system, called *ganglia* or *nuclei,* are the neural centers of the central auditory nervous system. A bundle of nerve fibers or axons in the periphery is

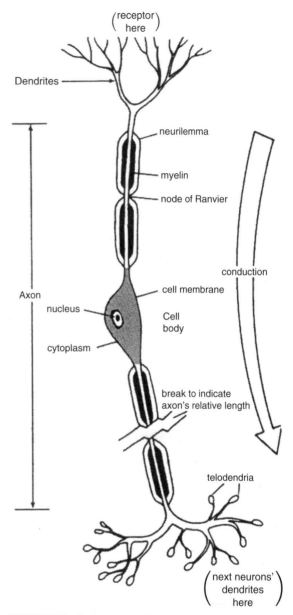

FIGURE E.2   Basic structure of a receptor neuron, such as found in the auditory system.

usually referred to as a *nerve*. In the central system, such a bundle may be called a *tract*.

PHYSIOLOGY

The study of the function of body structures is called *physiology*. This appendix deals primarily with *neurophysiology*, the physiology of nerves and nuclei, and explains how a nerve discharge begins in a nerve cell and how it is propagated down the nerve's axon to the next nerve.

NEURAL PHYSIOLOGY

The nerve's cell membrane separates the *intracellular* and *extracellular fluids*. The intracellular and extracellular fluids contain water and chemicals whose mixture causes *ions* to be formed. Ions take on positive or negative electric charges; the charges of the ions differ between the intracellular and extracellular fluids of the neuron. An electrical difference in charge between two ions produces an *electric potential*. That is, the potential exists for the flow of electric current. For instance, the two poles of a battery are of opposite charge because each pole consists of different chemicals with opposite ionic charges. Thus, a potential difference exists between the poles of the battery. Electric current will flow between the poles if a conductor, such as a metal wire, is connected between the poles of the battery.

Because a difference in the charge of the ions exists between the intracellular and extracellular fluids, a potential difference exists across the cell membrane. This potential difference always exists, whether or not the nerve is excited, and so this permanent potential difference is called a *resting potential*.

The intracellular fluid consists primarily of *potassium* and has a negatively charged *ionic field*; the extracellular fluid is primarily *sodium* and has a positively charged ionic field. The resting potential difference between the two fluids (across the cell membrane) is between −40 and −90 millivolts (mV). See Figure E.3.

The nervous system, thus, possesses the potential for the flow of electric current. The most widely accepted theory of how this flow is initiated concerns a change in the permeability of the cell membrane to potassium and sodium as a function of excitation of the nerve. The chain reaction is outlined as follows: First, some *adequate stimulus* (such as the shearing of the hair cell cilia) changes the permeability of the cell membrane that allows for sodium to flow into the cell. This exchange of chemicals, and, hence, of ions, changes the potential difference from a large negative value to a less negative value, i.e., to a positive value (this process is called *depolarization*). When the potential difference reaches a critical potential difference, then the cell membrane immediately in front of the initial point of change also changes in permeability. An ion exchange occurs at this point along the nerve. This ion exchange leads to the generation of an *action potential* (Figure E.4), which is the neural

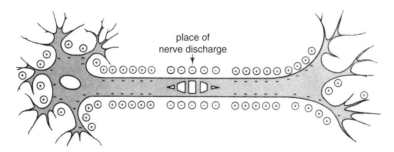

FIGURE E.3 Positive (outside of cell) and negative (inside of cell) ions and their charges as a function nerve stimulation. The ions are transported through the cell wall at the point of the nerve discharge.

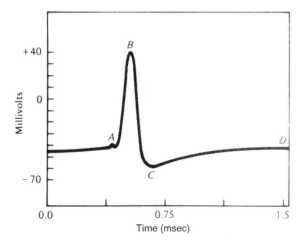

FIGURE E.4 Voltage changes during stimulation of nerve. From the resting potential there is an increase (*depolarization*), *A*, to a positive voltage, *B*, then a return to negative voltage (*hyperpolarization*) with a negative undershoot, *C*, and back to the resting potential, *D*. This is the voltage change that exists at the point of nerve discharge shown in Figure E.3. The time between *A* and *D* is the *total refractory period* of the neural discharge.

signal. Meanwhile, the ions move toward the resting state back at the initial region of excitation (the term *hyperpolarization* is used to describe the process whereby the cell returns to a more negative charge). At this initial place of excitation, the sodium begins to flow (sometimes referred to as a *sodium pump*) from the cell until the resting potential is reached at this point along the cell. An ion exchange is propagated down the nerve resulting in the propagation of the action potential down the axon in the direction away from the cell body. Meanwhile, the membrane behind the propagated chemical exchange is being restored to its initial resting state, allowing for the generation of another action potential. The ions flow through the membrane through *ion channels*, with each channel being specific for a particular ion (e.g., sodium channel or potassium channel).

This change in the transfer of ions and the resulting action potential can be measured by noting the electric potential change at <u>one point</u> along the nerve (see Figure E.4). In this example the resting potential

is approximately −45 mV. Next, a positive increase (*A*) in the potential occurs (depolarization) when the critical voltage is reached. The increase to +40 mV at time *B* is a result of the flow of sodium into the cell. Then, as the cell membrane goes back to its resting state and the ions flow the other way (hyperpolarization), there is a decrease in the potential, with some undershoot, to −70 mV at time *C*. Finally, at time *D* the potential difference is back at its resting state. The time between *B* and *C* is called the *absolute refractory period* of the nerve impulse. During this time, no new discharge can occur because the flow of ions must reach a resting state before they can move again. The time between *C* and *D* is the *relative refractory period,* because it is difficult (but possible) for a new discharge to occur during this period. Thus, the action potential is of limited duration (about 1.5 msec) measured at any one point along the axon. The action potential travels down the axon from the cell body to the dendrites at the end. The refractory periods indicate the limit as to how often a nerve impulse can be propagated down the nerve (the limit is about 1000 impulses a second, although this rate is rarely achieved). One important point concerning the nerve discharge should be emphasized. Once a discharge begins, it remains the same amplitude and has the same waveform shape (see Figure E.4), independent of the parameters of the stimulus that initially excited the nerve. This is referred to as the *all-or-none law of nerve conduction.* That is, the action potential either occurs or it does not occur. The all-or-none law poses a real challenge for understanding how the nervous system encodes the multitude of events occurring in the complex world.

Once the propagated discharge has reached the end foot of the axon, the discharge must cross the synapse before it can begin the chain of propagation down the next nerve fiber. Small chemical packets called *vesicles* (they rest in the end foot of the axon) aid in transferring the chemical action across the synapse. The vesicles help release *neurotransmitters*, chemicals that are transmitted across the synapse to the receiving dendrites, into the synapse. When the neurotransmitter reaches the receiving dendrite it either excites (depolarizes) or inhibits (hyperpolarizes) the cell membrane of the receiving dendrite, depending on whether or not the neurotransmitter has a chemical makeup that causes polarization (excitation) or hyperpolarization (inhibition). Thus, neurotransmitters can be excitatory or inhibitory.

ELECTROPHYSIOLOGY

Electrophysiology is the study of the electrochemical changes in the nervous system. Its main technique involves implanting an electrode into neural tissue and measuring the potential difference between the change in the tissue and some other point. The other point (reference electrode) might be another part of the nervous system or some neutral location. Each time an action potential is propagated down the nerve, the electrode will respond to the potential difference. This potential difference is then amplified and fed to a recording instrument. The electrode can rest outside of a nerve, and this form of *extracellular recording* measures the action potential, as described earlier. A more difficult recording technique calls for the measuring electrode to be implanted inside the nerve cell (*intercellular recording*). Intercellular recording measures the current or voltage changes inside the cell that lead to the action potential.

The auditory electrophysiologist is concerned with the potential differences existing not only in nerves but also in the structures of the inner ear. No matter where these differences exist, the electrode always measures the differences in electric charge between two points. As described earlier, this difference has the potential for electric current flow.

The physiological measures most often used are electrical. Sometimes electrical signals such as the cochlear microphonic (CM) can be recorded at a distance from the ear. However, because of the distance, the CM amplitude is very small relative to the other background electrical activity associated with other bodily functions. Presumably, most of this background activity is uncorrelated with the presentation of a signal to the ear and is thus considered noise. The CM, of course, is perfectly correlated with the occurrence of the acoustic signal because the CM always occurs when the signal occurs. Thus, if the signal is presented many times and the electrical responses of the distant electrode following each stimulus presentation are summed, the uncorrelated background noise should tend to cancel and the CM associated with the signal presentation is enhanced. This technique is called *signal averaging*. A computer is required for the sampling the CM waveforms and performing the addition. Many different types of weak electric potentials are recorded this way, especially those associated with auditory-evoked changes in the EEG (electroencephalogram), or brain waves recorded from the top of the head. The recording of the brainstem-evoked response (BSER; see Chapter 15) usually requires thousands of EEG waveforms to be averaged for the investigator to discern a definite pattern in the averaged response.

tissues with different speeds, thus differentially affecting its phase. The phase contrast microscope changes these phase differences (which are not visible to the eye) into amplitude differences, which appear as differences in brightness (i.e., light–dark contrast). The phase contrast microscope is often used in conjunction with the *whole-mount*, or *surface preparation, technique*. With this technique whole portions of the organ of Corti and basilar membrane of 1 to 5 mm in length can be placed in the microscope for observation, and a sizable number of adjacent hair cells can be viewed. Another advantage of this technique is that one can focus at different levels within the specimen. Thus, by adjusting the microscope to be in focus at various levels within the specimen, one can obtain a visual "slice" of the specimen without the inherent difficulties normally encountered in attempting mechanical slicing of the very delicate organ of Corti.

Since the 1950s, the *transmission electron microscope* has gained in popularity because of its remarkable resolving power. The specimen is sliced in sections and placed in the scope. Instead of passing light through the specimen, electrons are transmitted in a beam through the specimen in a manner similar to the way the light beam is diffracted in the light microscope. The reflected electronic beam is magnified by electromagnetic lenses and then directed toward a fluorescent screen, where the image is produced and photographed. By comparing the transmission electron micrographs in Figure 7.7 with the light micrograph of Figure 7.5a, you can obtain an idea of the resolving capabilities of this instrument. Figure 7.7 shows a great deal more detail than Figure 7.5a.

The *scanning electron microscope* (SEM) has a better resolving power than the light microscope, but it does not have the same level of capability as the transmission electron microscope. The SEM has the advantage of having a greater depth of field. This means that a larger portion of the viewed specimen will be in focus. The SEM does not use a beam of electrons transmitted through the specimen. Instead it uses an electron beam, focused on the specimen, that loosens electrons from the surface of the specimen. These loosened electrons and the reflected electron beam are col-

lected and used to form an image on a screen that resembles a television monitor. This process allows viewing of only the surface of the specimen. The SEM derives its name from the fact that the electron beam scans over the specimen in a systematic fashion. The specimen is usually prepared to emit electrons by prior coating with a very thin layer of gold or other soft metal. The scan of the microscope's electron beam is synchronized with the scan of the electron beam in the cathode-ray tube (similar to a TV picture tube). The collected electrons that are loosened from the specimen or reflected by it modulate the electron beam of the picture tube to create the image. Figures such as Figure 7.2 and Figure 7.6 are SEM photomicrographs.

NEURAL STAINS AND MARKERS

The anatomist, along with the physiologist and biochemist, has a large arsenal to probe the structure and function of neural tissue. In general terms, the tissue is exposed to some chemical, pharmacological, or radioactive agent. These agents may stain, mark, or label certain parts of the neural tissue (e.g., cell bodies as opposed to axons). The stained or marked parts can be differentiated from other tissue (for example, the axon from the cell body) under the microscope. An older technique involved destroying some part of a neural location (*lesions*). The nerves then die, and under the microscope the dead nerve fibers appear different from live nerves. Both the new chemical and the older lesion techniques allow the anatomist to trace the pathway of some particular part of the nervous system. In other preparations, the chemical agent may label the tissue (or part of the tissue) only when the neuron discharges. That is, the agent interacts with the chemistry of the neuron because of the chemical or metabolic changes that occur when an action potential is initiated. This interaction then causes the tissue to be labeled, and the labeled parts can be studied with a microscope or with some other instrument that is sensitive to the chemical or radioactive agent.

One example of such chemical agents is *horseradish peroxidase* (HRP). HRP is a protein that is taken

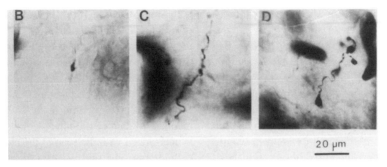

FIGURE F.2 Photomicrographs of HRP-injected brain slices showing individual nerve fibers in the cochlear nucleus of the hamster. From Schweitzer and Cecil (1992), used with permission.

up by a neural cell and goes to the cell body. After HRP is injected into some neural tissue in a live animal, the HRP is taken up by neural cells in the region of the injection. When this neural region is bathed in the proper chemicals and examined under a microscope, the fibers that have taken up the HRP can be seen by the dark stain the process gives to these fibers. Figure F.2 is an example of a fiber that has been marked via the HRP technique. Using HRP enables the neuroscientist to trace the path of fibers within a local region of the nervous system, and the fibers so labeled are ones that were neurally activated by a stimulus presentation.

Immunohistochemical techniques enable one to study how individual molecules are distributed in a section of neural tissue. For instance, an investigator may wish to determine which parts of some neural tissue have a certain type of neurotransmitter. In some cases, the investigator might want to know whether the neurotransmitter molecules in the tissue are ones that excite neurons to produce neural discharges or ones that inhibit neuronal discharging. The *immune system* of the body produces *antibodies* in response to *antigens,* which are *peptides,* such as those that reside on the surface of viruses. In normal function, when antibodies, produced by white blood cells, come in contact with the appropriate antigen, the antibody attaches to the antigen and seeks to destroy the virus. However, antibodies can be developed for a wide variety of

antigen molecules. When an antibody is made for a particular molecule (antigen), it will attach itself to that molecule in neural tissue. When a marker chemical is attached to the antibody and neural tissue is bathed in the substance, the antibody will attach itself to the antigen molecule (e.g., an excitatory neurotransmitter molecules), and the marker or dye that was mixed with the antibody will then show up on microscope under ultraviolet light, revealing those neural structures that contained the antigen molecule (e.g., the excitatory neurotransmitter). Figure 7.12 shows a photomicrograph from an immunohistochemical procedure.

Some techniques allow the scientist to determine those neural sites that were active for processing some particular stimulus condition. One such technique uses radioactive *2-deoxyglucose* (2-DG). 2-DG is like glucose (a sugar), which cells need to maintain their metabolism. If 2-DG is present in some neural tissue, those neurons that are active (are discharging) will take up the 2-DG to supply the energy necessary to maintain the firing rate. By marking the 2-DG with a radioactive substance, one can see those areas of the tissue that have taken up the 2-DG (i.e., have been neurally active) on an *autoradiograph* of the tissue. In an experiment, radioactive 2-DG is injected into the neural tissue of interest and the animal is presented with the test sound for a fairly long period of time. The animal is <u>sacrificed</u> and the tissue fixed and prepared for investigation. The autoradiograph will reveal which neural structures were involved with processing the information associated with the sound. Figure F.3 shows an autoradiograph from a 2-DG study. Today's neuroscientists have a wider range of markers and tracers that can be used to examine the anatomy and physiology of the nervous system, and more are being developed as more is learned about the nervous system.

ELECTROPHYSIOLOGY

Appendix E briefly outlines the way in which electrophysiological measurements are made. Most of the data shown in this textbook have been obtained with *extracellular recordings* made with single electrodes. That is, the electrode was near the neuron but not actually inside of it. *Intercellular* recordings, which

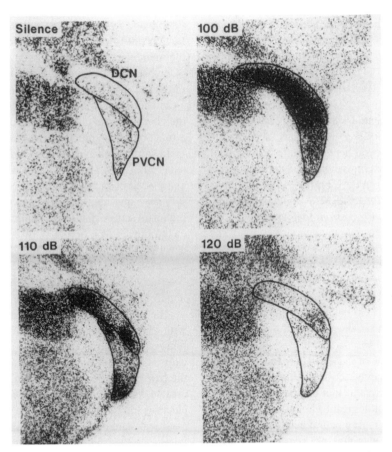

FIGURE F.3   Patterns of 2-DG uptake in the dorsal (DCN) and posterior ventral (PVCN) cochlear nucleus of a gerbil. The four panels indicate the level of uptake (the darker the area, the more 2-DG uptake and thus the more neurally active the area) to four intensity levels of two-octave noise (1414 to 5356 Hz). The amount of activity is greatest at 100 dB, decreases in some regions of the nucleus at 110 dB, and is much less at 120 dB. Some form of suppression might be occurring that results in the lowering of activity at high noise levels. From Ryan, Axelsson, and Wolf (1992), with permission.

involve implanting an extremely small electrode inside of a neuron, can be made (see Chapter 8), but they are much more difficult to perform.

Multi-electrode techniques are used for at least two reasons. In some experiments, a number of electrodes are implanted with some electrodes used for recording neural activity and others used to inject dye or chemicals (e.g., HRP) into the tissue. This makes it possible for the investigator to anatomically investigate the neurons that were recorded from, since the dyes would mark these neurons. In some cases, a multi-electrode can be used to record from and/or to stimulate a number of different neurons.

IMAGING

The evoked-potential technique was briefly described in Appendix E as one means of providing an "image" of the neural activity of the brain and/or brainstem. Other imaging techniques, such as *x-ray, computerized tomography* (CT), *magnetic resonance imaging* (MRI), *functional magnetic resonance imaging* (fMRI), and *positron emission tomography* (PET), have also been used to map the neural activity of the brain. X-ray, CT, fMRI, and MRI use either x-rays or magnetic fields to map the brain, with computer reconstruction of the image being an important part of the CT, MRI, and fMRI techniques. In PET the patient receives an injection of radioactive 2-DG, and, as explained earlier, the radiograph will reveal those areas of the brain that were active in processing information during the time of the test. These imaging techniques can measure large sections of the brain, but the resolution is not as great as that obtained with microscopic or electrophysiological techniques. Since brain imaging requires averaging neural activity over time, these techniques are also not very sensitive to events that will change over a short period of time. Figure 15.11 is a PET image. Functional MRI is currently the neural imaging technique most often used to study the human nervous system in awake human subjects. The fMRI technique is explained in Chapter 15, and an example is shown in Figure 15.12.

BIOPHYSICAL TECHNIQUES

Since such membranes as the tympanic membrane, oval and round window membranes, and basilar membrane all vibrate, techniques have been developed to study their vibrations. However, because the amplitude of vibration is so incredibly small, only recently has modern technology provided the means for direct measurement. Four of these tools are *holography*, the *Mossbauer technique, optical heterodyne spectroscopy,* and *laser interferometry*. Holography, laser interferometry, and spectroscopy take advantage of the laser beam to produce a light source that reflects off the membranes or off microscopic reflecting surfaces placed on the membranes so that the vibrations can be measured. The Mossbauer technique involves placing a radioactive source on the membrane and measuring the change in the emitted radioactivity that occurs as a function of the membrane's movement.

In very recent years, new biophysical techniques have allowed tissue to be excised from an organism and placed in an artificial environment for study. This *in vitro* experiment (as opposed to *in vivo,* or in the organism) allows the scientist to examine the anatomy, electrophysiology, or biochemistry of the tissue under a variety of controlled situations. The chemical and metabolic environment of the tissue can be varied to determine the interaction of these variables with neural action.

The study of isolated hair cells (Chapter 8) is done with in vitro procedures, in which the organ of Corti is removed from an animal and the hair cells chemically excised from this tissue and placed in a bath that allows the hair cells to remain biologically active. One powerful technique (*patch clamping*) involves attaching an electrode directly to the neural cell and controlling the electrical state of the neuron to allow one to carefully measure either the voltage or current flow within this isolated cell. Other manipulations of the hair cell are also possible, such as physiologically recording from a hair cell while individual stereocilia are moved. Such experiments are highly technical and require great experimenter technique and skill. When the tissue is taken from a developing organism, the in vitro study enables the experimenter to investigate the growth of neural tissue as well as aspects of its genetic code.

MOLECULAR AND CELL BIOLOGY AND GENETICS

All biological tissue (animal and plant) is made up of cells. The basic building blocks of cells are *proteins* and *enzymes*. *RNA* (*ribonucleic acid*) controls the way in which a cell's protein is established, and *DNA* (*deoxyribonucleic acid*) provides the genetic code for the cell by assisting in enzyme and protein control. DNA is located in the cell's nucleus, and DNA contains all the information the cell needs to sustain, grow, and reproduce itself. *Genes* are organized within the *chromosomes* of the DNA molecule. Genes control the traits (*alleles*) that the cells produce. For instance, brown-eye genes and blue-eye genes are alternative alleles for eye color. Each person has a particular catalog of genes, the *genotype*, and the genotype produces a particular physical, chemical, or behavioral characteristic of the organism called the *phenotype*. One phenotype is deafness, which is usually caused by a *mutation* of genes in a particular chromosome or set of chromosomes that describe the genotype, in that the normal genotype would not lead to deafness. Outer hair cell motility is another phenotype described in this book.

Cell and molecular biology is the study of the cells, their proteins and enzymes, and the RNA and DNA that control protein and enzyme production. To completely understand the full function of the cells that control the biology of hearing, one needs to be familiar with the cellular and molecular building blocks of the cells that make up the tissues of the auditory system. There is an ever-increasing number of molecular tools and methods available to the cell and molecular biologist to describe and explore the function of cells and their genetic control. A few proteins (e.g., prestin) and genes (e.g., *Atoh1*) are described in this book, and more are being discovered every day.

As described in Chapter 16, there is growing information about the genetic abnormalities that lead to several forms of inherited deafness. Information about what genes may be responsible for a particular phenotype, such as deafness, is often acquired by studying families that tend to have a propensity for a particular type of inherited disease or disorder. By tracing the "family tree" of such families, geneticists can narrow in on those in the family who are likely carriers of the genes that lead to the disorder or disease. The genetic makeup of these people can be compared to that of others in the family (via a simple blood test or by taking mouth swabs), and in this way the genes or their mutations that lead to the disease or disorder can be isolated. Often there may be an animal model for the same disease or disorder (or other genotypes and phenotypes, e.g., outer hair cell motility). In this case, it may be possible to produce an animal that is either provided a particular gene or is missing the gene of interest. Such animals are called *transgenic* animals (if the animal carries a foreign gene inserted into it) or *gene-knocked-out* animals (if the animal is missing a gene that it would normally have). Mice are often used in this case, and knockout mice can be used to test the original assumption that the gene in question was the one that caused the phenotype (e.g., was responsible for the deafness or in other cases for outer hair cell motility), and then other aspects of the cell biology and genetics of the knockout mouse can be studied to understand more thoroughly the underlying biology that is responsible for the phenotype (e.g., deafness or outer hair cell motility).

A more complete description of the cell and molecular biology of hearing and its genetic control are beyond the scope of this book, for understanding the recent developments in these areas requires knowledge of cell biology and genetics that we assume most readers of this book lack. For those who do have such backgrounds, a great deal of this book can be seen as providing a description of the structures of the parts of the auditory system responsible for hearing and their functions (often the phenotypes). As such, it is these structures and their functions whose molecular, cellular, and genetic descriptions are required to understand the hearing process more fully.

Terms, Measurements, Equations, and Conversions

This section contains the terms, symbols, equations, and measurements used through-out the book. Also see the Glossary for additional equations and the list of Abbreviations and Symbols.

Time

Term (t, T)	Symbol	Measurement	Equation/conversion
seconds	sec		
milliseconds	msec	$1/1000 = 0.001$ seconds	one one-thousandth of a second
microseconds	μsec	$1/1,000,000 = 0.000001$ seconds	one one-millionth of a second

Length (*L*) or Distance (*D*, *d*)

Term	Symbol	Measurement	Equation/conversion
meters	m		1 m = 39.36 inches = 3.28 feet; 1 foot = 0.3048 m
centimeters	cm	$1/100 = 0.01$ meters	one one-hundredth of a meter; 1 cm = 0.394 inches, 1 inch = 2.54 cm
millimeters	mm	$1/1000 = 0.001$ meters	one one-thousandth of a meter
micrometers	μm	$1/1,000,000 = 0.000001$ meters	one one-millionth of a meter
angstroms	Å	10^{-10} meters = 1/10,000,000,000 meters	1 Å = 10,000 μm

Area

Term	Symbol	Measurement	Equation/conversion
square centimeters	cm^2		
square millimeters	mm^2		
circle			πr^2; r = radius
area surface of sphere			$4\pi r^2$; r = radius

Volume (*V*, dry)

Term	Symbol	Measurement	Equation/conversion
cubic centimeters	cm^3		
cubic millimeters	mm^3		

Volume (liquid)

Term	Symbol	Measurement	Equation/conversion
liters	l		1 l = 2.11 pints, 1 pint = 0.473 l
milliliters	ml	1/1000 = 0.001 liters	one one-thousandth of a liter
microliters	μl	1/1,000,000 = 0.000001 liters	one one-millionth of a liter

Weight (m = mass, w = weight)

Term	Symbol	Measurement	Equation/conversion
grams	g		1 g = 0.035 ounces, 1 ounce = 28.35 g
milligrams	mg	1/1000 = 0.001 grams	one one-thousandth of a gram

Density

Term	Symbol	Measurement	Equation/conversion
density	p_o	grams/centimeter^3	mass/volume

Temperature

Term	Symbol	Measurement	Equation/conversion
Centigrade	C	degrees	$°C = (5/9)(°F - 32)$
Fahrenheit	F	degrees	$°F = 32 + (9/5)(°C)$

Motion

Term	Symbol	Measurement	Equation/conversion
velocity	v	meters/second	distance/time
acceleration	a	meters/second/second	distance/time/time = v/t

Mechanical-Electrical-Acoustic

Term	Symbol	Measurement	Equation/conversion
force	F	dynes, newtons	1 newton = 10^5 dynes; dyne = $(g \times cm)/sec^2$
potential difference, volts	V	V = volts; mV = millivolts; μV = microvolts	Volts is a pressure-like measure
pressure	p	pascals (Pa); micropascals (μPa)	$p = F/Ar$; 1 newton/cm^2 = 10^5 dynes/cm^2 = 10^4 Pa; 1 μPa = 10^{-6} Pa. F = force, Ar = area
instantaneous pressure	$p(t)$	pascals, micropascals	$p(t) = mv/tAr$, where m = mass, v = velocity, t = time, and Ar = area
energy	E	joules, ergs	force through distance; $E = P \times T$; 1 joule = 10^7 ergs; ergs = 10^7 dyne-cm = 1 newton-meter, where P = power, T = time
power	P	watts	$P = E/T$, 1 watt = 10^7 ergs/sec = 1 joule/sec, where E = energy, T = time
sound intensity	I	watts/cm^2	$I = p^2/p_oc$, where p = pressure, p_o = density of medium, c = speed of sound
decibels	dB		$10 \log (I_1/I_2)$, $10 \log (P_1/P_2)$, $10 \log(E_1/E_2)$, $20 \log(p_1/p_2)$, where P = power, E = energy, I = sound intensity, p = pressure
speed of sound	c	meters/second	approximately 345 m/sec
inverse square law		sound intensity or sound pressure	$I \propto 1/r^2$, $p \propto 1/r$, where r = distance between source and receiver, I = sound intensity, p = sound pressure
resonance frequency	f_r	hertz (Hz)	$f_r = \sqrt{[(s/m)/2\pi]}$, where s = stiffness, m = mass
resistance	R	ohms	
mass reactance	X_m	ohms	
stiffness reactance	X_s	ohms	
impedance	Z	ohms	$Z = \sqrt{\left[R^2 - (X_m - X_s)^2\right]}$
characteristic impedance	Z_c	ohms	$Z_c = p_oc$, where p_o = density of medium, c = speed of sound
wavelength	λ	meters, centimeters, millimeters	$\lambda = f/c$, where f = frequency, c = speed of sound
reverberation time	RT	seconds	RT $\propto$ Vol/Ab, where Vol = room volume, Ab = room absorption
fundamental mode (vibration)	f_o	hertz (Hz)	$f_o = c/2L$, open both ends; $f_o = c/4L$, open one end; where c = speed of sound, L = length of tube
period	Pr	time	Pr = 1/f, Pr in sec; Pr = 1000/f, Pr in msec; where f = frequency in hertz
frequency	f	hertz (Hz) kilohertz (kHz)	cycles/sec, kilohertz is frequency in units of 1000 hertz; f = 1/Pr, Pr in sec; f = 1000/Pr, Pr in msec; where Pr = period
peak amplitude	A	distance, pressure, sound intensity	
root-mean-square amplitude	A_{rms}	distance, pressure, sound intensity	$A_{rms} = \sqrt{1/T \int_0^T d^2(t)dt}$; where T = duration, t = time; for sinusoid: $A_{rms} = 0.707A$, where A = peak amplitude
starting phase tone, sinusoid	θ	degrees, angular	also ongoing phase $d(t) = A \sin(2\pi ft + \theta)$, $d(t)$ = instantaneous amplitude, where A = peak amplitude, θ = starting phase
sinusoidal amplitude modulation	SAM		$A(t) = A(1 + m \sin 2\pi F_m t) \sin 2\pi F_c t$, where $A(t)$ = instantaneous amplitude, m = depth of modulation, F_m = modulation rate or frequency, F_c = carrier frequency
sinusoidal frequency modulation	SFM		$A(t) = A \sin[(2\pi F_c t) + m/F_m \sin 2\pi F_m t]$; where $A(t)$ = instantaneous amplitude, m = modulation frequency range, F_m = modulation rate or frequency, F_c = carrier frequency

Psychoacoustics

Term	Symbol	Measurement	Equation/conversion
Weber fraction			$\Delta S/S$ = constant, where ΔS = just-noticeable difference (jnd), S = stimulus value
just noticeable difference	jnd		smallest perceived difference in a stimulus attribute between two sounds

Intensity Weber Fractions [I = intensity, ΔI = intensity jnd, P = power, V = amplitude (i.e., volts), s = signal, m = masker, α = phase angle of addition between s and m]

Measure of intensity discrimination for Weber fraction	Power	Amplitude	Weber fraction
increment power (ΔI)	$P_{m+s} - P_m$	$(1/2)V_s^2 + V_m V_s \cos \alpha$	$\Delta I/I = \Delta I$
relative increment power (Weber fraction, $\Delta I/I$)	$(P_{m+s} - P_m)/P_m$	$(1/2)V_s^2/V_m^2 + 2(V_s/V_m) \cos \alpha$	$\Delta I/I^b$
difference limen ("ΔI in dB")	$10 \log P_{m+s} - 10 \log P_m$	$10 \log [(1/2)V_s^2/V_m^2 + 2(V_s/V_m) \cos \alpha + 1]$	$10 \log(\Delta I/I + 1)^a = 10 \log[(\Delta I + I)/I]$
signal-to-masker ratio (s/m)	P_s/P_m	V_s^2/V_m^2	$[(\Delta I/I + \cos^2 \alpha)^{1/2} - \cos \alpha]^2$

Term	Symbol	Measurement	Equation/conversion
equivalent rectangular filter bandwidth—critical band	ERB	hertz (Hz)	ERB (Hz) = 24.73(4.37F + 1), where F = frequency in kHz
linear system			$y = ax + b$, where y = output, x = input, a and b = constants
nonlinear system			$y = ax + bx^2 + cx^3 + dx^4 + \ldots$, where y = output, x = input, $a, b, c, d, \ldots$ = constants
aural harmonics (harmonics)		hertz (Hz)	mf_0, where m = integer 1, 2, 3, $\ldots$, f_0 = base frequency
difference tone		hertz (Hz)	$mf_1 - nf_2$, where m and n = integer 1, 2, 3, $\ldots$, f_1, $m \neq n$; f_2 = base frequencies
cubic-difference tone		hertz (Hz)	$2f_1 - f_2$; where f_1 and f_2 = base frequencies, $f_1 < f_2$
summation tones		hertz (Hz)	$mf_1 + nf_2$, where m and n = integer 1, 2, 3, $\ldots$, $m \neq n$; f_1 and f_2 = base frequencies
octave		hertz (Hz)	doublings of a frequency, $2^n \times f_o$, where n = number of octaves, n = 1, 2, 3, $\ldots$, f_o = fundamental (base) frequency

[a] Refers to form used on left axis in Figure 10.7.
[b] Refers to form used on right axis in Figure 10.7.
All computations assume measurements made into a nominal 1-ohm load, such that $P = (1/T)\int x^2(t)dt$, where P is power, T (in units of seconds) is the signal duration, $x(t)$ is the time-domain waveform, and the integration is over the signal's duration.

Anatomical and Physiological Measurements

SUMMARY OF HUMAN OUTER AND MIDDLE EAR MEASUREMENTS

Most of the data listed here come from Wever and Lawrence's *Physiological Acoustics* (1954). Their Appendix D is a compilation of many authors' works, from which we have chosen the data to illustrate the range of measures. When available, a mean value is given. Additional data from recent investigations have also been added.

PINNA (MALE)

length: 60–75 mm, mean = 67 mm
breadth: 30–39 mm, mean = 34.5 mm
angle that length axis is inclined to head: 15°
concha volume: 2.5 cm^3
concha resonance frequency: 4.5 kHz

EXTERNAL AUDITORY MEATUS

cross section: 0.3–0.5 cm^2

EXTERNAL AUDITORY CANAL

cross section: 0.3–0.5 cm^2
length: 2.3–2.97 cm
diameter: 0.7 cm
volume: 1.0 cm^3
resonance frequency: 2.6 kHz

TYMPANIC MEMBRANE

diameter along the manubrium: 7.5–9 mm
diameter perpendicular to the manubrium: 7.5–9 mm
area: 0.5–0.9 cm^2
effective area: 42.9–55 mm^2
inward displacement of umbo: 2 mm
thickness: 0.1 mm
weight: 14 mg
breaking strength: 0.4–3.0×10^6 dynes/cm^2, mean = 1.61×10^6 dynes/cm^2
displacement amplitude for low-frequency tones at threshold of feeling: 10^{-2} cm
displacement amplitude for a 250-Hz tone: 125 Å at 75 dB SPL, 7.5 Å at 70 dB SPL, 5 Å at 65 dB SPL

MIDDLE EAR CAVITY

total volume: 2.0 cm^3
volume of ossicles: 0.5–0.8 cm^3

MALLEUS

weight: 23–32 mg
length from end of manubrium to end of lateral process: 5.8 mm
total length: 7.6–9.1 mm

INCUS

weight: 25–32 mg
length of long process: 7.0 mm
length of short process: 5.0 mm

STAPES

weight: 2.05–4.34 mg, mean = 2.86 mg
height: 2.50–3.78 mm, mean = 3.26 mm
length of footplate: 2.64–3.36 mm, mean = 2.99 mm
width of footplate: 1.08–1.66 mm, mean = 1.41 mm
area of footplate: 2.65–3.75 mm^2, mean = 3.2 mm^2
width of elastic ligament: 0.015–0.1 mm
amplitude of displacement for a constant eardrum
    pressure of 1 dyne/cm^2:
        125 Hz: 75×10^{-8} cm
        200 Hz: 28×10^{-8} cm
        400 Hz: 20×10^{-8} cm
        750 Hz: 18×10^{-8} cm
        1500 Hz: 10×10^{-8} cm
        2000 Hz: 6×10^{-8} cm
        2500 Hz: 2×10^{-8} cm
maximum displacement: 0.1 mm

SUMMARY OF INNER EAR MEASUREMENTS

Because most of the experimental work on the inner ear has been performed with animals, both animal and human data are listed. The principal sources for these data are Angelborg and Engstrom (1973), Rauch and Rauch (1974), Spoendlin (1966), and Wever and Lawrence (1954). These sources are often secondary, so the data given here actually represent the results of measurements by many authors.

OVAL WINDOW

dimensions: 1.2×3 mm to 2.0×3.7 mm *human*
area: 1.12–1.27 mm^2; mean = 1.20 mm^2 *cat*; mean: 1.4 mm^2 *guinea pig*

ROUND WINDOW

dimensions: 2.25×1.0 mm *human*
area: 2 mm^2 *human*; 3 mm^2 *cat*; 1 mm^2 *guinea pig*

COCHLEA

number of turns: 2–5/8 *human*
volume: 98.1 mm^3 (including the vestibule proper) *human*
length of cochlear channels: 35 mm *human*

HELICOTREMA

area: 0.08–0.04 mm^2 *human*

BASILAR MEMBRANE

length: 25.3–35.5 mm, mean = 34 mm *human*; 19.4–25.4 mm, mean = 22.5 *cat*; mean = 18.8 mm *guinea pig*; mean = 20.7 mm *squirrel monkey*, mean = 18.4 mm *chinchilla*
width, basal end: 0.08–0.16 mm *human*; 0.062 mm *guinea pig*
width, apical end: 0.423–0.651 mm, mean = 0.5 *human*; mean = 0.209 mm *guinea pig*

ORGAN OF CORTI

cross-sectional area, basal end: 0.00053 mm^2 *human*; 0.0055 mm^2 *cat*
cross-sectional area, apical end: 0.0223 mm^2 *human*; 0.0201 mm^2 *cat*

OUTER HAIR CELLS

number: 12,000 *human*
cell body length: 20 μm (basal end); 50 μm (apical end) *human*
cell body width: 5 μm *human*
cilium width: 0.05 μm at its base to 0.2 μm at tip *human*
cilium length: 2 μm in basal turn; 6 μm in apical turn *human*

arrangement: 100–150 stereocilia per outer hair cell
   human

cilia 6–7 rows in W or V pattern hair cell *human*

cilia 3 rows in W or V pattern per outer hair cell *cat and guinea pig*

cilia of outermost row have tips embedded in the tectorial membrane; angle in V shape 120° in the basal turn and 60° in the apical turn

INNER HAIR CELLS

number: 3500 *human*; 2600 *cat*

arrangement: 40–60 cilia per cell arranged in a shallow U shape, 204 rows of cilia per cell, length of cilia longer in apical turn than in basal turn, lengths and diameters vary among individual coils of the cochlea, and within a single cell

SPIRAL LIGAMENT

cross-sectional area: $0.543\,mm^2$ near basal end, $0.042\,mm^2$ at the apex *human*

SCALA VESTIBULI

volume: $54\,mm^3$ including vestibule proper *human*

SCALA TYMPANI

volume: $37.4\,mm^3$ *human*

COCHLEAR DUCT

volume: $6.7\,mm^3$ *human*

length: 35 mm *human*

PERILYMPH

volume: scala vestibuli, 10–15 µl, *human*

scala tympani, 6–8 µl *human*

total, 16–23 µl *human*

K^+ concentration: 4 mEq/liter* (scala vestibuli) *human*

Na^+ concentration: 139 mEq/liter (scala vestibuli) *human*

pH: 7.4–7.8 *human*; 7.9 *guinea pig*; 7.3–7.87 *cat*

viscosity: 1.030–1.050, in relation to H_2O at 27°C = 1 *human*

surface tension: 49.6 dynes/cm *guinea pig* (at 23°C)

protein: 70–100 mg/100 ml *human*; 142 mg/100 ml *cat*; 70–107 mg/100 ml *guinea pig*

ENDOLYMPH

volume: scala media, 2.7 µl *human*

K^+ concentration: 144 mEq/liter *human*

Na^+ concentration: 13 mEq/liter *human*

pH: 7.5 *human* (postmortem); 7.4 *guinea pig*; 7.82 *cat*

viscosity: saccule, 1.030–1.050 in relation to H_2O at 27°C = 1 *human*

surface tension: 52 dynes/cm *guinea pig* (at 23°C)

protein: 20–30 mg/1000 ml *human*; 118 mg/100 ml *cat*; 25 mg/100 ml *guinea pig*

* mEq/liter: milliequivalents per liter

Abbreviations and Symbols Used in the Text

Symbols used uniquely in the appendixes are defined in those appendixes. Also see the Glossary for additional definitions, and see Terms, Measurements, Equations, and Conversions.

CHAPTER 1

Au.D.	Doctor of Audiology
Ph.D.	Doctor of Philosophy
CV	confounding variable
DV	dependent variable
ENT	ear, nose, and throat
IV	independent variable
S	speed of ball
SL	slope of incline

CHAPTER 2

a, x	acceleration
A	peak amplitude
A_{rms}	root-mean-square (rms) amplitude
d	distance
$D(t)$	instantaneous amplitude [sometimes a_i or $a(t)$]
F	force
f	frequency in hertz
Hz	hertz
m	mass
Pr	period (sometimes T)
rms	root mean square
s	stiffness
t	time
v	velocity
w	$\theta t = 2\pi f$; angular velocity
θ	starting phase angle

CHAPTER 3

Ar	area
Ab	absorption
a	acceleration
c	speed of sound
dB SL	decibels in sensation level
dB SPL	decibels in sound pressure level
E	energy
F	force
f	frequency
f_o	fundamental frequency
I	sound intensity
l, L	length
m	mass
P	power
p	pressure
$p(t)$	instantaneous pressure
p_o	density of a medium
R	resistance
RT	reverberation time
r	radius
s	stiffness
T	duration
t	time
V	velocity
Vol	volume
v	voltage
x	distance
X	reactance
X_m	mass reactance
X_s	stiffness or spring reactance

Z	impedance	
Z_c	characteristic impedance	
λ	wavelength	
λ_o	wavelength of f_o	

CHAPTER 4

$A, A(t), a_i$	amplitude
AM	amplitude modulation
α	standard deviation
BW	bandwidth
D	duration
$D(t)$	instantaneous amplitude
ERB	equivalent rectangular bandwidth
$e(t)$	envelope function
f_x	frequency number x
$f(t)$	fine-structure function
F_c	carrier frequency
$F_c \pm F_m$	sidebands
F_m	modulation frequency
FM	frequency modulation
m	modulation depth
N_o	spectrum level (noise power per unit bandwidth)
$P(a_i)$	Gaussian probability
Pr	period
SAM	sinusoidal amplitude modulation
TP	total power
$x(t)$	complex sound function
β	modulation depth for frequency modulation, m/F_m

CHAPTER 5

Atten_{db}	attenuation in decibels
BW	bandwidth
CF	center frequency
cut	cutoff frequency
ERB	equivalent rectangular bandwidth
f	frequency
f_i	different frequencies, where $i = 1, 2, 3, 4, \ldots$

f_r	resonant frequency
in	input
m	mass
out	output
Q	indicator of relative bandwidth, CF/BW
Q_{10}	Q at 10-dB downpoints
roll	roll-off in db/octave
s	stiffness

CHAPTERS 6–9 (ANATOMY)

an	auditory nerve
A	afferent nerve
BC	border cell
BM	basilar membrane
C	Claudius' cell
COCB	crossed olivocochlear bundle
Cn	cochlear nerve
CP	cuticular nerve
D	Deiters cell
E	efferent nerve fibers
Fn	facial nerve
Gc	ganglion cell
H	Hensen's cell
HC	hair cell
HP	habenula perforata
HS	Hensen's stripe
IAM	internal auditory meatus
IHC	inner hair cell
IP	inner pillar
IS	inner spiral bundle
ISC	inner sulcus cell
m	microvillus
M	modiolus
Mc	mitochondria
MNF	myelinated nerve fibers
n	nerve
N	nucleus
OC	organ of Corti
OCB	olivocochlear bundle
OHC_1	outer hair cell, row 1
OHC_2	outer hair cell, row 2

OHC_3	outer hair cell, row 3
OP	outer pillar
OS	outer spiral fibers
OW	oval windows
PC	pillar cell
PP	phalangeal process
PST	poststimulus time histogram
R	radial fibers
Rm	Reissner's membrane
RW	round window
S	stapes
Sc	stereocilia
Sl	spiral ligament
SL	spiral lamina
Sm	scala media
SM	stapedial muscle
SN	space of Nuel
St	scala tympani
Sv	stria vascularis
TB	temporal bone
TC	tunnel of Corti
TL	tympanic layer
Tm	tectorial membrane
TR	tunnel radial fibers
TSB	tunnel spiral bundle
tt	tensor tympani
UCO-CB	uncrossed olivocochlear bundle
VIIIth nerve	eighth cranial nerve

CHAPTERS 6–9 (PHYSIOLOGY)

ac	alternating current
ALSR	average localized synchronized rate
AP	action potential
BF	best frequency
CF	characteristic frequency
CM	cochlear microphonic
dc	direct current
DPOAE	distortion product otoacoustic emission
EP	endolymphatic potential
EOAE	evoked otoacoustic emission
f_1, f_2	frequencies

HRTF	head-related transfer function
kHz	kilohertz
OAE	otoacoustic emission
PST	poststimulus time histogram
SOAE	spontaneous otoacoustic emission
SP	summating potential
TEOAE	transient evoked otoacoustic emission

CHAPTER 10

AM	amplitude modulation
ANSI	American National Standards Institute
dB HL	decibels in hearing level
E	energy
f	frequency
F_m	modulation frequency
I	intensity
I_∞	intensity, $T > 500$ msec
jnd	just-noticeable difference
m	depth of amplitude modulation, and masker [subscript of P (power) or V (voltage)]
M	masker
MAF	minimal audible field
MAP	minimal audible pressure
$n(t)$	noise waveform
$P(C)$	percent correct
s	signal [subscript of P (power) or V (voltage)]
Δf	frequency difference (usually a jnd)
ΔI	temporal difference (usually a jnd)
ΔT	temporal difference (usually a jnd)
P	power
RETFL	reference equivalent threshold force level
RETSPL	reference equivalent threshold sound pressure level
SAM	sinusoidal amplitude modulation
S	signal
SPL	sound pressure level
T	time (duration)
TMTF	temporal modulation transfer function

PRIMARY REFERENCES

Abel, S. M. (1971). Duration discrimination of noise and tone bursts. *J. Acoust. Soc. Amer.* **51**, 1219–1224. (*Fig. 10.8*) 10

Ades, H. W. (1959). Central auditory mechanisms. In *Handbook of Physiology, Vol. 1, Neurophysiology*. J. Field, H. W. Magoun, and V. E. Hall, eds. American Physiological Society, Washington, DC (*Fig. 15.1*) 15

Ades, H. W., and Engstrom, H. (1974). Anatomy of the inner ear. In *Handbook of Sensory Physiology, Vol. 5*. W. D. Keidel and W. D. Neff, eds. Springer-Verlag, New York. (*Fig. 6.1*) 6

Adrian, E. D. (1931). The microphonic action of the cochlea in relation to theories of hearing: Report of a discussion on audition. London. *Physical Society*, 5–9. 8

Angelborg, C., and Engstrom, H. (1973). The normal organ of Corti. In *Basic Mechanisms in Hearing*. A. Moller, ed. Academic Press, London. Measures

Bacon, S. P., and Viemeister, N. F. (1985). Simultaneous masking by gated and continuous sinusoidal maskers. *J. Acoust. Soc. Amer.* **78**, 1220–1230. (*Fig. 10.10*) 10

Bekesy, G. von. (1936). Zur Psychik des Mittelohres und uber das Horen bei fehlerhaftem Trommelfell. *Akust. Zeits* **1**, 13–23. (*Fig. 6.7*) 6

Bekesy, G. von. (1941). Uber die Messung der Schwingungsamplitude der Gehorknochelchen mittels einer kapazitiven Sonde. *Akust. Zeits.* **6**, 1–16. (*Fig. 6.7*) 6

Bekesy, G. von. (1947). The variation of phase along the basilar membrane with sinusoidal vibrations. *J. Acoust. Soc. Amer.* **19**, 452–460. (*Fig. 7.17*) 7

Bendor, D., and Wang, X. (2005). The neuronal representation of pitch in primary auditory cortex. *Nature* **426**, 1161–1165. 15

Bilger, R. C., Matthies, M. L., Hammel, D. R., and Demorest, M. E. (1990). Genetic implications of gender differences in the prevalence of spontaneous otoacoustic emissions. *J. Speech Hear. Res.* **33**, 418–433. 8

Bilsen, F. A., and Raatgever, J. (2000). On the dichotic pitch of simultaneously presented interaurally delayed white noises: Implications for binaural theory. *J. Acoust. Soc. Amer.* **108**, 272–284. 13

Brownell, W. E., Bader, C. R., Bertrand, D., and Ribaupierre, Y de. (1985). Evoked mechanical responses of isolated cochlear outer hair cells. *Science* **227**, 194–196. 8

Brugge, J. F., and Merzenich, M. M. (1973). Patterns of activity of single neurons of the auditory cortex in monkey. In *Basic Mechanisms in Hearing*. A. G. Moller, ed. Academic Press, New York. (*Fig. 15.20*) 15

Brugge, J. F., Kitzes, L. M., and Javel, E. (1981). Postnatal development of frequency and intensity sensitivity of neurons in the anteroventral cochlear nucleus of kittens. *Hear. Res.* **5**, 217–229. 15

Buus, S., Florentine, M., and Poulsen, T. (1999). Temporal integration of loudness in listeners with hearing losses of primarily cochlear origin. *J. Acoust. Soc. Amer.* **195**, 3464–3480. 13

Campbell, K. C. M. (2003). Developing overprotective agents for ototoxic noise-induced hearing loss: D-Methionine and other compounds. *NHCA Spectrum* **19**, 12–14. 16

Canlon, B., Borg, E., and Flock. A. (1988). Protection against noise trauma by pre-exposure to a low level acoustic stimulus. *Hear. Res.* **34**, 197–200. 16

Cant, N. B. (1992). The cochlear nucleus: Neuronal types and their synaptic organization. In *The Auditory Pathway: Neuroanatomy*. D. Webster, R. R. Fay, and A. N. Popper, eds. Springer-Verlag, New York. (*Fig. 15.4*) 15

Carder, H. M., and Miller, J. D. (1972). Temporary threshold shifts from prolonged exposure to noise. *J. Speech Hear. Res.* **15**, 603–623. 16

Carlyon, R. P. (1991). Discriminating between coherent and incoherent frequency modulation of complex tones. *Hear Res.* **41**, 223–236. 14

Carlyon, R. P., and Datta, A. J. (1997). Excitation produced by Schroeder-phase complexes evidence for fact-acting compression in the auditory system. *J. Acoust. Soc. Amer.* **101**, 3636–3647. 11

Chandler, D. W., and Grantham, D. W. (1992). Minimum audible movement angle in the horizontal plane as a function of stimulus frequency and bandwidth, source azimuth, and velocity. *J. Acoust. Soc. Amer.* **91**, 1624–1636. 12

Cherry, C. (1953). Some experiments on the recognition of speech with one and with two ears. *J. Acoust. Soc. Amer.* **25**, 975–981. 12

Cheveigne, A., de. (2005). Pitch perception models. In *Pitch: Neural Coding and Perception*. C. J. Plack, A. J. Oxenham, R. R. Fay, and A. N. Popper, eds. Springer-Verlag, New York. 13

Clark, W. W. (1991a). Noise exposure from leisure activities: A review. *J. Acoust. Soc. Amer.* **90**, 175–182. 16

Clark, W. W. (1991b). Recent studies of temporary threshold shift (TTS) and permanent threshold shift (PTS) in animals. *J. Acoust. Soc. Amer.* **90**, 155–164. 16

Colburn, H. S., and Kulkarni T. (2005), Models of sound localization. In *Sound Source Localization*. A. N. Popper and R. R. Fay, eds. Springer-Verlag, New York, 272–317. 12

Dallos, P., Santos-Sacchi, J., and Flock, A. (1982). Intercellular recordings from cochlear outer hair cells. *Science* **218**, 582–584. 9

Darwin C. J. (1981). Perceptual grouping of speech components differing in fundamental frequency and onset time. *Quart. J. Exp. Psychol.* **33A**, 185–207. 14

Darwin, C. J., and Ciocca V. (1992). Grouping in pitch perception: Effects of onset asynchrony and ear of presentation of a mistuned component. *J. Acoust. Soc. Amer.* **91**, 3381–3391. 14

Dau, T., Kollmeier, B., and Kohlraush, A. (1997). Modeling auditory processing of amplitude modulation: II. Spectral and temporal integration in modulation detection. *J. Acoust. Soc. Amer.* **102**, 2906–2919. 10

Davis, H. (1956). Initiation of nerve impulses in the cochlea and other mechanoreceptors: Physiological triggers and discontinuous rate processes. Bullock, T. D., ed.. *American Physiolog. Soc.* 60–71. (*Fig. 8.1*) 8

Davis, H. (1960). Mechanism of excitation of auditory nerve impulses. In *Neural Mechanisms of the Auditory and Vestibular Systems.* T. Rasmussen and W. F. Windle, eds. Thomas, Springfield, IL. (*Fig. 8.5*) 8

Diamond, I. T. (1973). Neuroanatomy of the auditory system: Report on a workshop. *Arch. Otolaryng.* **98**, 397–413. (*Fig. 15.1*) 15

Durlach, N. I. (1972). Binaural signal detection: Equalization and cancellation theory. In *Foundations of Modern Auditory Theory, Vol. II.* J. V. Tobias, ed. Academic Press, New York. 12

Durlach, N. I., Mason, C. R., Shinn-Cunningham, B. G., Arbogast, T. L., Colburn, H. S., and Kidd, Jr., G. (2002). Informational masking: Counteracting the effects of stimulus uncertainty by decreasing target-masker similarity. *J. Acoust. Soc. Amer.* **114**, 368–372. 14

Elliott, D. N., and Trahiotis, C. (l972). Cortical lesions and auditory discrimination. *Psychol. Bull.* **77**, 198–222. (*Fig.15.19*) 15

Fettiplace, R., and Crawford, A. C. (1980). The origin of tuning in the turtle cochlear hair cells. *Hear. Res.* **2**, 447–454. 8

Fletcher, H. (1924). The physical criterion for determining the pitch of a musical tone. *Physic. Rev.* **23**, 427–437. 13

Fletcher, H., and Munson, W. A. (1933). Loudness: Its definition, measurement, and calculation. *J. Acoust. Soc. Amer.* **5**, 82–108. 13

Formby, C., Sherlock, L. P., and Li. S. (1998). Temporal gap detection measured with multiple sinusoidal markers: Effects of maker number, frequency, and temporal position. *J. Acoust. Soc. Amer.* **104**, 984–998. 10

Glasberg, B. R., and Moore, B. C. J. (1990). Deviation of auditory filter shapes from notched-noise data. *Hear. Res.* **47**, 133–138. 11

Grantham, D. W., and Yost, W. A. (1982). Measures of intensity discrimination. *J. Acoust. Soc. Amer.* **72**, 406–411. 10

Green, D. M. (1971). Temporal auditory acuity. *Psychol. Rev.* **78**, 542–551. 10

Green, D. M. (1993). Intensity processing. In *Human Psychoacoustics.* W. A. Yost, A. N. Popper, and R. R. Fay, eds. Springer-Verlag, New York. 10

Green, D. M., and Yost, W. A. (1975). Binaural analysis. In *Handbook of Sensory Physiology: Hearing.* W. D. Keidel and W. Neff, eds. Springer-Verlag, New York. 12

Greenwood, D. D. (1990). A cochlear frequency-position function for several species—29 years later. *J. Acoust. Soc. Amer.* **87**, 2592–2605. (*Fig. 9.13*) 9

Griffiths, T. D., Buchel, C., Frachowiak, R. S. J., and Patterson, R. P. (1998). Analysis of temporal structure in sound by the human brain. *Nat. Neurosci.* **1**, 422–427. (*Fig. 15.11*) 15

Griffiths, T. D., Uppenkamp, S., Johnsrude, I., Josephs, O., and Patterson, R. D. (2001). Encoding of temporal regularity of sound in the human brain. *Nat. Neurosci.* **4**, 633–637. (*Fig. 15.12*) 15

Guinan, J., and Peake, W. T. (1967). Middle ear characteristics of anesthetized cats. *J. Acoust. Soc. Amer.* **41**, 1237–1261. 6

Hall, J. L. (1975). Nonmonotic behavior of distortion product $2f_1$–f_2: Psychophysical observations. *J. Acoust. Soc. Amer.* **58**, 1046–1050. (*Fig. 13.6*) 13

Hall. J. W., Haggard, M., and Fernandes, M. A. (1984). Detection in noise by spectrotemporal pattern analysis. *J. Acoust. Soc. Amer.* **76**, 50. (*Fig. 14.7*) 14

Harrison, J. M., and Howe, M. E. (1974a). Anatomy of the afferent auditory nervous system of mammals. In *Handbook of Sensory Physiology, Vol. 5.* W. D. Keidel, and W. D. Neff, eds. Springer-Verlag, New York. (*Fig. 15.1*) 15

Harrison, J. M., and Howe, M. E. (1974b). Anatomy of the descending auditory system (mammalian). In *Handbook of Sensory Physiology, Vol. 5.* W. D. Keidel and W. D. Neff, eds. Springer-Verlag, New York. (*Figs. 15.1, 15.3*) 15

Hartmann, W. M. (1987). Temporal fluctuations and the discrimination of spectrally dense signals by human listeners. In *Auditory Processing of Complex Sounds.* W. A. Yost and C. S. Watson, eds. Erlbaum, Hillsdale, NJ. 4

Hartmann, W. M., and Zhang, P. (2003). Binaural models and the strength of dichotic pitches. *J. Acoust. Soc. Amer.* **114**, 3317–3326. 13

Hartmann, W. M., McAdams, S., and Smith, B. K. (1990). Hearing a mistuned harmonic in an otherwise periodic complex tone. *J. Acoust. Soc. Amer.* **88**, 1712–124. 13

Henning, G. B. (l977). Detectability of interaural delay in high-frequency complex waveforms. *J. Acoust. Soc. Amer.* **55**, 84–90. 12

Hind, J., Anderson, D., Brugge, J., and Rose, J. (1967). Coding of information pertaining to paired low-frequency tones in single auditory nerve fibers of the squirrel monkey. *J. Neurophysiol.* **30**, 794–816. (*Fig. 9.9*) 9

Hofman, P. M., Van Ryswick, J. G. A., and Van Opstal, A. J. (1998). Relearning sound localization with new ears. *Nat. Neurosci.* **1**, 417–422. (*Fig. 15.13*) 15

Hudspeth, A. J. (l983). The hair cells of the inner ear. *Scientific American* **183**, 54–65. 8

Hudspeth, A. J. (2005). How the ear's works work: Mechanoelectrical transduction and amplification by hair cells. *C. R. Biol.* **328**, 155–162. 7, 8

Irino, T., and Patterson, R. D. (1997). A time-domain, level-dependent auditory filter: The gammachirp. *J. Acoust. Soc. Amer.* **101**, 412–419. 9

Izumikawa, M., Minoda, R., Kawamoto, K., Abrashkin, K. A., Swiderski, D. L., Dolan, D. F., and Raphael, Y. (2005). Auditory hair cell replacement and hearing improvement after *Atoh1* gene therapy in deaf mammals. *Nat. Med.* **11**, 271–276. 16

Jeffress, L. A. (1948). A place theory of sound localization. *J. Comp. Physiolog. Psychol.* **41**, 35–39. 12

Jerger, J., and Hays, D. (1980). Diagnostic applications of impedance audiometry: Middle ear disorders; sensorineural disorders. In *Clinical Impedance Audiometry,* 2nd ed. J. Jerger and J. Northern, eds. American Electromedics Corp., Acton, MA. 6

Jesteadt, W. (1980). An adaptive procedure for subjective judgments. *Percep. Psychophys.* **28**, 85–88. 13

Jesteadt, W., and Bilger, R. C. (1974). Intensity- and frequency-discrimination one-tone and two-tone interval paradigms. *J. Acoust. Soc. Amer.* **55**, 1266–1279. 11

Jesteadt, W., Weir, C. C., and Green, D. M. (1977). Intensity discrimination as a function of frequency and sensation level. *J. Acoust. Soc. Amer.* **61**, 169–177. (*Fig. 10.7*) 10

Kemp, D. T. (1978). Stimulated acoustic emissions from within the human auditory system. *J. Acoust. Soc. Amer.* **64**, 1386–1391. 8

Kiang, N. Y-S. (1965). Stimulus coding in the auditory nerve and cochlear nucleus. *Acta Otolaryngol.* (Stockholm) **59**, 186–200. (*Fig. 15.6*) 15

Kiang, N. Y-S., and Moxon, E. C. (1972). Physiological considerations in artificial stimulation of the inner ear. *Ann. Oto. Rhin. Laryn.* **81**, 725. (*Fig. 9.5*) 9

Kiang, N. Y-S., Watanabe, T., Thomas, E. C., and Clark, L. F. (1965). *Discharge Patterns of Single Fibers in the Cat's Auditory Nerve.* M.I.T. Press, Cambridge, MA. (*Figs. 9.7, 9.10*) 9

Killion, M. C. (1978). Revised estimate of minimum audible pressure: Where is the "Missing 6 dB"? *J. Acoust. Soc. Amer.* **63**, 1501–1505. 10

Klein, A. J., and Teas, D. C. (1978). Acoustically dependent latency shifts of BSER (wave V) in man. *J. Acoust. Soc. Amer.* **63**, 1887–1892. (*Fig. 15.10*) 15

Knudsen, E. I. (2004). Sensitive periods in the development of the brain and behavior. *J. Cogn. Neurosci.* **8**, 1412–1425. 15

Konishi, T., and Nielsen, D. W. (1978). The temporal relationship between basilar membrane motion and nerve impulse initiation in auditory nerve fibers of guinea pigs. *Jpn. J. Physiol.* **28**, 291–307. 8

Konishi, M., Takahashi, T. T., Wagner, H., Sullivan, W. E., and Carr, C. E. (1988). Neurophysiological and anatomical substrates of sound localization in the owl. In *Auditory Function: Neurobiological Bases of Hearing.* G. W. Edelman, W. E. Gall, and W. M. Cowan, eds. Wiley & Sons, New York. 15

Kubke, M. F., and Carr, C. E. (2005). Development of the auditory centers responsible for sound localization. In *Sound Source Localization.* A. N. Popper and R. R Fays, eds. Springer-Verlag, New York, 179–238. 12

Kuhn, G. F. (1987). Physical acoustics and measurements pertaining to directional hearing. In *Directional Hearing.* W. A. Yost and G. Gourevitch, eds. Springer-Verlag, New York. (*Fig. 12.3*) 12

Langner, G. (1992). Periodicity coding in the auditory system. *Hear. Res.* **60**, 115–143. 15

Liberman, M. C. (1978). Auditory-nerve response from cats raised in a low-noise chamber. *J. Acoust. Soc. Amer.* **63**, 442–455. (*Fig. 9.1*) 9

Liberman, M. C. (1980). Morphological differences among radial afferent fibers in the cat cochlea: An electron-microscope study of serial sections. *Hear. Res.* **3**, 45–63. 8

Liberman, M. C. (1982). Single-neuron labeling in the cat auditory nerve. *Science* **216**, 1239–1241. 8

Liberman, M. C. (1991). Effects of chronic de-efferentation on auditory-nerve response. *Hear. Res.* **49**, 209–223. 9

Liberman, M. C., and Brown, M. C. (1986). Physiology and anatomy of single olivocochlear neurons in the cat. *Hear. Res.* **24**, 17–36. 8

Liberman, M. C., Gao, J., He, D., Wu, X., Jia, S., and Zuo. J. (2002). Prestin is required for electromotility of the of the outer hair cells and for the cochlear amplifier. *Nature* **419**, 300–304. 8

Licklider, J. C. R. (1954). Periodicity by "pitch" and place "pitch." *J. Acoust. Soc. Amer.* **26**, 945–951. 13

Lippe, W., and Rubel, E. (1983). Development of the place principle: Tonotopic organization. *Science* **219**, 514–516. 15

Litovsky, R., Colburn, S., Yost, W. A., and Guzman, S. (1999). The precedence effect. *J. Acoust. Soc. Amer.* **106**, 1633–1654. 12

Lonsbury-Martin, B. L., and Martin, G. K. (1990). The clinical utility of distortion-product otoacoustic emissions. *Ear Hear.* **11**, 144–154. 8

Lutfi R. A. (1988). Complex interactions between pairs of forward maskers. *Hear. Res.* **35**, 71–78. 11

Margolis, R. H., and Hunter, L. L. (2000). Acoustic immittance measurements. In *Audiological Diagnosis.* R. Roeser, R. J. Valente, and M. H. Hosford-Dunn, eds., Chap. 17, Thieme Press, New York. 3

Martin, G. K., Probst, R., and Lonsbury-Martin, B. L. (1990). Otoacoustic emissions in human ears: Normative findings. *Ear Hear.* **11**, 106–120. (*Fig. 8.8*) 8

May, B. J., Budelis, J., and Niparko, J. K. (2004). Behavioral studies of the olivocochlear efferent system: Learning to listen in noise. *Arch. Otolaryng. Head Neck Sur.* **130**, 660–664. 9

McFadden, D., and Passenan, E. G. (1975). Binaural beats at high frequencies. *Science* **190**, 394–397. 12

Meddis, R. (1986). Simulation of mechanical to neural transduction in the auditory receptor. *J. Acoust. Soc. Amer.* **79**, 702–711. 9, 14

Melnick, W. (1991). Human temporary threshold shifts (TTS) and damage risk. *J. Acoust. Soc. Amer.* **90**, 147–155. (*Fig. 16.5*) 16

Miller, J. D., Watson, C. S., and Cosell, W. (1963). Deafening effects of noise on the cat. *Acta Otolaryng. Suppl.* **176**. 16

Miller, J. D. (1970). Audibility curve of the chinchilla. *J. Acoust. Soc. Amer.* **48**, 513–523. 16

Mills, A. W. (1972). Auditory localization. In *Foundations of Modern Auditory Theory, Vol. 2.* J. V. Tobias, ed. Academic Press, New York. (*Fig. 12.7*) 12

Moller, A. R. (1970). The middle ear. In *Foundations of Modern Auditory Theory, Vol. 2*. J. V. Tobias, ed. Academic Press, New York. (*Fig. 6.4*) 6

Moody, D. B., Stebbins, W. C., and Hawkins, J. R. (1976). Noise-induced hearing loss in the monkey. In *Effects of Noise on Hearing*. D. Henderson, D. Hamernik, D. Dosanjh, and J. Mills, eds. Raven Press, New York. (*Fig. 16.6*) 16

Moore, B. C. J.; see Glasberg; see Patterson.

Moore, B. C. J. (1978). Psychophysical tuning curves measured in simultaneous and forward masking. *J. Acoust. Soc. Amer.* **63**, 524–532. (*Fig. 11.13*) 11

Moore, B. C. J. (1992). Frequency processing. In *Human Psychoacoustics*. W. A. Yost, A. N. Popper, and R. R. Fay, eds. Springer-Verlag, New York. 11

Moore, B. C. J., and Glasberg, B. R. (1982). Interpreting the role of suppression in psychophysical tuning curves. *J. Acoust. Soc. Amer.* **72**, 1374–1379. 11

Moore, B. C. J., Peters, R. W., and Glasberg, B. R. (1985). Thresholds for the detection of inharmonicity in complex tones. *J. Acoust. Soc. Amer.* **77**, 1861–1867.

Moore, E. J. (1983). *Bases of Auditory Brainstem-Evoked Responses*. Grune & Stratton, New York. 15

Morest, D. K., and Oliver, D. L. (1984). The neuronal architecture of the inferior colliculus in the cat: Defining the functional anatomy of the auditory midbrain. *J. Com. Neurol.* **222**, 209–236. 15

Moushegian, G., Rupert, A., and Whitcomb, M. (1972). Processing of auditory information by medial superior olivary neurons. In *Foundations of Modern Auditory Theory*. J. Tobias, ed. Academic Press, New York. (*Fig. 15.17*) 15

Mulroy, J. J., Altmann, D. W. ,Weiss, T .F., and Peake, W. T. (1974). Intracellular electrical response to sound in a vertebrate cochlea. *Nature* **249**, 482–485. 9

Naunton, R. F., and Fernandez, C., eds. (1978). *Evoked Electrical Activity in the Auditory Nervous System*. Academic Press, New York. (*Fig. 8.9*) 8

Nedzelnitsky, V. (1980). Sound pressures in the basal turn of the cat cochlea. *J. Acoust. Soc. Amer.* **68**, 1676–1680. (*Fig. 6.8*) 6

Neff, D. L., and Green, D. M. (1987). Masking produced by spectral uncertainty with multicomponent maskers. *Percep. Psychophys.* **41**, 409–415. 14

Neti, C., Young, E. D., and Schneider, M. H. (1992). Neural network models of sound localization based on directional filtering by the pinna. *J. Acoust. Soc. Amer.* **92**, 3140–3157. 15

Nuttal, A. L., and Dolan, D. F. (1996). Steady-state sinusoidal velocity response of the basilar membrane in guinea pig. *J. Acoust. Soc. Amer.* **99**, 1556–1565. 8

Oliver, D. L., and Huerta, M. F. (1992). Inferior and superior colliculi. In *The Auditory Pathway: Neuroanatomy*. D. Webster, R. R. Fay, and A. N. Popper, eds. Springer-Verlag, New York. (*Fig. 15.4*) 15

Osborne, M., Comis, S. D., and Pickles, J. O. (1988). Further observations on the fine structure of tip links between stereocilia of the guinea pig cochlea. *Hear. Res.* **35**, 99–108. (*Fig. 7.11*) 7

Patterson, J. H. (1991). Effects of peak pressure and energy of impulses. *J. Acoust. Soc. Amer.* **90**, 205–209. 16

Patterson, R. D., Allerhand, M., and Giguere, C. (1995). Time-domain modeling of peripheral auditory processing: A modular architecture and a software platform. *J. Acoust. Soc. Amer.* **98**, 1890–1895. (*Figs. 9.15, 14.1*) 9, 11, 14

Patterson, R. D., and Moore, B. C. J. (1989). Auditory filters and excitation patterns as representations of frequency resolution. In *Frequency Selectivity in Hearing*. B. C. J. Moore, ed. Academic Press, London. (*Figs. 11.7, 11.8*) 11

Pestalozza, G., and Davis, H. (1956). Electric responses of the guinea pig ear to high audio frequencies. *Amer. J. Physiol.* **185**, 595–600. (*Fig. 8.3*) 8

Pickles, J. O., Comis, S. D., and Osborne, M. (1984). Cross-links between stereocilia in the guinea pig organ of Corti, and their possible relation to sensory transduction. *Hear. Res.* **15**, 103–112. 8

Plack, C. J., and Oxenham, A. J. (1998). Basilar membrane nonlinearity and the growth of forward masking, *J. Acoust. Soc. Amer.* **103**, 1598–1608. (*Fig.11.15*) 11

Postman, L. J., and Egan, J. (1949). *Experimental Psychology: An Introduction*. Harper & Row, New York. (*Fig. 16.4*) 16

Ranke, O. F. (1942). Das Massenverhaltnis zwischen Membrane und Flussigkut im Innenohn. *Akust. Zeits.* 7, 1–11. (*Fig. 7.14*) 7

Rauch, S., and Rauch, I. (1974). Physicochemical properties of the inner ear, especially ironic transport. In *Handbook of Sensory Physiology. Vol. 5*. W. D. Keidel and W. D. Neff, eds. Springer, New York. Measures

Reed, C. M., and Bilger, R. C. (1973). A comparative study of S/N and E/No. *J. Acoust Soc. Amer.* **53**, 1039–1045. (*Figs. 11.4, 11.5*) 11

Riesz, R. R. (1928). Differential intensity sensitivity of the ear for pure tones. *Phys. Rev.* **31**, 867–875. 10

Robles, L., Ruggero, M. A., and Rich, N. C. (1986). Basilar membrane mechanics at the base of the chinchilla cochlea: I. Input–output functions, tuning curves, and response phase. *J. Acoust. Soc. Amer.* **80**, 1363–1374. (*Fig. 7.18*) 7

Rose, J. E., Brugge, J. F., Anderson, D. J., and Hind, J. E. (1967). Phase-locked response to low-frequency tones in single auditory nerve fibers of the squirrel monkey. *J. Neurophysiol.* **30**, 769–793. (*Fig. 9.8*) 9

Rose, J. E., Galambos, R., and Hughes, J. R. (1959). Microelectrode studies of the cochlear nuclei of the cat. *Bull. Johns Hopkins Hosp.* 104, 211–251. (*Fig. 15.15*) 15

Rose, J. E., Hind, J. E., Anderson, D. J., and Brugge, J. F. (1971). Some effects of stimulus intensity on response of auditory nerve fibers in the squirrel monkey. *J. Neurophysiol.* **34**, 685–699. (*Fig. 9.4*) 9

Subject Index and Glossary

The definitions of some of these terms are from the American National Standards Institute (ANSI). These definitions are reproduced with permission from American National Standard S.3.20–1974 (R 1978), copyright 1974 by the American National Standards Institute (copies of which may be purchased from the Acoustical Society of America, 335 East 45th St., New York, NY 10017). Note that certain ANSI definitions do not agree in detail with the uses of terms in this book. The first page listed for a term most likely is the page where the term is defined within the context of this book.

A

AI, AII, 15

abscissa, 6

absolute limen. *See* absolute threshold

absolute pitch, 199

absolute refractory period, 121, 285

absolute threshold, 27, 143–147. The absolute threshold is the minimum stimulus that evokes a response in a specified fraction of the trials.

absorption (Ab), 31

acceleration (a, x), 12, 20, 34

accidents (auditory damage), 249

acetylcholine (ACh), 230

acoustic echoes, 112–114, 180

acoustic impedance (Z), 28, 78–79

acoustic nerve (an), 67, 113–118, 121–138. The acoustic nerve is the eighth cranial nerve. It consists of two sets of fibers: the anterior branch, or cochlear nerve, and the posterior branch, or vestibular nerve. The acoustic nerve conducts neural signals from the internal ear to the brain.

acoustic properties of speech, 216

acoustic reflex, 77, 79

acoustics, 1

actin, 90, 96

action potential, 107–108, 121–122, 284–286

    auditory action potential (AP), 103, 107–108, 119, 135

active process/system, 63, 112–113

adaptation, 127, 191

adequate stimulus (neural), 284

afferent fibers (A), 113–119, 121–125

auditory nerve, 113–119

    outer spiral (OS, type II), 115–117

    radial (R, type 1), 115–117

    function of, 121–125

aging auditory system, 249, 254

air conduction, 75, 79. Air conduction is the process by which sound is conducted to the internal ear through the air in the external acoustic meatus (ear canal) as part of the pathway.

air molecules, 21–23

air pressure (p), 24–27

all-or-none law of nerve conduction, 122, 285

alleles, 293

alternating binaural loudness balance (ABLB), 198

alternating current (ac), 103

amino acid, 230

aminoglycosides, 230, 254

    kanamycin, 254

    neomycin, 254

    streptomycin, 254

amplification hearing aid, 259

amplitude (A, $A(t)$, a_i), 12–14, 17–18, 20, 22–24, 50–51, 153–154, 212–215, 264

    distortion. *See* distortion

    instantaneous, 17, 264

    modulation (AM), 43, 50–51, 153–154, 212–215

    spectrum. *See* spectrum

    peak (A), 13, 17–18

    peak to peak, 17–18

    root mean square (A_{rms}), 17–18, 20

analog-to-digital converter (A-to-D converter, or ADC), 287

analytic (listening), 208

anatomy, 2, 281–284

anechoic room, 30. An anechoic room is a room in which the boundaries absorb nearly all the sound incident thereon, thereby effectively affording free-field conditions.

angle, degrees of, 13, 15, 263

angular velocity(ω), 19, 271

annoyance, 249

annular ligament, 71

anterior, 281

anterior ligament of the malleus, 70–71

anteroventral cochlear nucleus (AVCN), 238, 241

antibodies, 96, 290–291

antigens, 290–291

antinodes, 31–33

apex of cochlea, 85, 95–96, 106–107

area under ROC curve, 277–278

articulators (speech), 216–218

artificial ear. *See also* coupler. An artificial ear is a device for the measurement of earphones that presents an acoustic impedance to the earphone equivalent to the impedance presented by the average human ear. It has a microphone that measures the sound pressures developed by the earphone.

ascending pathways, 113, 223–229

asymptotic threshold shift (ATS), 251, 260

Atoh1, 258, 261

attack, 212, 219

attention, 204

attenuation, 56–58

attributes of sound, 1, 14, 203

audibility, 11, 143–146

audiogram, 146. An audiogram is a graph showing hearing threshold level as a function of frequency.

audiology, 3, 249. Audiology is the study of hearing.

audition, 1–3. Audition is the sense of hearing.

auditory action potential. *See* action potential

auditory adaptation. *See* auditory fatigue and temporary threshold shift

auditory brainstem response (ABR), 235

auditory cortex, 67, 226–227, 243–246

auditory-evoked response (AER), 233–235

auditory fatigue. *See* temporary threshold shift. Auditory fatigue is the temporary increase in the threshold of audibility resulting from a previous auditory stimulus. It may be considered a mild temporary threshold shift lasting up to several minutes.

auditory flutter, 197. Auditory flutter is the wavering auditory sensation produced by periodically interrupting a continuous sound at a sufficiently slow rate.

auditory fusion, 181–204. Auditory fusion is the phenomenon in which a series of (primary) sounds of short duration with successive arrival times at the ear(s) produce the sensation of a single (secondary) sound.

auditory image model (AIM), 138, 204

auditory induction. *See* pulsation threshold.

auditory lateralization, 14, 173–180. Auditory lateralization is the determination by a subject that the apparent direction of a sound is either left or right of the frontal-medial plane of the head.

auditory localization. Auditory localization is the determination by a subject of the apparent direction and/or distance of a sound source.

auditory nerve, *See* acoustic nerve, (an)

auditory ossicles. *See also* incus; malleus; stapes. The auditory ossicles are the three small bones in the middle ear: the malleus, the incus, and the stapes. These bones transmit the sound vibrations from the tympanic membrane to the oval window.

auditory scene analysis, 7, 220

auditory sensation area. *See* dynamic range. The auditory sensation area is the region enclosed by the curves defining the threshold of pain and the threshold of audibility as functions of frequency.

auditory streams, 210
  stream fusion, 210
  stream segregation, 210

auditory threshold, 26, 144, 276

auditory tube. *See* eustachian tube. The auditory tube, or eustachian tube, is a canal that connects the middle ear with the nasal part of the pharynx. It serves to equalize the air pressure on the two sides of the tympanic membrane, i.e., the middle ear pressure and the ambient pressure.

auditory virtual environments, 183, 196

aural harmonic, 161, 169, 196, 265. An aural harmonic is a harmonic generated in the auditory mechanism.

auricle. The auricle, or pinna, the most visible part of the ear, is an ovid-formed, skin-covered, fibrocartilaginous plate attached to the head. The auricle is believed to be useful in the localization of sounds in the front–back and vertical dimensions.

autoradiograph, 299

average localized synchronized rate (ALSR), 137

average noise power, 47–48

average power, 47

axial ligaments, 71
  anterior, 71
  posterior, 71

axon, 223, 283

azimuth, 173–178, 190, 229, 241

B

backward fringe masking, 166

backward masking, 166. Backward masking describes the condition in which the masking sound appears after the masked sound.

band narrowing, 163

band-reject filter, 55–56

banded cells, 225, 229

bandpass filter, 55–58, 61–61, 95, 126, 132, 163. A bandpass filter is a wave filter that has a single transmission band extending from a lower cutoff frequency greater than zero to a finite upper cutoff frequency.
  of the auditory nerve, 126
  of the cochlea, 99

bandwidth (BW, Q), 62

basilar membrane (BM), 79, 85–102, 107, 109, 212, 125. The basilar membrane is a fibrous plate extending from the osseous spiral lamina to the spiral ligament on the outer wall of the cochlea. It separates the scala media from the tympanum and supports the organ of Corti.

basilar membrane tuning, 99

basilar papilla, 258

beating tones, 41–42, 156, 160–162

beats, 41, 156, 160–162, 187. Beats are periodic variations that result from the superposition of two simple harmonic quantities of different frequencies f_1 and f_2. They involve the periodic increase and decrease of amplitude at the beat frequency $(f_1 - f_2)$.
  best beats, 160
  binaural beats, 187
  measuring ΔI, 156
  measuring ΔF, 156

behavioral neuroscience, 3

bel, 26. The bel is a unit of level when the base of the logarithm is 10. Use of the bel is restricted to levels of quantities proportional to power.

best frequency (BF), 125. *See* characteristic frequency

beta (β), 52

bias (response), 275–276

bilateral, 225

binaural, 30, 173–175, 225–227. Binaural pertains to the use of two ears.

binaural beats, 187

binaural masking, 184–186

binaural masking level difference (BLMD). *See* masking level difference

biochemistry, 87, 292

biophysical techniques, 292–293

bipolar cells, 229

blood oxygenation level-dependent (BOLD) response, 237

bone conduction, 75, 79–80, 155. Bone conduction is the process by which sound is conducted to the internal ear through the cranial bones.

bone vibrator, 155
border cells (BC), 88. The border cells are a single row of supporting cells lying on the inward side of the inner hair cells in the organ of Corti. The upper part of the border cells partially encloses the cuticular plates of the inner hair cells.
brain images, 225–226, 247, 292
brainstem-evoked response (BSER), 235
Brownian motion, 34
bushy cells, 225, 229

C

Cajal, 4
cancellation method, 106, 196–197
cancellation tone, 196–197
capitulum, 69
carrier frequency (f_c), 43–46
cartwheel cells, 229
case of missing fundamental. *See* missing fundamental
catch trial, D. *See* false alarm
categorical perception, 218
cell and molecular biology, 293
cell body, 283, 289
cell membrane, 283–284
cells of Claudius, 86. The cells of Claudius are cells that lie on the outward side of the cells of Hensen in the organ of Corti.
cells of Deiters, 86. The cells of Deiters comprise several rows of supporting cells that extend from the basilar membrane and support the outer hair cells in the organ of Corti. Processes from the cells of Deiters form part of the reticular lamina.
cells of Hensen, 86. The cells of Hensen comprise several rows of supporting cells lying on the outward side of the cells of Deiters in the organ of Corti. Processes from the cells of Hensen form part of the reticular lamina.
center or critical or characteristic frequency (CF), 62, 100, 122–123, 164, 169
central, 281
central auditory nervous system (CANS), 67–68, 223–225
central nucleus (of the inferior colliculus), 242
cents, 192

cephalic, 281
characteristic delay, 242
characteristic frequency (CF). *See* best frequency
characteristic impedance (Z_c), 28, 53
characteristic of logarithm, 269
chirp-gammatone filter, 240
choppers, 230–231
chromosome, 293
cilia, 85, 88–90
circumaural headphones, 145
classical psychophysics, 275–276
Claudius' cells (C). *See* cells of Claudius
click stimulus, 39–41, 112, 131
    condensation, 41, 131
    rarefaction, 41, 131
clinical audiology. *See* audiology
CM. *See* cochlear microphonic
cochlea, 83–87. The cochlea is a spirally coiled, tapered bony tube of about $2\frac{3}{4}$ turns located within the internal ear. It contains the receptor organs essential to hearing.
cochlear amplifier, 112, 119
cochlear duct (sac), 86, 104. The cochlear duct is the portion of the membranous labyrinth contained within the cochlea. It is an endolymph-filled duct following the spiral shape of the cochlea, and it contains the organ of Corti. The cavity of the cochlear duct is called the *scala media*.
cochlear emission, 112–114
    DPOAE, 112–114
    OAE, 112
    SOAE, 112
    TOAE, 112, 114
cochlear hearing loss, 250
cochlear implant (cochlear prosthesis), 238, 259
cochlear map, 135, 140
cochlear microphonic (CM), 103–107, 134, 286. The cochlear microphonic is an ac electric potential generated within the cochlea in response to a sound stimulus. At low and moderate sound pressure levels, the amplitude of the cochlear microphonic is proportional to the instantaneous sound pressure of the stimulus and is a faithful reproduction of the stimulus waveform. The source of the microphonic is believed to be the

cuticular plates of the hair cells in the organ of Corti.
cochlear nerve (Cn). *See also* acoustic nerve. The cochlear nerve is the anterior branch of the acoustic nerve. It arises from the nerve cells of the spiral ganglion of the cochlea and terminates in the dorsal and ventral cochlear nuclei in the brainstem.
cochlear nucleus, 118, 223, 225, 227, 238–241
cochlear partition, 86. The cochlear partition is the term used collectively to describe the partitions of the scala media, the most significant of which are the basilar membrane, the tectorial membrane, and the organ of Corti.
cochlear potentials, 103–104
cochlear sac. *See* cochlear duct
cochleogram, 256
cocktail party effect, 185, 187, 208
codes (neural) for sound, 4, 204
coefficient of synchrony, 128, 131, 244
    vector strength, 244
collaterals, 283
combination tone, 59–60, 62, 161, 199, 265. A combination tone is a (secondary) tone that can be perceived when two loud (primary) tones are presented simultaneously. The secondary tone may be a difference tone or a summation tone. Several combination tones may be produced from a single pair of primary tones.
    difference tones, 51–60, 101–102, 134
    summation tones, 59–60, 199
commissure of inferior colliculus, 224
commissure of Probst, 224
communication system, 3–4
comodulation masking release (CMR), 212–213
complex math, 273
complex number, 273
complex pitch, 193–195, 208, 236
complex stimuli, 37–51
complex tone, *See* complex stimuli. (1) A complex tone is a sound wave containing simple sinusoidal components of different frequencies. (2) A complex tone is a sound sensation characterized by more than one pitch.

complex vibration. *See* complex stimuli

complex waveform. *See* complex stimuli

compliance, 78

compound threshold shift (CTS), 251

compression, 100, 169, 172

  compressive nonlinearity, 100, 169

computational models, 287

computerized axial tomography (CAT), 236, 292

computers in audition, 5, 287

concha, 67–68

condensation, 21–23, 28–29, 34, 41

condensation click, 41

conductive hearing loss, 225

cones of confusion, 177–178

confounding variable (CV), 6

consonance, 197. Consonance is the phenomenon in which tones presented together produce a blended or pleasant sensation.

constant energy, 148–149

  temporal integration, 149–150

constant stimuli (method of), 275

constructive interference, 283

continuous spectrum, 39. A continuous spectrum is a spectrum of a wave, the components of which are continuously distributed over a frequency region.

contralateral, 116, 134, 140, 223, 242

control experiments, 6

correct detection (hit), 276–277. A correct detection is the event that occurs in the detection situation, during a specified observation interval, when a "signal-plus-noise" stimulus (output) follows a "signal-plus-noise" stimulus (input).

correct dismissal (correct rejection), 276–277. A correct dismissal is the event that occurs in a detection situation, during a specified observation interval, when a "noise-along" response (output) follows a "noise-alone" stimulus (input).

correct hit. *See* correct detection

correct rejection. *See* correct dismissal

cortex, 67, 223, 243–246

Corti, 4

Corti's organ. *See* organ of Corti

cortical cell types, 228

cortilymph, 88

cosine (cosinusoid, cos), 17, 263–265

coupler, 144–145. A coupler is a device for acoustic loading of earphones. It has a specified arrangement of acoustic elements and is provided with a microphone for measurement of the sound pressure developed in a specified portion of the device.

  artificial ear, 145

  2-cm^3 coupler, 145

  6-cm^3 coupler, 145

  Zwislocki coupler, 145

cranial, 281

criterion (bias), 276–277

critical band, 163–166, 171–172, 191, 198, 205. The critical band (for loudness) is that frequency band within which the loudness of a band of continuously distributed sound of constant sound pressure level is independent of its bandwidth.

  critical band filter, 164

  critical bandwidth, 164

  equivalent rectangular bandwidth (ERB), 164–165, 171

  power in the critical band (P_{ncb}), 163, 172

critical potential difference, 284

critical ratio (CR), 172

cross bridges, 90–95

cross-modality matching, 278

cross-sectional, 287

crossed olivocochlear bundle (COCB), 116–117, 134, 140

crura (crus). *See* stapes

cubic-difference tone, 113–114, 134, 162, 196–199

cuticular plate (CP), 91, 96

cutoff frequency, 55–57

cycle, 11–15. A cycle is the complete sequence of values of a periodic quantity that occurs during one period.

cytocochleogram. *See* cochleogram

cytoplasm, 283

D

damage risk criterion, 260. A damage risk criterion for hearing is the level of sound to which a population may be exposed for a specified time with a specified risk of hearing loss.

damped vibration, 18, 34–35, 53

decay, 51, 212

decibel (dB), 25–27, 190. The decibel is one-tenth of a bel. Thus, the decibel is

a unit of level when the base of the logarithm is the 10th root of 10, and the quantities concerned are proportional to power.

  dBA, 190

  of energy, 26

  of power, 26

  of pressure, 26

  of sound intensity, 26

Deiters' cells. *See* cells of Deiters

Δf, 150–151

ΔI, 151–152

ΔT, 152–153

dendrites, 283

density (p_o), 28

density (subjective tonal), 197. Density is that attribute of auditory sensation in terms of which sound may be ordered on a scale extending from diffuse to compact.

dependent variable (DV), 5

depolarization, 110, 284

depth of modulation (m), 43–45, 153–154, 214–215

  AM, 43

  FM, 45, 52

destructive interference, 28

development of the auditory system, 237–238

diaphragm, 216

dichotic, 184. Dichotic refers to the condition in which the sound stimulus presented at one ear differs from the sound stimulus presented at the other ear.

dichotic pitch, 195

difference limen. *See* differential threshold

difference threshold, 150–156, 275

difference tone, 58–60, 161–162, 169, 196–199. *See* cubic-difference tone. A difference tone is a combination tone with a frequency equal to the difference between the frequencies of two primary tones or of their harmonics.

  primary-difference tone, 162

  secondary-difference tone, 162

differential electrode technique, 106

differential equation, 272

differential sensitivity, 150

differential threshold. *See* difference threshold. The differential threshold, or difference limen, is the minimum change in stimulus that can be correctly judged as different from a reference stimulus in a specified fraction of the trials.

diffracted wave, 29. A diffracted wave is a wave for which the wavefront has been changed in direction by an obstacle or other nonhomogeneity in a medium, other than by reflection or refraction.

diffraction, 29, 145

diffuse field, 30

digital signal processing, 287

digital-to-analog converter (D-to-A converter, or DAC), 287

diotic, 184. Diotic refers to the condition in which the sound stimuli presented at each ear are identical.

direct current (dc), 103, 272

direct scaling, 193, 278–279

discharge (neural), 284–285

discharge rate, 285

discrimination, 143, 275

diseases (auditory), 254–255

displacement (distance, D), 12, 17–18
  instantaneous, 12
  maximal (A), 17–18

dissonance, 197. Dissonance is the phenomenon in which tones presented together produce a harsh or unpleasant sensation.

distal, 281

distance (range) perception, 173–174, 179

distortion, 59. Distortion is an undesired change in waveform. Noise and certain desired changes in waveform, such as those resulting from modulation or detection, are not usually classified as distortion.

distortion-product otoacoustic emission (DPOAE), 112–114, 120

diuretics, 254
  ethacrynic acid, 254
  furosemide, 254

DNA (deoxyribonucleic acid), 292

Doppler shift, 35

dorsal, 281

dorsal cochlear nucleus (DCN), 238–239

dorsal cortex of inferior colliculus, 242

driving frequency, 53–56

drugs, 249, 254
  ototoxic, 249, 254

duplex theory of localization, 176, 183

duty cycle, 45

dynamic range. See auditory sensation area
  basilar membrane response, 100
  neural, 123

E

$E–E$ cells, 230, 242

$E–I$ cells, 230, 242

ear canal. See external acoustic meatus

ear, nose, throat (ENT), 3

eardrum. See tympanic membrane

echo, 180. See otoacoustic emission. An echo is a wave that has been reflected or otherwise returned with sufficient magnitude and delay to be detected as a wave distinct from that directly transmitted.

echolocate, 187

efferent fibers (E), 110, 113, 116–120, 134, 140
  auditory nerve, 113, 116–120, 134, 140

eighth (VIIIth) cranial nerve. See acoustic nerve

elasticity, 11

electric potential, 103, 105, 121, 284–285
  neural, 121, 284–285

electroacoustic (impedance) bridge, 78–79

electrocochleograph, 119

electrodes, 104, 223, 259, 291–292

electroencephalogram (EEG), 119, 233–234, 286

electrophysiology, 286–287, 291–292

empirical method, 5

encoding, 1, 113, 118, 134–135

endocochlear potential (EP) (endolymphatic potential), 104–105. The endocochlear potential is a resting electric polarization of the endolymph of the scala media, positive relative to the perilymph in the scala vestibular and scala tympani and also to tissues outside of these canals.

endolymph, 86–87, 95, 103–104. Endolymph is a watery fluid contained within the membranous labyrinth. It is thought to be secreted by the stria vascularis.

energetic masking, 211, 221

energy (E), 25–26, 34, 51, 147–149, 162, 165, 252. Energy is a measure of the capacity of a body to do work or of work that is done. The unit of measure is the erg, 1 erg being expended when a mass of 1 g is accelerated 1 cm per second per second.

ENT. See ear nose throat

envelope, 40, 49–51, 96–98, 182, 193–194, 212–213, 246
  amplitude, 49–51
  function ($e(t)$), 51
  neural, 246
  pitch, 193–194
  spectral, 40, 51
  of the traveling wave, 96–98

enzymes, 293

epitympanic recess, 69

epitympanum, 69

equal energy rule (3-dB rule), 252
  4-db, 5-dB rules, 252

equal-loudness contour, 189–191

equal temperament scale, 192

equalization-cancellation (EC), 187

equivalent rectangular bandwidth (ERB), 52, 164–165, 171
  critical band, 164–165, 171

eustachian tube, 69, 71, 225

evoked acoustic potential (EAP), 235

evoked otoacoustic emissions, 112

evoked potentials, 235

excitation pattern, 164–165, 170
  masking, 164–165, 170

excitatory and inhibitory cells, 230
  connections, 230. See $E–E$ cells, $E–I$ cells

external acoustic meatus, 68. The external acoustic meatus, or ear canal, is the canal that conducts sound vibrations from the auricle to the tympanic membrane.

external auditory canal, 38

external auditory meatus. See external acoustic meatus.

external ear. See outer ear. The external ear consists of the auricle and external acoustic meatus.

external hair cells. See hair cells, outer.

extracellular fluids, 284

extracellular recording, 108, 113, 286, 291

extratympanic electrocochleography, 119

F

false alarm, 276–278. A false alarm is the event that occurs in a detection situation, during a specified observation interval, when a "signal-plus-noise" response (output) follows a " noise-along" stimulus (input).

fast Fourier transform (FFT), 273, 287

Fechner, 4, 150
fibers of passage, 225
filters, 54–58, 99, 126, 157, 164–166, 183
    critical band, 164–166, 183
    in the cochlea, 99
    internal, 165–166
    modulation filter bank, 157
    neural, 126
    shaping sounds, 57–58
    spectral analysis, 57
    types of, 55–56
fine structure, 49–52
first-order fibers, 223
fissure of Sylvius, 243
flutter. *See* auditory flutter
following response. *See* phase-locked
        response
footplate (stapes), 70–71, 76–78
force (F), 11–12, 19–20, 25
forced vibration, 53
formant frequency (F_n, $n = 1, 2, ...$),
        136–138, 217–218
formant peaks, 217–218
formant shift or formant transition, 217–218
forward fringe masking, 166–167
forward masking, 166–167. Forward
        masking describes the condition in
        which the masking sound appears
        before the masked sound.
Fourier analysis, 13, 19, 38, 271–273
Fourier integral, 271–273
Fourier series, 271–272
Fourier theorem, 13, 272
fourth ventricle, 134
free field. *See* free sound field
free sound field, 30, 73. A free sound field
        is a field in a homogeneous, isotropic
        medium free from boundaries. In
        practice, it is a field in which the
        effects of the boundaries are
        negligible over the region of interest.
free vibration, 12, 19–20
frequency. *See* frequency of a periodic
        quantity
    cutoff frequency, 55
    driving frequency, 53–54
    formant frequency, 217–218
    frequency discrimination, 150–151
    frequency domain, 37–39
    frequency-modulated stimuli, 45–46
    fundamental frequency, 33, 39, 56
    fundamental frequency of the speech, 216
    repetition frequency, 14–15

resonance frequency, 53–55
sinusoidal frequency, 14–15
frequency of a periodic quantity, 1, 14–15,
        33, 37–39, 53–56, 150–151, 216–218.
        The frequency of a periodic quantity,
        in which time is the independent
        variable, is the number of periods
        occurring in unit time. Unless
        otherwise specified, the unit is the
        cycle per second.
friction (R), 12, 18–19, 28, 35, 78
front–back confusions (back–front
        confusions), 177–178
functional and integrative neuroscience, 3
functional MRI (fMRI), 237, 255, 292
fundamental frequency (f_0), 33, 39, 56.
        The fundamental frequency of a
        periodic quantity is the frequency of
        the sinusoid that has the same period
        as the periodic quantity.
fundamental frequency of the speaking
        voice, 216
fundamental mode of vibration, 33
fused image. *See* auditory fusion
fusiform (F) cell, 228, 239, 241
fusion. *See* auditory fusion

G

gamma-aminobutyric acid (GABA), 230
gammatone filter, 140, 171
ganglia, 283
ganglion cells (Gc), 283
gas laws, 21, 34
Gaussian noise, 47–50, 52, 162. Gaussian
        noise is noise for which the
        amplitudes of some measure follow a
        Gaussian distribution.
    normal distribution [$P(a_i)$], 52
generator potential, 121
genetics, 283
    gene therapy, 293
    genes, 293
genotype, 293
giant cells, 228
globular (G) cells, 228, 239, 241
globular bushy (GB) cells, 228, 229
glutamate, 121
glycine, 230
granule cells, 228

H

habenula perforate (HP), 115, 117, 120–121
hair cell regeneration, 238, 258–261

hair cells (HC), 83, 85, 88–92, 94, 96, 102,
        108–112, 115–116, 120, 139,
        249–251, 254–259. Hair cells are the
        sensory receptor cells for hearing.
        They are ciliated epithelial cells
        located within the organ of Corti and
        are subdivided into the inner hair cells
        and the outer hair cells. Several dozen
        hairlike processes are attached to a
        cuticular surface at the free end of
        each hair cell; the cuticular surface
        forms part of the reticular lamina. The
        bases of the hair cells are in contact
        with the dendritic processes of the
        neurons of the spiral ganglion of the
        cochlea.
    damage, 249–251, 254–259
    motility, 110–113, 119–120
    inner hair cells (IHC), 88–90, 92, 94,
        108, 110–112, 115–117, 120, 139,
        251, 256–258
    outer hair cells (OHC), 85, 88–92, 94,
        108–116, 119, 251, 256–258
half-octave shift, 253
half-wave rectification, 127, 130–131, 140
harmonic, 39, 56, 59–60, 101, 134,
        161–162, 193–197, 208, 265, 272. A
        harmonic is a sinusoidal quantity
        having a frequency that is an integral
        multiple of the fundamental frequency
        of a periodic quantity to which it is
        related.
harmonic motion. *See* simple harmonic
        motion
head of stapes, 70–71
head-related transfer function (HRTF), 72,
        174, 178–179, 183–184, 186
headphones, 145–146, 184–185
    calibration, 145
    circumaural, 145
    insert, 145
    supra-aural, 145
hearing aids. *See* amplification hearing
        aids
hearing level (HL), 146
helicotrema, 85–86. The helicotrema is the
        narrow aperture within the apex of the
        cochlea that allows communication
        between the scala vestibuli and the
        scala tympani.
Helmholtz, 4, 7, 73, 80, 143
Hensen's cells. *See* cells of Hensen
Hensen's stripe (HS), 89, 94

method of cross-modality matching, 278. The method of cross-modality matching is a psychophysical method used primarily to scale sensations; in this procedure, the subject adjusts a stimulus along some dimension until that stimulus appears equal to another stimulus received via a different send modality.

method of limits, 275. The method of limits is a psychophysical method used primarily to determine thresholds; in this procedure, some dimension of a stimulus, or of the difference between two stimuli, is varied incrementally until the subject changes his response.

method of magnitude estimation, 278. The method of magnitude estimation is a psychophysical method used primarily to scale sensations; in this procedure, the subject assigns to a set of stimuli numbers that are proportional to some subjective dimension of the stimuli.

method of theory of signal detection, 276–277

methods (psychophysical), 275–279

microanatomy, 281

microscope, 281, 287–288

microvillus (m), 93

middle ear (tympanic cavity), 68, 75–80. The middle ear, or tympanic cavity, is the air-filled chamber within the mastoid portion of the temporal bone that contains the three auditory ossicles. It communicates with the auditory tube and the mastoid cells.

muscles, 77, 79–80

ossicles, 70

middle ear cavity. *See* middle ear

middle ear reflex. *See* stapedial muscle, tensor tympani muscle

middle latency-evoked potentials, 235

mid-sagittal plane, 177

minimal audible angle (MAA), 176, 182

minimal uncertainty task, 211

minimum audible field (MAF), 144–145. The minimum audible field is the sound pressure level of a tone at the threshold of audibility measured in a free sound field for a subject facing the sound source. The value of the sound pressure level is determined

after the subject is removed from the field.

minimum audible pressure (MAP), 144–145. The minimum audible pressure is the sound pressure of a tone at the threshold of audibility that is presented by an earphone and measured or inferred at the tympanic membrane.

miss, 277

missing fundamental, 193–196

tonal complex, 193–196

missing 6 dB, 134, 145

mitochondria (Mc), 116

models, 6, 12, 88, 137–138, 187, 204, 261

computational models, 137–138, 204, 287

modiolus, 85, 88, 104. The modiolus is the conically shaped central core of the cochlea. It contains the spiral ganglion of the cochlea and forms the inner wall of the scala vestibuli and the scala tympani.

modulation depth (m), 153–154, 157, 214–215

modulation detection interference (MDI), 214–216

modulation filter bank, 157, 215

modulation frequency or rate (f_m), 43, 153–154

monaural. *See* monotic. Monaural pertains to the use of only one ear.

monotic, 184–185. Monotic refers to the condition in which a sound stimulus is presented at only one ear.

morphology, cell morphology, 225

Mossbauer technique, 99, 292

motility (hair cells), 108–109

motor neurons, 282

moving sound sources, 186

multi-electrode, 232, 292

multipolar (M) cells, 228, 239, 241

music, 2, 46, 192, 197, 199, 219–220

musical scale, 192. A musical scale is a series of notes (symbols, sensations, or stimuli) arranged from low to high by a specified scheme of intervals, suitable for musical purposes.

equal temperament, 192

just intonation, 192

mel, 192–193

Pythagorean, 192

mutation, 238, 293

myelin sheath, 117, 120–121, 237, 250, 283

myelinated nerve fibers (MNF), 250, 283

myosin, 90

N

narrowband noise, 49–51, 163, 212–213

nasal, 75, 216, 255

nasopharynx (nose cavity), 69

near miss to Weber law, 152

nerve. *See* acoustic nerve

neural code, 1, 204

neural map for auditory space, 229

neural synchrony, 128, 131, 133, 137

neural temporal modulation transfer function, 244

neural transduction, 83, 108–109

neurilemma, 283

neuroanatomy, 282

neuronal dynamic range, 123

neurophysiology, 284

neurotransmitter, 230, 283, 285–286, 290

nodes, 31–33, 283

nodes of Ranvier, 283

noise, 34, 49–51, 249. *See* random noise. Noise is any undesired sound. By extension, noise is any unwanted disturbance within a useful frequency band, such as undesired electric waves in a transmission channel or device.

exposure, 249–252

waveform ($n(t)$), 51

noise-induced hearing loss (NIHL), 249. Noise-induced hearing loss is the cumulative permanent hearing loss that is due to repeated exposure to intense noise.

noise-induced permanent threshold shift (NIPTS), 249. *See* permanent threshold shift

noise-induced temporary threshold shift (NITTS), 251

noise-induced threshold shift (NITS), 251

noise power per unit band width (N_o). *See* spectrum level

nonlinear system, 59–60, 62, 161, 265

nonlinear tones, 196–197

nonlinearity, 59–61, 63, 100, 161, 169–170

compressive, 61, 100, 169–170

normal equation. *See* Gaussian noise

nucleus/nuclei (N), 283

O

observational method, 5

occluded-ear simulator, 154

occlusion effect, 155
Occupational Safety and Health
    Administration (OSHA), 260
octave, 55–56, 192, 219, 253. (1) An
    octave is the interval between two
    sounds having a basic frequency ratio
    of 2. (2) An octave is the pitch
    interval between two tones such that
    one tone may be regarded as
    duplicating the basic musical import
    of the other tone at the nearest
    possible higher pitch.
octopus cell (O), 239, 241
off-frequency listening, 171
off response, 230
olivary complex, 116–117
olivarycochlear bundle (OCB), 116–117,
    134–136, 140
on–off response, 230
on response, 231
optical heterodyne spectroscopy, 292
ordinate, 6
organ of Corti (OC), 85–90, 92, 96, 99,
    106, 109–110, 115–116. The organ of
    Corti is a series of neuroepithelial hair
    cells (receptor cells for hearing) and
    their supporting structures lying
    against the osseous spiral lamina
    and the basilar membrane within the
    scala media of the cochlea. It extends
    from the base of the cochlea to its
    apex.
oscillation (vibration), 12, 15, 34, 132.
    Oscillation is the vibration, usually
    with time, of the magnitude of a
    quantity with respect to a specified
    reference when the magnitude is
    alternately greater and smaller than
    the reference.
osseous spiral lamina, 85–87, 108–109.
    The osseous spiral lamina is the bony
    ledge that projects from and winds
    around the modiolus for $2^{3}/_{4}$ turns
    from the base of the cochlea to the
    apex. The basilar membrane is
    attached to its free border and runs
    parallel to it.
ossicular chain, 71, 73, 75–80
otitis media, 75, 254–255
    with effusion, 254
otoacoustic emission (OAE), 112–113
otolaryngology. See ear, nose, throat
    (ENT)

otology, 3. Otology is the branch of
    medicine dealing with the ear.
otorhinolaryngology, 3
otosclerosis, 255
ototoxic (drugs), 249, 254, 258.
outer ear, 67, 68. See external ear.
outer hair cells. See hair cells
outer pillar cells (OP), 116
outer spiral fibers (OS, Type II), 115, 120
oval window (OW), 71, 75–80, 83, 85–86,
    255. The oval window is an opening
    through the bone that separates the
    middle ear from the scala vestibuli of
    the cochlea. It is closed by the
    footplate of the stapes, which is
    attached to it by the annular ligament.
    membrane, 6
overshoot, 167
overtones, 219

P

pain threshold, 145, 147
palette, 216
paracentral nuclei (of the IC), 242
pars flaccida, 69
pass band, 55, 57
patched clamping, 110, 292
pausers, 230
peak amplitude. See amplitude
peak-to-peak value, 15, 18, 24. The peak-
    to-peak value of an oscillating
    quantity is the algebraic difference
    between the extremes of the quantity.
peptides, 290
perceived location, 14, 143, 180
percent correct [$P(C)$], 144, 278
perception, 2, 143, 203
perilymph, 86, 87, 103, 105. Perilymph is a
    clear, watery fluid contained within
    the osseous labyrinth.
period (P), 13–16. The period of a periodic
    quantity is the smallest increment of
    the independent variable for which the
    function repeats itself.
period histograms, 128
periodicity pitch, 194
peripheral, 2, 281
peripheral auditory nervous system, 281
permanent hearing loss. See permanent
    threshold shift. Permanent hearing
    loss of an ear is the permanent
    impairment of sensitivity of hearing of
    that ear.

permanent threshold shift (PTS), 251.
    Permanent threshold shift is a
    permanent increase in the threshold of
    audibility for an ear at a specified
    frequency above a previously
    established reference level. The
    amount of permanent threshold shift is
    customarily expressed in decibels.
perstimulatory fatigue. See loudness
    adaptation
phalangeal cells, 87–88
phalangeal process, 88
phase, 12–17, 37, 72, 95–98, 195–197
    instantaneous, 17
    interaural, 195, 197
    sensitivity to, 12, 37
    spectrum, 37
    starting, 15–17
    of traveling wave, 95–98
phase angle, 12–13
phase contrast light microscope, 287
phase of cubic-difference tone, 196
phase lag, 17
phase lead, 17
phase-locked PST histograms, 128
phase-locked response, 126, 128, 131, 195
phase spectrum, 37
phenotype, 293
phon. See loudness level. The phon is the
    unit of loudness level.
phoneme, 216
photomicrographs, 287
physical attributes (of sound), 1–2, 14
physiology, 3, 284–296
pillar cells, 92–94, 115
pillars of Corti. See rods of Corti
pink noise, 48, 50
pinna. See auricle
pitch, 4, 14, 191–196, 198. Pitch is that
    attribute of auditory sensation in terms
    of which sounds may be ordered on a
    scale extending from low to high. The
    unit of pitch is the mel.
    of the missing fundamental, 13
pitch scale, 192
pitch shift of the residue, 195
place of articulation, 216
place theory, 4, 135, 254, 256
plasticity (neural plasticity), 237–239,
    259
population response, 136
positron emission tomography (PET), 236,
    292

posterior, 83, 281

posterior crus, 70

posterior ligament of the incus, 71

posteroventral cochlear nucleus (PVCN), 238, 240

poststimulus time (PST) histogram, 127–129, 133, 135, 138, 232

potassium (K), 87, 103, 111, 284–285

potential difference, 284–285

power (P), 25–27. Power is the rate at which energy is expended or work is done. The unit of measure is the watt.

power function. *See* psychophysical power law

power spectrum, 37

power value (constant), 279

precedence effect, 180. The precedence effect is the phenomenon that occurs during auditory fusion when two (primary) sounds of the same order of magnitude are presented dichotically and produce localization of the secondary sound toward the ear receiving the first (primary) sound stimulus.

   fusion, 180

   localization dominance, 180

   suppression discrimination, 180

preolivary nuclei, 241–242

presbycusis, 147, 254

pressure (p), 21–22, 25–27. Pressure is a measure of force divided by the area to which the force is applied. It is usually measured in dynes per square centimeter.

   instantaneous, 25

prestin, 90, 102, 110, 120, 293

primary difference tone. *See* difference tone

primary fibers, 230

probe microphone, 78

probe tone, 166, 214–215

profile analysis, 206–207, 215

promontory, 119

propagate, 23

proteins, 90, 110, 255, 293

proximal, 281

PST histogram. *See* poststimulus time histogram

psychoacoustics, 14. Psychoacoustics is the science that deals with the psychological correlates of the physical parameters of acoustics.

Psychoacoustics is a branch of psychophysics.

psychometric function, 143–144, 147, 153, 275–276, 278. A psychometric function is a mathematical relationship in which the independent variable is a measure of a stimulus and the dependent variable is a measure of response.

psychophysical power law, 279. The psychophysical power law describes the relationship between stimulus magnitude and resulting sensation magnitude.

psychophysical suppression, 171–172

psychophysical techniques, 275–279

psychophysical tuning curves, 160–162, 164, 167

psychophysics, 14, 275. Psychophysics is the science that deals with the quantitative relationship between physical and psychological events. Psychophysics is a branch of psychology.

pulsation threshold. 220

Pythagorean scale, 192

Q

Q (of a filter), 62

qualitative aspects of pitch, 193

quinine, 254

R

radial fibers (R, type I), 115, 120

radians, 12, 15

range (localization), 174, 179

random noise, 47, 52. Random noise is an oscillation for which the instantaneous magnitude is not specified for any given instant of time. The instantaneous magnitudes of a random noise are specified only by probability distribution functions giving the fraction of the total time that the magnitude, or some sequence of magnitudes, lies within a specified range.

   pink noise, 48

   thermal noise, 34

rarefaction, 22–24

rarefaction click, 41, 131–132

rate-level function. *See* input–output functions

rate suppression, 133

ratio scale, 26, 55

Rayleigh, 4, 52, 176

   Rayleigh distribution, 52

reactance (X), 28, 35, 54, 76, 78–79

   mass (X_m), 28, 54, 78

   spring (stiffness, X_s), 28, 54

real-ear measurement, 72

real-time holography. *See* holography.

real value of complex number, 273

receiver, 3–4

receiver operator characteristic (ROC), 277–278. A receiver operator characteristic is a graphical summary of the performance of a detector. Detection probability is plotted on the ordinate, and false-alarm probability is plotted on the abscissa. These are conditional probabilities, that is, the probability that the condition (signal present or signal absent) is true. A family of nonintersecting curves is often plotted with either constant detectability index or constant signal-to-noise ratio as the parameter. Each curve shows how detection probability and false-alarm probability vary monotonically as a function of the decision criteria (operating point) of the detector.

receptor neurons, 283

receptor potential, 121

recruitment, 190–191, 259. Recruitment is the otological condition in which weak sounds are not heard while strong sounds are heard as loud as by a normal ear. The function that relates loudness to sound pressure level is steeper than normal and is often nonlinear. In recruitment, the dynamic range of hearing is narrowed.

rectified, 131

reference equivalent threshold force level (RETFL), 145–146, 155–156

reflection, 30–32, 179–180

refractory period, 126–127, 285

   absolute, 285

   relative, 285

regenerated hair cells, 257–260, 261

regular interval stimuli (RIS), 199

reinforcement (reinforce), 28–31, 36

Reissner's membrane (RM), 86–87, 105. Reissner's membrane is a delicate cellular membrane attached to the inner part of the spiral limbus and to the spiral ligament. It separates the scala media from the scala vestibuli and forms one wall of the cochlear duct.

reject band, 55

relative pitch, 199

relative refractory period, 285

repetition frequency, 15, 192

repetition (periodicity) pitch, 194

resistance (R), 12, 18, 28, 35, 54, 78

resolution (spectral), 112, 218, 257

resonance, 54–55, 62, 73, 77–78, 145, 216, 219. Resonance is the property of a mechanical or electrical system of oscillating at a particular frequency with minimum dissipation of energy.
of concha, 73, 77
of external auditory canal, 77

resonance frequency (f_r), 54–55, 73. A resonance frequency is a frequency at which resonance exists.

resonator, 54–55

response area, 124–125

response bias, 275

response criterion, 277

response proclivity, 275

response table, 277

resting potential, 284–285

resting state, 11

restoring force, 11–12, 20

reticular lamina, 90–91, 106. The reticular lamina is a stiff membrane formed by processes of the supporting cells in which are incorporated the cuticular plates of the hair cells. The tectorial membrane, within the scala media, is in contact with the reticular lamina.

reticular membrane. See reticular lamina.

reverberation, 30–32. (1) Reverberation is the persistence of sound in an enclosed space as a result of multiple reflections after the sound source has stopped. (2) Reverberation is the sound that persists in an enclosed space as a result of repeated reflection or scattering after the source of the sound has stopped.

reverberation room, 30

reverberation time (RT), 30–31. The reverberation time of a room is the

time that would be required for the mean-square sound pressure level therein, originally in a steady state, to decrease 60 dB after the source has stopped.

rhino-otolaryngology. See ear, nose, throat (ENT).

rhythm (music), 219

ribonucleic acid (RNA), 293

rise–decay time, 51–52

rods of Corti, 88, 199. The rods of Corti are two rows of stiff rodlike structures (inner and outer rods) supported by the basilar membrane. Each rod consists of a base, a striated body, and a head. The heads of the inner and outer rods are in contact and form part of the reticular lamina. The rods and the basilar membrane enclose the inner tunnel of Corti. The openings between successive rods (both inner and outer) allow communication among the inner and outer tunnels of Corti, the space of Nuel, and the internal spiral sulcus.

roex (rounded exponential) filter, 165, 177

roll-off, 50, 55–57

root-mean-square (rms), 18, 20

rostral, 281

roughness, 197

round window (RW), 79, 85, 106, 119. The round window is an opening through the bone that separates the middle ear from the scala tympani of the cochlea. It is located behind and below the oval window and is closed by the round window membrane (secondary tympanic membrane).
electrode, 119
recording, 119

S

saccule, 83

salicylate, 254

SAM stimuli (sinusoidal amplitude modulation), 43, 51, 153

scala (ducts), 85

scala media (Sm), 85–88. The scala media is the cavity of the cochlear duct, filled with endolymph and containing also the tectorial membrane. The scala media is separated from the scala

vestibuli by Reissner's membrane and from the scala tympani by the basilar membrane and the cellular structures attached to it. The scala media has a closed end at the helicotrema.

scala tympani (St), 85–88. The scala tympani is the perilymph-filled passage of the cochlear canal that extends from the round window at the base to the helicotrema at the apex. It is separated from the scala media by the basilar membrane and the cellular structures attached to it.

scala vestibuli (Sv), 85–88. The scala vestibuli is the perilymph-filled passage of the cochlear canal that extends from the oval window at the base to the helicotrema at the apex. It is separated from the scala media by Reissner's membrane.

scales, 192, 278–279
musical, 192
psychophysical, 278–279

scaling procedure, 278–279

scanning electron microscope (SEM), 288–289

Schroeder tones, 172

second filter, 120

secondary-difference tones. See cubic-difference tone

segregation (source), 204

semicircular canals, 83–84

semitone, 192

sender, 3–4

sensation 6, 143, 203. Sensation is the element of reaction resulting from the action of a stimulus on a sensory receptor.

sensation level (SL), 27. The sensation level of a sound is the pressure level of the sound, in decibels, above its threshold of audibility for the individual subject or for a specified group of subjects.

sensitivity, 275

shearing force, 108–109

short-term spectrum, 46–47

sidebands, 43–44

signal (s), 140, 147, 159, 172, 278. A signal is (1) a disturbance used to convey information; (2) the information to be conveyed over a communication system.

signal averaging, 235, 286, 292

signal-to-masker ratio, *See* signal-to-noise ratio
signal-to-noise ratio, 140, 162, 171. Signal-to-noise ratio is the ratio of the signal to the corresponding noise, where the signal and noise may be electric energy, electric power, voltage, current, and the acoustic correlates thereof, i.e., sound energy, sound power, sound pressure, and sound particle velocity, especially.
simple harmonic motion, 13
simple sound. *See* tone
simultaneous masking (SM), 166–170
sine, 13
single neuron threshold, 122
single unit, 122, 125
    response 122
    threshold, 125
sinusoid. *See* tone
sine wave, 13
sinusoidal amplitude modulation (SAM), 43, 153, 182
    in lateralization, 182
sinusoidal frequency, 15, 43
sinusoidal frequency modulation, 45
sinusoidal vibrations, 13, 15, 19
sodium (Na), 87, 103, 108, 284–285
sodium pump, 285
soma, 283
sone, 190–193, 198. The sone is a unit of loudness. One sone is the loudness of a sound for which the loudness level is 40 phons. The loudness of a sound that is judged by a subject to be *n* times that of a 1-sone tone is *n* sones.
sound, 1, 11, 21. Sound is an oscillation in pressure, stress, particle displacement, particle velocity, and so on, in a medium with internal forces (for example, elastic, viscous) or the superposition of such propagated oscillations.
sound analysis, 53–63
sound field, 30–33, 145
sound intensity (I), 25–28, 35. The sound intensity in a specified direction at a point is the average rate of sound energy transmitted in the specified direction through a unit area normal to this direction at the point considered.
sound intensity level, 26

sound localization, 72, 173–184, 241–243
sound power level, 25, 252. Sound power level, in decibels, of a sound is 10 times the logarithm to the base 10 of the ratio of the power of this sound to the reference power. The reference power should be explicitly stated.
sound pressure level (SPL), 26, 144 Sound pressure level, in decibels, of a sound is 20 times the logarithm to the base 10 of the ratio of the pressure of this sound to the reference pressure. The reference pressure should be explicitly stated.
sound shadow, 29–30, 174, 176–178. A sound shadow is a region in which a sound field is reduced in magnitude relative to the free-field value as a result of its incidence on an obstacle.
sound source determination, 7, 204
sound transmission, 21–36
space of Nuel (SN), 91
spectral cues (in localization), 178
spectral pitch, 194
spectral profile, 205–208
spectrogram/spectrograph, 46, 49, 217
spectrum, 37–39, 46. (1) The spectrum of a function of time is a description of its resolution into components, each of different frequency and (usually) different amplitude and phase. (2) Spectrum is also used to signify a continuous range of components, usually wide in extent, within which waves have some specified common characteristic; e.g., audio-frequency spectrum.
    amplitude spectrum, 37–38
    continuous spectrum, 39
    line spectra, 39
    long-term spectrum, 46
    phase spectrum, 37–38
    short-term spectrum, 46
    spectral envelope, 40, 51
spectrum level (N_o), 47–48, 50, 52, 162–163, 172. The spectrum level of a specified signal at a particular frequency is the level of that part of the signal contained within a band of unit width and centered at the particular frequency. Ordinarily this

has significance only for a signal having a continuous distribution of components within the frequency range under consideration. The words *spectrum level* cannot be used alone but must appear in combination with a prefatory modifier; e.g., pressure, velocity, voltage power.
speech, 2, 4, 136–137, 215–219
speed of sound, 23, 25, 27, 30, 33–35, 173
speech perception, 217–219
speech production, 215–217
sphere (area of), 27
spherical bushy (SB) cells, 228, 239, 241
spikes (neural spikes), 121
spiral ganglion of the cochlea, 116. The spiral ganglion of the cochlea is composed of the cell bodies of the neurons of the cochlear nerve. It is located within the modiolus. The dendritic processes of these bipolar neurons make synaptic contact with the hair cells. The axons terminate in the cochlear nucleus in the medulla.
spiral lamina (SL), 85–87. The spiral lamina consists of the osseous spiral lamina and the basilar membrane (membranous spiral lamina).
spiral ligament (Sl), 85, 109. The spiral ligament is the periosteum-like outer wall of the scala media. It is attached to the outward border of the basilar membrane at the basilar crest. The spiral ligament is covered by the stria vascularis within the cochlear duct.
spiral limbus, 83, 108–109. The spiral limbus is an extension of the osseous spiral lamina toward the scala vestibuli. Near its inner edge it is attached to Reissner's membrane; and on its outer edge, which also forms the internal spiral sulcus, it is attached to the tectorial membrane.
spontaneous activity, 122–123
spontaneous otoacoustic emissions (SOAEs), 112, 254
spontaneous rate, 122–125
spread of energy, 51, 148–151
spring (s), 11–12
spring reactance (X_s), 28, 54
square wave, 43–45, 156, 194, 272
standing wave, 31
stapedectomy, 255

stapedial muscle (SM), stapedius, 71, 85. The stapedius is the intra-aural muscle attached to the neck of the stapes. Its reflex response to an intense sound stimulus is to swing the footplate of the stapes outward and backward from the oval window. The combined action of the stapedius and the tensor tympani muscles is to limit the motion of the auditory ossicles and thereby help protect the internal ear from damage by intense sound, especially at low frequencies.

stapes (S), 69–71, 75–78. The stapes is the innermost and smallest of the three auditory ossicles located in the middle ear. Its shape resembles a stirrup. The head of the stapes is attached to the lenticular process of the incus, and the footplate nearly fills the oval window and is attached there by the annular ligament.

starting phase (θ), 12–13, 15–17

state of equilibrium. *See also* resting state

static air pressure, 22–24, 34

steady-state speech (vowels), 217

stellate (S) cells, 225, 228–229, 239, 241

stereocilia (Sc), 88–96

Stevens, S. S., 176, 197–198, 275

Stevens and Newman, 176, 182

stiffness, 11, 20, 28, 78, 95
  membranes, 95

stimulus–response table, 277

streams (auditory), 209–210
  fusion, 210
  segregation, 210

stria vascularis, 86–88, 104–105, 250. The stria vascularis is a vascularized epithelial structure that covers the spiral ligament within the scala media. It is thought that the stria vascularis is the source of the endolymph and of its electrical polarization within the cochlea.

strychnine, 243

subjective attributes, 197, 278–279

subjective evaluation, 278–279

summating potential (SP), 103–105, The summating potentials are positive and negative changes in the dc polarization of the cochlea in response to a sound stimulus.

summation tone, 59–60, 199. A summation tone is a combination tone with a frequency equal to the sum of the frequencies of two primary tones or of their harmonics.

superior, 281

superior olive, 225–226, 241–242

superposition, 62

supporting cells, 88–90. The supporting cells are a group of cells extending from the basilar membrane that support the organ of Corti. The free ends of these cells form the reticular lamina. The supporting cells consist of the (a) inner rods of Corti, (b) outer rods of Corti, (c) inner phalangeal cells, (d) outer phalangeal cells (cells of Deiters), (e) border cells, and (f) cells of Hensen.

suppression, 131–135, 140, 166–168, 172
  neural, 131–135, 141
  masking, 166–169, 172

suppression tone (SU), 168–169

supra aural, 145

surface preparation technique, 289

synapse, 110, 223, 229–230, 283

synchrony-level function, 131

synchrony suppression, 133

synthetic (listening), 208

T

tangent function, 263

tectorial membrane (Tm), 88–89, 92, 94 108–109. The tectorial membrane is a soft, semigelatinous, ribbon-like structure attached along one edge to the spiral limbus and along the other edge to the outer border of the organ of Corti. It is in intimate contact with the cilia of the hair cells.

telodendria, 283

temporal acuity, 157

temporal bone (TB), 79, 83

temporal discrimination, 152–153

temporal gap, 157

temporal integration, 149–150, 156

temporal masking, 166–170

temporal modulation transfer function (TMTF), 154, 156–157, 214, 246
  neural temporal modulation transfer function, 246

temporal theory, 4, 136

temporary hearing loss, 251

temporary threshold shift (TTS), 251–254. A temporary threshold shift is a temporary increase in the threshold of audibility for an ear at a specified frequency. The amount of temporary threshold shift is customarily expressed in decibels.
  half-octave shift, 253

tensor tympani muscle (tt), 71, 85. The tensor tympani is the intra-aural muscle attached to the handle of the malleus. Its reflex contraction, in response to intense sound or to tactile stimulation to parts of the face, draws the malleus inward, which increases tension on the tympanic membrane. The combined action of the tensor tympani and the stapedius muscles is to limit the motion of the auditory ossicles and thereby help protect the internal ear from damage by intense sounds, especially at low frequencies.

theories of hearing, 4, 135–136, 254
  temporal type theory, 4, 136
  place theories of hearing, 4, 135, 254
  volley, 4

theory of signal detection (TSD), 276–278

thermal noise, 34

three-dB rule, 252
  4- or 5-dB rule, 252

threshold, 25, 77, 122, 143–144

threshold of audibility, 143–144. The threshold of audibility for a specified signal is the minimum effective sound pressure level of the signal that is capable of evoking an auditory sensation in a specified fraction of the trials. The characteristics of the signal, the manner in which it is presented to the subject, and the point at which the sound pressure level is measured must be specified.

threshold of discomfort, 147. The threshold of discomfort for a specified signal is the minimum effective sound pressure level of that signal at the entrance to the external acoustic meatus that, in a specified fraction of the trials, will stimulate the ear to a point that is uncomfortable.

threshold of pain, 147. The threshold of pain for a specified signal is the minimum effective sound pressure